T0259495

Companion Animal Medicine: Evolving Infectious, Toxicological, and Parasitic Diseases

Guest Editor

SANJAY KAPIL, DVM, MS, PhD

VETERINARY CLINICS OF NORTH AMERICA: SMALL ANIMAL PRACTICE

www.vetsmall.theclinics.com

November 2011 • Volume 41 • Number 6

SAUNDERS an imprint of ELSEVIER, Inc.

W.B. SAUNDERS COMPANY
A Division of Elsevier Inc.

1600 John F. Kennedy Blvd. • Suite 1800 • Philadelphia, PA 19103-2899

http://www.vetsmall.theclinics.com

VETERINARY CLINICS OF NORTH AMERICA: SMALL ANIMAL PRACTICE Volume 41, Number 6
November 2011 ISSN 0195-5616, ISBN-13: 978-1-4557-7998-7

Editor: John Vassallo; j.vassallo@elsevier.com

Veterinary Clinics of North America: Small Animal Practice (ISSN 0195-5616) is published bimonthly (For Post Office use only: volume 41 issue 6 of 6) by Elsevier Inc., 360 Park Avenue South, New York, NY 10010-1710. Months of issue are January, March, May, July, September, and November. Business and Editorial Offices: 1600 John F. Kennedy Blvd., Ste. 1800, Philadelphia, PA 19103-2899. Customer Service Office: 3251 Riverport Lane, Maryland Heights, MO 63043. Periodicals postage paid at New York, NY and additional mailing offices. Subscription prices are $262.00 per year (domestic individuals), $427.00 per year (domestic institutions), $128.00 per year (domestic students/residents), $347.00 per year (Canadian individuals), $525.00 per year (Canadian institutions), $385.00 per year (international individuals), $525.00 per year (international institutions), and $186.00 per year (international and Canadian students/residents). To receive student/resident rate, orders must be accompanied by name of affiliated institution, date of term, and the signature of program/residency coordinator on institution letterhead. Orders will be billed at individual rate until proof of status is received. Foreign air speed delivery is included in all *Clinics* subscription prices. All prices are subject to change without notice. **POSTMASTER:** Send address changes to *Veterinary Clinics of North America: Small Animal Practice*, Elsevier Health Sciences Division, Subscription Customer Service, 3251 Riverport Lane, Maryland Heights, MO 63043. Customer Service (orders, claims, online, change of address): Elsevier Periodicals Customer Service, Elsevier Health Sciences Division, Subscription Customer Service, 3251 Riverport Lane, Maryland Heights, MO 63043. Tel: 1-800-654-2452 (U.S. and Canada); 314-447-8871 (outside U.S. andCanada). Fax: 314-447-8029. E-mail: journalscustomerservice-usa@elsevier.com (for print support); journalsonlinesupport-usa@elsevier.com (for online support).

Reprints. For copies of 100 or more of articles in this publication, please contact the Commercial Reprints Department, Elsevier Inc., 360 Park Avenue South, New York, NY 10010-1710. Tel.: 212-633-3812; Fax: 212-462-1935; E-mail: reprints@elsevier.com.

Veterinary Clinics of North America: Small Animal Practice is also published in Japanese by Inter Zoo Publishing Co., Ltd., Aoyama Crystal-Bldg 5F, 3-5-12 Kitaaoyama, Minato-ku, Tokyo 107-0061, Japan.

Veterinary Clinics of North America: Small Animal Practice is covered in *Current Contents/Agriculture, Biology and Environmental Sciences, Science Citation Index, ASCA, MEDLINE/PubMed (Index Medicus), Excerpta Medica,* and *BIOSIS.*

Printed and bound by CPI Group (UK) Ltd, Croydon, CR0 4YY

Transferred to Digital Print 2011

Contributors

GUEST EDITOR

SANJAY KAPIL, DVM, MS, PhD
Diplomate, American College of Veterinary Microbiology (Virology and Immunology); Professor of Clinical Virology, Department of Veterinary Pathobiology, Oklahoma Animal Disease Diagnostic Laboratory, Center for Veterinary Health Sciences, Stillwater, Oklahoma

AUTHORS

ANA ALCARAZ, DVM, PhD
Diplomate, American College of Veterinary Pathologists; Associate Professor, College of Veterinary Medicine, Western University of Health Sciences, Pomona, California

KELLY E. ALLEN, MS, PhD
Lecturer and Researcher, Department of Veterinary Pathobiology, Oklahoma State University Center for Veterinary Health Sciences, Stillwater, Oklahoma

FRANK J. BOSSONG, DVM
Assistant Professor, College of Veterinary Medicine, Western University of Health Sciences, Pomona, California

JILL BRUNKER, DVM
Diplomate, American College of Veterinary Internal Medicine; Assistant Professor of Small Animal Internal Medicine, Center for Veterinary Health Sciences, Department of Veterinary Clinical Sciences, Oklahoma State University, Stillwater, Oklahoma

CANIO BUONAVOGLIA, DVM
Dipartimento di Sanità Pubblica e Zootecnia, Università degli Studi Aldo Moro di Bari, Bari, Italy

JAMIE M. BUSH, DVM, MS
Diplomate, American College of Veterinary Pathologists; IDEXX Laboratories, Memphis, Tennesee

LEAH A. COHN, DVM, PhD
Diplomate, American College of Veterinary Internal Medicine (Small Animal Internal Medicine); Professor, Veterinary Medicine and Surgery, Department of Veterinary Medicine and Surgery, University of Missouri-Columbia, Columbia, Missouri

ELLEN W. COLLISSON, PhD
Professor, College of Veterinary Medicine, Western University of Health Sciences, Pomona, California

NICOLA DECARO, DVM, PhD
Department of Veterinary Public Health, Faculty of Veterinary Medicine of Bari, Valenzano, Bari, Italy

PEDRO PAULO V.P. DINIZ, DVM, PhD
Assistant Professor, College of Veterinary Medicine, Western University of Health Sciences, Pomona, California

YVONNE DRECHSLER, PhD
Assistant Professor, College of Veterinary Medicine, Western University of Health Sciences, Pomona, California

JAMES F. EVERMANN, PhD
Professor, Department of Veterinary Clinical Sciences and Washington Animal Disease Diagnostic Laboratory, College of Veterinary Medicine, Washington State University, Pullman, Washington

CLAUDE FAVROT, PhD, DVM
Dermatology Department, Clinic for Small Animal Internal Medicine, Vetsuisse Faculty, University of Zurich, Switzerland

LYNDI L. GILLIAM, DVM
Diplomate, American College of Veterinary Internal Medicine; Assistant Professor of Equine Internal Medicine, Center for Veterinary Health Sciences, Department of Veterinary Clinical Sciences, Oklahoma State University, Stillwater, Oklahoma

EILEEN M. JOHNSON, DVM, MS, PhD
Clinical Associate Professor, Department of Veterinary Pathobiology, Oklahoma State University Center for Veterinary Health Sciences, Stillwater, Oklahoma

SANJAY KAPIL, DVM, MS, PhD
Diplomate, American College of Veterinary Microbiology (Virology and Immunology); Professor of Clinical Virology, Department of Veterinary Pathobiology, Oklahoma Animal Disease Diagnostic Laboratory, Center for Veterinary Health Sciences, Stillwater, Oklahoma

CHRISTIAN E. LANGE, DVM, MS
Dermatology Department, Clinic for Small Animal Internal Medicine; Institute of Virology, Vetsuisse Faculty, University of Zurich, Zurich, Switzerland

ERIC C. LEDBETTER, DVM
Diplomate, American College of Veterinary Ophthalmologists; Department of Clinical Sciences, College of Veterinary Medicine, Cornell University, Ithaca, New York

SUSAN E. LITTLE, DVM, PhD
Diplomate, European Veterinary Parasitology College; Professor and Krull-Ewing Endowed Chair in Veterinary Parasitology, Department of Veterinary Pathobiology, Oklahoma State University Center for Veterinary Health Sciences, Stillwater, Oklahoma

ROGER K. MAES, DVM, PhD
Diagnostic Center for Population and Animal Health, Michigan State University, Lansing, Michigan

CHELSEA L. MAKLOSKI, DVM, MS
Diplomate, American College of Theriogenologists; Veterinarian, JEH Equine Reproduction Specialists, Whitesboro, Texas

VITO MARTELLA, DVM
Dipartimento di Sanità Pubblica e Zootecnia, Università degli Studi Aldo Moro di Bari, Bari, Italy

PASCHALINA MOSCHIDOU
Dipartimento di Sanità Pubblica e Zootecnia, Università degli Studi Aldo Moro di Bari, Bari, Italy

JACQUELINE M. NORRIS, BVSc, PhD
Faculty of Veterinary Science, University of Sydney, New South Wales, Australia

NOEL OPITZ, DVM
Medical Director and Staff Veterinarian, The Gabriel Foundation, Elizabeth, Colorado

PIERFRANCESCO PINTO, DVM
Dipartimento di Sanità Pubblica e Zootecnia, Università degli Studi Aldo Moro di Bari, Bari, Italy

BRIAN SPEER, DVM
Diplomate, American Board of Veterinary Practitioners-Avian; Diplomate, European College of Avian Medicine and Surgery; Medical Center for Birds, Oakley, California

ALISON STICKNEY, BVSc, MVs, MACVSc
Massey University, Veterinary Teaching Hospital, Institute of Veterinary, Animal, and Biomechanical Sciences, Massey University, Palmerston North, New Zealand

JOANNA WHITE, BVSc, MACVSc
Massey University, Veterinary Teaching Hospital, Institute of Veterinary, Animal, and Biomechanical Sciences, Massey University, Palmerston North, New Zealand

TERESA J. YEARY, PhD
Ames, Iowa

Contents

Sanjay Kapil and Teresa J. Yeary

> Canine distemper virus (CDV) causes a major disease of domestic dogs
> that develops as a serious systemic infection in unvaccinated or
> improperly vaccinated dogs. Domesticated dogs are the main reservoir
> of CDV, a multihost pathogen. This virus of the genus *Morbillivirus* in the
> family Paramyxoviridae occurs in other carnivorous species including
> all members of the Canidae and Mustelidae families and in some
> members of the Procyonidae, Hyaenidae, Ursidae, and Viverridae
> families. Canine distemper also has been reported in the Felidae family
> and marine mammals. The spread and incidences of CDV epidemics in
> dogs and wildlife here and worldwide are increasing.

Vito Martella, Paschalina Moschidou, and Canio Buonavoglia

> Canine astroviruses appear to be widespread geographically. The
> prevalence may be significantly higher in pups with gastroenteric
> disease than in asymptomatic animals and virus shedding has been
> shown to correlate with gastroenteric signs in naturally infected dogs.
> Animal experiments are required to understand better the pathogenic
> role of astroviruses in dogs.

James F. Evermann, Eric C. Ledbetter, and Roger K. Maes

> This review documents how clinical inquiry expands as our knowledge
> base about canine herpesvirus (CHV) increases. We must understand
> the various forms of CHV infection that may occur in the dog popula-
> tion. This has prompted the veterinary community to develop more
> sensitive diagnostic assays. CHV is more common than we considered
> a decade ago. Up to 70% of some high-risk dog populations have been
> infected with and are latent carriers of CHV. Recognition of the various
> forms of CHV-induced disease, availability of diagnostic assays with
> increased sensitivity, and the formation of reliable biosecurity measures
> will allow for better control steps.

This article reviews the currently available literature on pantropic canine coronavirus (CCoV), providing a meaningful update on the virologic, epidemiologic, clinical, diagnostic, and prophylactic aspects of the infections caused by this emerging pathogen of dogs. It also describes pantropic CCoV-induced disease reproduced under experimental conditions.

Feline infectious peritonitis (FIP), a fatal disease in cats worldwide, is caused by FCoV infection, which commonly occurs in multicat environments. The enteric FCoV, referred to as feline enteric virus (FECV), is considered a mostly benign biotype infecting the gut, whereas the FIP virus biotype is considered the highly pathogenic etiologic agent for FIP. Current laboratory tests are unable to distinguish between virus biotypes of FCoV. FECV is highly contagious and easily spreads in multicat environments; therefore, the challenges to animal shelters are tremendous. This review summarizes interdisciplinary current knowledge in regard to virology, immunology, pathology, diagnostics, and treatment options in the context of multicat environments.

Noroviruses are recognized as emerging enteric pathogens of humans and have been identified in recent years in a number of mammalian species. The role of noroviruses as pathogens in immune-competent animals and under natural conditions remains uncertain, although both homologous and heterologous animal models are now available to investigate the pathogenesis, the immune response, and the molecular mechanism regulating norovirus infection. Recently, evidence has been gathered that noroviruses may also circulate in domestic carnivores. The zoonotic implications of these novel viruses deserve more attention, due to the strict social interactions between humans and pets.

Papillomaviruses can infect epithelia and induce proliferative disorders. Different types of canine papillomaviruses have been found to be associated with distinct pathologies including exophytic warts as in canine oral papillomatosis, endophytic warts, and pigmented plaques and, in some cases, squamous cell carcinomas. Virus infection is followed by a phase of subclinical infection before the onset of symptoms. A diagnosis can in some cases be made clinically but should be verified if there are any doubts. Most papillomas do regress spontaneously within a few months. Preventative vaccination is possible but not on the market.

Feline Immunodeficiency Virus: Disease Association Versus Causation in Domestic and Nondomestic Felids

Joanna White, Alison Stickney, and Jacqueline M. Norris

Feline immunodeficiency virus (FIV) is an important infection in both domestic and nondomestic cats. Although many studies have provided insight into FIV pathophysiology and immunologic responses to infection in cats, questions remain regarding the association of FIV with specific disease syndromes. For many diseases, both association and causation of disease with FIV remain to be confirmed and clarified. The use of experimental infection models is unlikely to yield answers about naturally infected domestic cats and is not feasible in nondomestic felids, many of which are endangered species. Researches might consider further study of naturally occurring disease with an emphasis on confirming which diseases have a likely association with FIV.

Canine Brucellosis Management

Chelsea L. Makloski

Infertility in dogs is a growing concern in breeding kennels. There are a number of bacteria, viruses, and husbandry practices that must be considered to determine the cause of decreased litter sizes, abortions, weak puppies, and lack of pregnancy, but brucellosis should be at the top of the differential list.

Hepatozoon spp Infections in the United States

Kelly E. Allen, Eileen M. Johnson, and Susan E. Little

Two *Hepatozoon* spp are recognized as parasites of domestic dogs in the United States, *H canis* and *H americanum*. *H canis* was first described in India in 1905 and has been documented in many areas of the world, although not definitively identified in North America until recently. *H americanum*, causing American canine hepatozoonosis, was first documented in a coyote in 1978 and is now considered an emerging etiologic agent of disease in domestic dogs throughout the United States. The authors review current knowledge of canine hepatozoonosis caused by *H canis* and *H americanum* and elaborate on more recent research findings.

> Snake envenomation can be a cause of significant morbidity in dogs and cats in North America. Being familiar with the venomous snakes in your area and understanding the mechanisms of action of their venom will allow for successful treatment of envenomation cases. Treatment of snake envenomation revolves around supportive care in mild to moderate cases and venom neutralization with antivenom in severe cases. Dogs and cats envenomated by North American snakes have a good prognosis if treated appropriately.

> A number of common misconceptions exist regarding the degree of transmission from companion parrots to dogs and cats. Concern regarding bacterial, viral, fungal, and parasitic transmission is generally unfounded, because disease transmission between companion parrots and dogs and cats is not well-documented. Infections with *Mycobacterium* spp, *Aspergillus* spp, *Giardia* spp, *Chlamydophila psittaci*, *Salmonella* spp, *Yersinia pseudotuberculosis*, *Cryptococcus neoformans*, *Histoplasma capsulatum*, *Cryptosporidium* spp, and avian influenza are often considered possible transmissible diseases, causing pet caregivers unwarranted concerns.

> Feline respiratory disease complex (FRDC) refers to the characteristic acute presentation of a contagious respiratory or ocular disease caused by one or multiple pathogens. Environmental and host factors impact the transmission, clinical presentation, preventive strategy, and treatment of affected cats. The FRDC is especially problematic in settings where large numbers of cats cohabit, including animal shelters, catteries, and semi-feral colonies. Although elimination of FRDC is an unrealistic goal, improved understanding can lead to strategies to minimize disease impact.

FORTHCOMING ISSUES

January 2012

Hematology
Joanne Messick, VMD, PhD,
Guest Editor

March 2012

Small Animal Toxicology
Stephen B. Hooser, DVM, PhD and
Safdar A. Khan, DVM, MS, PhD,
Guest Editors

May 2012

Small Animal Theriogenology
Catherine Lamm, DVM, MRCVS, and
Chelsea Makloski, DVM,
Guest Editors

RECENT ISSUES

September 2011

Surgical Complications
Christopher A. Adin, DVM,
Guest Editor

July 2011

Organ Failure in Critical Illness
Timothy B. Hackett, DVM, MS,
Guest Editor

May 2011

Palliative Medicine and Hospice Care
Tamara S. Shearer, DVM,
Guest Editor

RELATED INTEREST

Veterinary Clinics of North America: Exotic Animal Practice
September 2011 (Vol. 14, No. 3)
Zoonoses, Public Health and the Exotic Animal Practitioner
Marcy J. Souza, DVM, MPH, Dipl. ABVP–Avian, Dipl. ACVPM,
Guest Editor

THE CLINICS ARE NOW AVAILABLE ONLINE!

Access your subscription at:
www.theclinics.com

Preface

Companion Animal Medicine: Evolving Infectious, Toxicological, and Parasitic Diseases

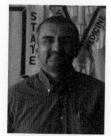

Sanjay Kapil, DVM, MS, PhD
Guest Editor

Expansion of growing human populations into wilderness has increased the opportunity of exposure to infectious agents because of contact between companion animals with urban wildlife. Most newly emerging RNA viruses jump species from wildlife exposure. Moreover, there has been an increase in sensitivity in the detection of novel canine viruses in the last few years with the application of metagenomics and newer sequencing methods on canine samples.

In this issue, I have invited experts who have made significant contributions to emerging infectious disease, parasitic, and biologic poison issues that affect the health of companion animals. I thank all of the authors for writing their articles and providing color pictures in a timely manner. I also thank John Vassallo and the Elsevier staff for help. I hope this issue will be helpful to practicing veterinarians and animal owners.

Sanjay Kapil, DVM, MS, PhD
Department of Veterinary Pathobiology
Oklahoma Animal Disease Diagnostic Laboratory
Center for Veterinary Health Sciences
Farm and Ridge Road
Stillwater, OK 74078, USA

E-mail address:
sanjay.kapil@okstate.edu

Vet Clin Small Anim 41 (2011) xiii
doi:10.1016/j.cvsm.2011.09.002
0195-5616/11/$ – see front matter © 2011 Elsevier Inc. All rights reserved.

Canine Distemper Spillover in Domestic Dogs from Urban Wildlife

Sanjay Kapil, DVM, MS, PhD[a],*, Teresa J. Yeary, PhD[b]

KEYWORDS
- Canine distemper virus genetics • Transmission
- Pathogenicity • Wildlife • Vaccines

Canine distemper virus (CDV) causes a major disease of domestic dogs that develops as a serious systemic infection in unvaccinated or improperly vaccinated dogs.[1] Domesticated dogs are the main reservoir of CDV, which is a multihost pathogen. This virus of the genus *Morbillivirus* in the family Paramyxoviridae occurs in other carnivorous species including all members of the Canidae (fox, coyote, wolf) and Mustelidae families (ferret, skunk, badger, mink, weasel, otter) and in some members of the Procyonidae (raccoon, lesser panda, kinkajou), Hyaenidae (hyenas), Ursidae (bear), and Viverridae (palm civet) families.[2] Canine distemper also has been reported in the Felidae family (lions, tigers) and marine mammals (river otters).[3–9] In the United States, spillover of infection from domestic dogs with spillback from raccoons, which may serve as intermediate hosts,[10] and other susceptible wildlife is well documented.[11] The spread and incidences of CDV epidemics in dogs and wildlife here and worldwide are increasing due to the rise in dog populations associated with growing human populations and widespread urbanization.

VIRUS PROPERTIES

CDV is a small, enveloped, nonsegmented single-stranded, negative-sense RNA virus (about 15,000 bases long) that encodes 6 structural proteins: the nucleocapsid (N) protein, 2 transcriptase-associated proteins (phosphoprotein P and large protein L), the envelope stabilizing matrix (M) protein, and 2 transmembrane glycoproteins embedded in the viral envelope, which are important immunogens of CDV, the hemagglutinin (H) and fusion (F) proteins.[12] CDV has an affinity for many cell types including epithelial, lymphocytic, neuroendocrine, and mesenchymal cells. The viral

The authors have nothing to disclose.
[a] Department of Veterinary Pathobiology, Oklahoma Animal Disease Diagnostic Laboratory, Center for Veterinary Health Sciences, Farm and Ridge Road, Stillwater, OK 74078, USA
[b] Ames, IA, USA
* Corresponding author.
E-mail address: sanjay.kapil@okstate.edu

attachment factor, protein H, controls the host specificity and cell tropism and induces the majority of CVD-neutralizing antibodies.[13-15] Humoral immunity due to the presence of neutralizing antibodies to CDV, elicited by either immunization or natural infection, is detectable within 10 to 14 days, providing protection against infection or reinfection. Viral infection of a susceptible host cell begins when the H protein of CDV binds to the signaling lymphocyte activation molecule (SLAM; CD150) receptor site of the cell.[16] A conformational change of the H protein occurs on binding, which signals the F protein–mediated fusion of the CDV envelope with the host cell membrane. Binding between SLAM and the H protein is a high-affinity, host–virus specific interaction.[14,17] The H and F glycoproteins may mediate fusion activity between neighboring cells leading to syncytium formation and, ultimately, to cell lysis.[16] Host cell surface sites CD46 and a heparin-like receptor have been suggested as putative H protein receptors in SLAM-negative cells, but strong supporting evidence is lacking at this time.[18,19]

DISEASE

Distemper is a highly contagious disease that poses a threat mainly to concentrated populations of previously unexposed or unvaccinated, susceptible species. In these populations, distemper is almost always fatal. The disease is complex in that it presents varying clinical symptoms and may run varying clinical courses. Outcomes of CDV infection range from complete recovery to persistent disease to death depending on the age and immune status of the animal infected.[12] Robustness of the humoral immune response correlates with the disease outcome. Canine distemper virus replicates initially in the lymphoid tissues of the upper respiratory tract followed by immune-mediated progression of the disease over a period of 1 to 2 weeks. A diphasic fever is a characteristic feature of the disease, occurring 7 or 8 days after infection, that drops rapidly and again climbs by day 11 or 12. Clinical signs of distemper are often unapparent or initially mild during this time, and disease is characterized by mucopurulent oculonasal discharges, conjunctivitis, respiratory distress, anorexia, vomiting, diarrhea and dehydration, and cutaneous rash. Anti-CDV antibody titers that develop 10 to 14 days postinfection contribute to viral elimination and recovery when a vigorous humoral response occurs characterized by highly specific anti–H protein antibodies. Cell-mediated immunity also plays a role in recovery from CDV infection, and a strong T-cell–mediated CDV-specific immune response causes viral elimination in convalescing dogs.[20]

Weak humoral and cell-mediated responses lead to systemic intracellular spread of virus to the epithelial cells of the gastrointestinal and urinary tracts, skin, and the endocrine and central nervous systems causing direct virus-mediated damage. Additional clinical signs that may occur are localized twitching, ascending paresis/paralysis, and/or convulsions. Hyperkeratosis of the foot pads and nose may be seen. The infection may either prove fatal or persist resulting in subacute or chronic central nervous system (CNS) signs. Delayed lymphocytolysis correlates with persistence of CDV in the CNS.[21] Within 1 to 3 weeks after recovery from gastrointestinal and respiratory signs, depression and neurologic signs indicating CNS involvement are often evident, although sometimes neurologic impairment does not occur until months later, even without a history of systemic signs.[12] Dogs that recover from acute disease with persistent infection may shed virus in urine and through the skin on the foot pads. These animals should be isolated from contact with unvaccinated animals, especially puppies.

DIAGNOSIS

Canine distemper infection can be challenging to diagnose because many diseases can cause symptoms resembling canine distemper. The respiratory symptoms of canine distemper may be mistaken as canine respiratory disease complex. Canine parvovirus, coronavirus, bacterial, and internal parasite infections should be ruled out as causes of vomiting and diarrhea. Often, CDV-infected animals that exhibit neurologic signs are mistaken as having rabies. Neurologic symptoms must be differentiated from other infections, trauma, and ingestion of toxins. Vaccination history of the affected animal, clinical symptoms, and laboratory testing support a probable diagnosis of CDV infection. State and commercial veterinary diagnostic laboratories offer testing for canine distemper and advice practitioners on appropriate specimens to submit, tests to order and the limitations of test results given the circumstances of each individual case submitted. The following 5 diagnostic methods are commonly offered:

- IFA (immunofluorescence assay) of antemortem specimens detects CDV inclusion bodies in cells from conjunctival scrapes, buffy coat (peripheral blood lymphocytes [PBL]), urine sediment, traumatic bladder catheterization, transtracheal washes, cerebrospinal fluid, and biopsies of footpads or nose when callusing is present. This test is most reliable within the first 3 weeks of infection in acute disease. Virus often persists in the CNS for 60 days or longer.
- Serology for the following:
  ○ IgM, present as serum antibodies, is measured by enzyme-linked immunosorbent assay (ELISA). A high IgM titer indicates recent infection or recent vaccination and may last for 3 months after detection.
  ○ IgG serum antibodies are measured as serial titers on 2 samples taken 14 days apart to detect rising titers. In unvaccinated dogs, rising titers indicate CDV infection. A greater than 4-fold titer increase indicates infection even in recently vaccinated dogs.
  ○ Distemper antibodies in cerebrospinal fluid (CSF) are highly indicative of distemper infection. Vaccine-induced antibodies do not cross the blood-brain barrier into the CSF fluid.
- Cell culture may not yield timely results as virus isolation may take up to 3 weeks. However, newer cell lines, Vero cells expressing the canine SLAM receptor (Vero.DogSLAMtag or Vero-DST cells), can provide results in few days.[22,23] Specimen quality and origin are other limitations of this technique.
- Reverse transcription–polymerase chain reaction (RT-PCR) can detect virus in respiratory secretions, CSF, feces, urine, whole blood, and conjunctival or ocular samples. A negative result does not rule out distemper. Immunization for CDV with modified live virus (MLV) vaccine interferes with PCR testing for approximately 3 to 4 weeks, creating a false-positive result.
- Necropsy/histopathology of post-mortem specimens including spleen, tonsil, lymph node, stomach, kidney, lung, duodenum, bladder, and brain tissues are processed with conventional stains, IFA, or immunohistochemistry (IHC).

Diagnostic testing for CDV and anti-CDV antibodies presents a special challenge because results do not distinguish between naturally acquired CDV disease (wild-type strains), infection with attenuated virus vaccine strains used in modified-live (MLV) vaccines, or immune response due to the recombinant, virus-vectored vaccine. Canine distemper viruses are of a single serotype (monotypic), thus the various genotypes cannot be distinguished using classic serologic techniques with polyclonal antibodies.[15] Use of monoclonal antibodies to differentiate recent field isolates from older field isolates and vaccine strains of CDV has met with limited success and the reagents developed are not widely available.[24,25] Currently, 2 in-clinic serologic test kits are licensed for sale in the United States, the TiterCHEK CDV/CPV ELISA-based assay (Synbiotics, San Diego, CA, USA) and the ImmunoComb Canine VacciCheck (Modern Veterinary Products, Coral Gables, FL, USA).[26] Both kits evaluate an immune response to CDV from vaccination or infection but neither differentiates between titers to the vaccine or infection with wild-type CDV strains.

Licensed RT-PCR kits for detection of CDV are not available in the United States. Among the commercial and state veterinary diagnostic laboratories that perform RT-PCR testing of their own design to detect CDV, one of the challenges is differentiating between vaccine strains and wild-type isolates that may be present concurrently in samples. The RT-PCR assays are typically designed to amplify a portion of the H, F, M, or N gene to verify the presence of CDV RNA in specimens. Absolute identification of strains and differentiation between vaccine and wild-type CDV may be performed by sequence analysis of the cloned RT-PCR amplified H gene region.[10] Rapid methods have been designed to differentiate CDV strains as either wild-type or vaccine derived without the need to perform time-consuming gene sequencing. Two popular methods are based on RT-PCR of a specific CDV structural protein genes followed either by a restriction fragment length polymorphism (RFLP) analysis of the amplified nucleic acid or by a second round of nested PCR with analyses by electrophoresis.[10,27–29] Other unique approaches that have been developed are multiplex RT-nested PCR (RT-nPCR) of the M protein and amplification refractory mutation system (ARMS)-PCR of the CDV M-F intergenic and untranslated, prepeptide regions of the F gene followed by RFLP.[30,31]

VACCINATION AND PREVENTION

Most CDV vaccines in the United States, Canada, and Europe are of the American-1 (Onderstepoort) lineage with the exception of the Vanguard vaccine (Pfizer Animal Health, Madison, NJ, USA), which is of the America-2 genotype.[27,32] The major vaccine strains were isolated in the 1930s and it is not known if they continue to circulate in nature as they have not been detected for many years.[33,34] Although CDV vaccine strains have not changed in the past 60 years, there is potential for newer antigenic variants of CDV to emerge around the world.[23] However, the current vaccines have largely provided adequate protection against clinical disease when properly administered to healthy domesticated dogs in this country.

Core vaccination guidelines, including canine distemper MLV and recombinant canarypox vectored canine distemper virus (rCDV) vaccines, recommended by the American Animal Hospital Association Canine Vaccine Guidelines, were revised in 2006.[35] Recommendations for administering the rCDV and MLV vaccines are similar. Advantages of the rCDV vaccine is that it does not contain live virus that replicates and spreads from vaccinees and it is more likely to produce immunity in puppies that have passively acquired maternal antibodies. Vaccination failures can occur when MLV vaccines are used to immunize puppies that have not cleared maternal antibodies.[36] Maternal antibodies are adsorbed in the intestine from colostrum during the first 2 days of life and are cleared 6 to 12 weeks later. It is recommended that puppies receive a series of 3 vaccinations beginning at 6 to 16 weeks of age to achieve complete immunity to CDV followed by a booster at 1 year of age. Canine distemper virus vaccines impart long-term immunity in dogs.[37] Duration of immunity of 3 years has been reported for both MLV and rCDV vaccines.[38,39] In animal shelters and high-risk environments, one dose of MLV or rCDV vaccine has been reported to be protective in puppies already exposed to CDV.[40] Ferrets are also highly susceptible to CDV and the disease is virtually 100% fatal. The American Ferret Association recommends vaccinating ferrets with PureVax Ferret Distemper Vaccine (Merial Inc, Athens, GA, USA), the only USDA-licensed vaccine product labeled for use in ferrets, following the product label for kits or adults.[41]

Reasons that a vaccine may fail, in addition to the presence of maternal antibodies in puppies, are incomplete immunity due to failure to complete the puppy booster vaccination series, stressors in the physical environment, the animal's immune competence and specific responsiveness to CDV antigen or intercurrent exposure to other virulent viruses such as canine parvovirus or coronavirus or even parasites, and improper storage and handling of vaccine.[36,42–44] A concern voiced by scientists is that new genetic CDV variants may be associated with pathogenesis changes or immune evasion in dogs vaccinated with current vaccines.[45] In infected dogs with a history of recent vaccination with MLV vaccine, exposure to wild-type CDV prior to vaccination is usually assumed to be the source of the CDV infection.[10] However, CDV infections reported in previously vaccinated dogs in Japan, Mexico, and the United States were caused by novel CDV lineages distantly related to the America-1 vaccine group.[10,44,46–49] Variation of key amino acid residues and the addition or loss of N-glycosylation sites on the H and F proteins may alter interaction between the H and F proteins during binding and fusion with susceptible cells, leading to changes in antigenicity, virulence, and tissues targeted by CDV variants.[50,51] Continued surveillance, study of genetic and antigenic drift in circulating CDV strains, and molecular analysis of emerging CDV variants are warranted to ensure that vaccines for prevention of distemper continue to be potent and efficacious in preventing infection in domestic dogs.

In addition to immunization of domestic dog populations, hygienic measures are necessary. Unvaccinated puppies should be isolated from dogs other than their bitches. Strict isolation of dogs infected with CDV is the most important step in controlling the disease. Virus is shed in all body secretions and excretions during the acute systemic disease. Direct dog-to-dog contact and indirect aerosol transmission are the main routes of viral spread, but CDV can be transmitted from fomites at room temperature or lower for several hours. Disinfection of CDV in the environment, particularly in shelters and kennels, is important. Inactivation of canine distemper virus with benzalkonium chloride (0.05%), a quaternary ammonium compound, occurs in 10 minutes at room temperature.[52] Similarly, 70% ethanol is effective against CDV.[53]

GENOTYPES AND GENOTYPING

Nucleic acid sequence analysis of the H gene is the gold standard for phylogenetic analysis, classification, and genotyping of CDV because it has the greatest heterogeneity (about 10% amino acid variation) of the 6 structural proteins of CDV.[54] Studies of complete H gene sequences have identified 12 distinct geographically separated clusters of CDV genotypes: American-1 (including most vaccine strains), American-2 (North America), Arctic (Arctic region and Europe), Asia-1, Asia-2, Asia-3, Europe, European wildlife, South Africa, Argentina, Rockborn-like, and a new genotype of primarily Mexican strains.[28,48,55–57] Serengeti isolates are distinctive from CDV isolates from other parts of the world.[5] In the United States, genotypes that have been identified in dogs and wildlife in addition to the American-1 and America-2 strains are the European wildlife, EdoMex, and Arctic strains in domestic dogs.[10,49,55] Amino acid sequence variation between the genotypes is greater than 4% and strains within each genotype have less than 2% amino acid variation.[12] Characterization of

CDV strains from South America may be of special interest. Scientific archivists point to documentation of distemper-like epizootics occurring in Peruvian dogs in the mid-1700s that may have spread to Europe circa 1760 with the importation of diseased dogs by Spanish colonials.[58]

Sequence analysis of CDV strains from different geographical locations and animal species indicates that the H protein gene undergoes genetic drift.[59] Viral recombination in CDV has been documented in an isolate recovered from a giant panda.[60] Recently, a CDV genotype designated "Wildlife Europe 2006–2009 (WE/06–09)" found exclusively in wild carnivores was described that evolved and spread over a wide geographical area in Northern Italy in 10 months following its initial detection in 2006.[61] Bavarian wildlife isolates collected during the 2008 distemper outbreak in the Southern Alps were 99.7% to 100% similar to the Italian isolates.[62] The evolutionary origin of the group was estimated to have diverged from its most recent ancestor 5 months prior to identification of the first virus CDV.[63] The mean nucleic acid substitution rate in the new CDV genotype was estimated to be 10.53×10^{-4} subs per site per year, which was within the range typically observed for CDV.[63] Phylogenetic analysis of 73 CDV H gene and H protein sequences from dog and non-dog hosts indicated that amino acid residues 530 and 549 are under positive selection, and these residues are located in the regions of the H protein that are important in binding to the host cell SLAM receptor and triggering activation of the F protein cellular entry.[17,59,64] This provides compelling evidence that repeated evolution at known functional sites of emerging strains of CDV is associated with multiple independent occurrences of disease emergence in a range of novel host species.

Facilitation of large-scale diagnostic and molecular epidemiologic studies of CDV requires rapid molecular-based methods that accurately differentiate among the genotypes and between vaccine and wild-type strains of CVD without the need to perform either full-length or partial sequencing of the H gene for each isolate. A hemi-nested PCR system was developed that can genotype 5 of the 12 CDV lineages (America-1, Europe, Asia-1, Asia-2, and Arctic) using specific primers targeted to the H gene.[32] The ARMS-PCR method followed by RFLP also differentiates a broad variety of lineages.[31] Further development of rapid protocols for distinguishing among all CDV genotypes is needed to advance epidemiologic studies of this important pathogen. Genotyping is important for tracing the relatedness of CDV isolates and cross-transmission between and within species of carnivores.

NONCANID HOSTS OF CDV

Distemper outbreaks in Rhesus monkeys (Macaca culatta) have occurred since 2006 at the largest monkey breeding farm in mainland China that supplies breeding stock for biomedical research facilities and zoos.[65] Over 10,000 monkeys contracted the disease and more than 4,250 died at the farm and at the facilities it serves. The entire genome of the isolated virus was sequenced. Phylogenetic analysis of the H gene places it within the larger clade of Asian genotypes yet it is unique in the number of amino acid changes to its structural proteins. Although monkeys and monkey-derived cell cultures have been experimentally infected with CDV, only one other natural CDV outbreak of monkeys (Macaca fuscata) occurring in Japan was reported in 1989.[66]

Canine distemper is not a clinically recognized entity in domestic cats; however, large felids are susceptible to infection with CDV. Most of the large cats are threatened or endangered species; thus surveillance of pathogens that have the potential to cause their extinctions is critical. Where CDV has caused widespread distemper outbreaks in nondomestic cats, domestic dogs, raccoons, or wild canids have been implicated as reservoirs of the disease. CDV outbreaks with multiple mortalities were reported in lions, tigers, jaguars, and leopards in zoos and wildlife safari parks in the 1980s.[67] Raccoons living in the area surrounding one suburban zoo had increased numbers of fatal distemper cases and may have transmitted the disease to the large cats. CDV isolated from large felids in the zoo was of the America-2 genotype circulating in the local feral raccoons.[64] A retrospective immunohistochemistry study of paraffin tissues from 42 necropsy cases of lions and tigers from Swiss zoo and circus cats collected from 1972 through 1992 indicated that 19 were CDV positive.[4] Of 56 Asiatic lions from 6 captive breeding centers in western India tested in 2007 for antibodies against CDV, 88% were positive.[68] In addition to domestic dogs, urban wildlife in the United States such as raccoons, foxes, and skunks may play a role in direct transmission of distemper to large felids and other carnivores in zoos, wildlife parks, circuses, and captive breeding facilities.

Many studies of canine distemper in free-ranging large felids have been reported.[69–75] African lions of the Serengeti are the most intensively studied of the large felids with regard to the prevalence of CDV. In 1994, a CDV epidemic in Serengeti lions caused fatalities in 30% of the population with only an estimated 2,000 lions remaining in 1996.[69] Prior to 1994, disease-related mortality due to CDV infection of lions had not been documented, although retrospective serology tests indicated that 29% of lions that were living in the area from 1984 to 1989 had titers to CDV. A single CDV genotype was common among the susceptible animal species living in the Serengeti during the 1994 CDV outbreak that included lions, hyenas, bat-eared foxes, domestic dogs, and jackals.[5] Unowned, feral domestic dogs living in or near the Serengeti are not vaccinated, experience periodic distemper outbreaks, and likely serve as a primary reservoir of CDV. Jackals and hyenas may be amplifying species that spread CDV throughout the park to lions and other felids.[6,76,77] A Brazilian study was performed in 2 state parks with the goal of determining the prevalence of CDV titers in wild felid populations (jaguars, pumas, and ocelots) and correlating it with the prevalence of CDV titers in, and density of, domestic dogs in the areas adjacent the parks.[72] Dog owners in small rural settlements surrounding the parks were questioned about the CDV vaccination status of their dogs. Unvaccinated dogs were tested for CDV titers. Jaguars (60%) and pumas (11%) from one park had titers to CDV and 100% of the dogs living adjacent to the park were seropositive for CDV. None of the large felids tested at the second park had CDV titers and only 35% of the local unvaccinated dog population was seropositive for CDV. The occurrence of CDV in wild felids appears to be related with home range and close association with unvaccinated, infected domestic dogs living nearby.

PREVENTION OF CDV INFECTION IN WILDLIFE

Vaccine coverage of 95% of domesticated dogs is needed to control canine distemper in these pets.[78] Currently the best means for breaking the circulation of CDV between susceptible wildlife populations and domestic dogs is through regular vaccination of pet dogs and preventing them from roaming freely and interacting with unvaccinated dogs and wildlife that may harbor the virus. Free roaming wildlife are not vaccinated in the United States unless federal and state authorities determine that an endangered species may benefit from vaccination in captive breeding programs designed to stabilize and increase existing populations for release back into the wild. One study reported the vaccination of wild raccoons with MLV canine distemper vaccine prior to 1997 in a forest preserve near a Chicago area zoo.[64] In the 1960s through the 1980s, primarily killed vaccines (KV) were used to vaccinate endangered wildlife and zoo animals against CDV.[79,80] Virus-neutralizing titers developed postvaccination to the KV were generally quite low, and several exotic species that had been vaccinated died from outbreaks of CDV infection. Use of MLV CDV vaccines is often fatal to many wildlife and zoo animals; thus they have only been used in rare situations in the United States to control disease in endangered species and display animals in zoologic parks.[1,79–82] After the univalent canarypox vectored recombinant distemper vaccine, Purevax Ferret (Merial Inc), was licensed and marketed in 2001, many North American zoological institutions began using the rCDV vaccine to vaccinate numerous at-risk species.[83] Currently, the American Association of Zoo Veterinarians' Distemper Vaccine subcommittee recommends the extralabel use of the rCDV PureVax Ferret Distemper Vaccine (Merial, Inc) in all susceptible zoological display animals where CDV is endemic in local wildlife.[84]

Vaccination of endangered species that are susceptible to CDV has been an important in the success of recovery programs. Initially, commercial KV and MLV CDV vaccines were used to vaccinate the endangered black-footed ferret but these products proved to be nonprotective or fatal.[80,85,86] In 1988, an experimental canarypox vectored rCDV vaccine (Merial Inc) used to vaccinate ferrets in the captive breeding program successfully prevented distemper, one of several diseases that had threatened the species with extinction.[87] All wild-born black-footed ferrets are trapped and vaccinated. After the 1999 CDV outbreak on Santa Catalina Island, California, the native island fox population plummeted from 1,300 to less than 100 individuals. Infected domesticated dogs or stowaway raccoons from boats anchoring on the island mingling with the foxes may have caused the outbreak.[88] The federally endangered island fox was vaccinated with the rCDV vaccine to reestablish the population beginning in 1999 with permission from the California Department of Fish and Game.[89,90] Wildlife rescue and research organizations also vaccinate CDV-susceptible animals in areas where distemper is endemic. The rCDV vaccine, PureVax, is used prevent disease in captive southern sea otters at California institutions.[9] Free-ranging sea otters are susceptible to CDV.

Immune-stimulating complexes (ISCOMs), a novel form of adjuvant that, combined with antigens, generally induces strong activation of both the cell-mediated and humoral immunity. African wild dogs (*Lycaon pictus*), which are on the International Union for Conservation of Nature Red List of Threatened Species, cannot be vaccinated with MLV CDV vaccines, which are always fatal.[91] One study reported the use of ISCOMs incorporating the F and H proteins to vaccinate African wild dogs.[92] The dogs initially vaccinated at the beginning of the captive breeding program in 1995 developed protective immunity. However, in 2000, when the 49 of 52 dogs in the colony succumbed to distemper, neutralizing anti-CDV antibodies were not measurable despite a recent vaccination. Although the use of ISCOMs appeared to be promising for control of CDV in a variety of wildlife, the successes have been limited.[82]

Oral bait vaccines to control zoonotic diseases like rabies and plague in wildlife are currently in use. Oral vaccines to control wildlife distemper are not yet available. Two major issues in developing an efficacious oral bait vaccine for distemper are achieving an adequate mucosal immune response in the gut and overcoming interference from maternal antibodies in infant animals. Attempts at inducing mucosal immunity using vaccinia and canarypox vectored CDV vaccines have been reported using ferrets as model animals.[80,93–95] Highly attenuated vaccinia and canarypox virus strains expressing the H and F proteins of CDV were administered by parenteral, intranasal, and intradoudenal routes. Juvenile ferrets receiving either vaccine intramuscularly or intranasally had 100% survival rates, but intradoudenal vaccination protected only 60%.[93] In studies of infant ferrets with and without maternal antibody, the vaccinia and canarypox vectored vaccines were administered parenterally or intranasally. All infant ferrets vaccinated parenterally with either vaccine in the absence of maternal antibody survived challenge. Parenteral vaccination with either vaccine in the presence of maternal antibody did not protect against death from CDV challenge. Intranasal vaccination with either vaccine, in ferrets with or without maternal antibody, was not protective against CDV.[94] Other studies have shown low efficiency in producing a protective immune response with the nonparenteral delivery of CDV canarypox vectored vaccines.[80,95] As with the Raboral V-RG (Merial, Inc), the CDV vaccinia vectored vaccines stimulate a stronger protective mucosal immune response.[93] If an efficacious CDV oral bait vaccine can be developed for wildlife, vigorous domestic dog vaccination programs here and abroad will continue to be the primary means to control the disease.

DISEASE SURVEILLANCE AND CONTROL IN THE UNITED STATES

In the United States, several federal agencies are tasked with surveillance of animal diseases of wildlife. The U.S. Department of Agriculture–APHIS Wildlife Services' administers the National Wildlife Disease Program (NWDP), which participates in wildlife disease monitoring and surveillance in all regions of the United States.[96] Additionally, NWDP assists state, federal, tribal and international agencies, and nongovernment organizations, with development of local wildlife disease monitoring programs and nationally coordinated wildlife surveillance systems. Canine distemper is among diseases of interest to the surveillance program, although minor.[97] Over the past 10 years, the NWDP has assisted in distemper surveillance monitoring and research activities with state agencies and veterinary colleges.[96,98,99] The USDA National Wildlife Research Center is currently assisting the Zambian Wildlife Authority and the African Wild Dog Conservation Trust in the development of conservation management plans for several critically endangered species including African wild dogs, African lions, bat-eared foxes, and leopards. It has been postulated that diseased village dogs are the reservoirs of distemper, rabies, parvovirus, and a number of parasites that are infecting African wildlife.[100,101] Three programs within the U.S. Department of the Interior also monitor threats to wildlife and wildlife health in the United States: the Fish and Wildlife Service (FWS), National Park Service (NPS), and U.S. Geological Survey (USGS).[102] The FWS administers health monitoring programs for endangered and threatened terrestrial and freshwater species under the Endangered Species Act of 1973. In 1988, in association with state and private organizations, the FWS began a captive breeding and vaccination program of black-footed ferrets, which were nearly extinct due to outbreaks of canine distemper and sylvatic plague.[86,103] The FWS was involved in the captive breeding and vaccination program and continuing surveillance of the Santa Catalina Island fox population after the 1999 canine distemper outbreak. By the end of 2010, the fox population rebounded from 100 foxes to 1,008 Individuals.[88,104,105] Grey wolves reintroduced by the FWS to Yellowstone National Park are monitored for canine distemper, which caused population declines in 1999, 2005, and 2008.[106] The NPS Biological Resource Management Division performs surveillance and disease management of wildlife health within the federal park system. The USGS National Wildlife Health Center, which provides wildlife health and disease investigative, research, and training support to federal, state, local, and international conservation agencies, was designated as an OIE Collaborating Centre for Research and Diagnosis of Emerging and Existing Pathogens of Wildlife, by the World Organization for Animal Health (OIE) in July of 2011.

SPREAD OF CANINE DISTEMPER AMONG DOMESTIC DOGS AND WILDLIFE

The epidemiology and transmission of CDV are complicated by the wide host range of animals susceptible to distemper.[2] Canine distemper virus is present on all continents wherever there are carnivores. Domestic dogs are considered to be the primary reservoir of CDV, which disseminates between free-ranging, unvaccinated or incompletely vaccinated dogs (pets and feral) and urban or rural wildlife.[1] Raccoons, foxes, and skunks have adapted well to urban environments and, in the United States, raccoons, a secondary reservoir of CDV, are among the most common wildlife species found in cities and towns. Cyclical outbreaks of distemper commonly occur in North America among raccoons associated with an increase in their populations. The periodic increase in distemper outbreaks in raccoons leads to spillback to domestic and feral dogs and spillover to other wildlife (skunks, foxes, badgers, coyotes, wolves, etc.). Over the past decade, many outbreaks of canine distemper in urban wildlife have been reported in the United States and Canada, prompting health officials to issue advisories to the public to avoid feeding or otherwise attracting wildlife to their property, keep dogs current on CDV vaccinations, and confine their pets in fenced enclosures or on a leash.[11,107]

Infection with CDV also is an important conservation threat to many carnivore species in their natural habitats, especially for small, endangered populations that already face environmental insults.[108,109] Distemper has contributed to population declines in black-footed ferrets, Catalina Island foxes, native Florida mink, gray wolves, coyotes, sea otters, pumas, and ocelots in the United States and many other wild carnivores worldwide. Often, multiple competent hosts for CDV exist within a region, allowing localized persistence of disease.[110] Susceptible captive animals that are held in high densities are especially vulnerable to infection; thus quarantine, vaccinations, and meticulous hygiene are important measures to take, as is reducing the potential for contact with free roaming wildlife that serve as reservoirs of disease.[4,64–68]

Transmission of CDV between animals is via aerosol or respiratory secretions (coughing, sneezing, barking, licking) and bodily excretions (urine and feces) or through direct contact with shared, virus-contaminated food and water bowls, garbage, compost piles, and other organic materials. Other disease-causing contacts include chasing, mating, fights, simultaneous and sequential feeding events at carcasses, and grooming.[76] Wild animals with distemper have similar symptoms as infected dogs. They are often mistaken as rabid because they display unusual behavior, disorientation, aimless wandering, and/or aggression and walk with an unusual gait due to CNS involvement. The majority of cases in wildlife are most often observed in spring and summer since juveniles are more susceptible to infection, but cases occur year round.

EPIDEMIOLOGY

Studies of threatened, endangered, or reintroduced carnivore species in the Greater Yellowstone Ecosystem and in the Serengeti National Park, Tanzania, have supplied a wealth of information on the epidemiology of CDV in these expansive natural habitats over many decades.[69,76,77,88,110,111] However, little is known of the overall health status and disease problems in free-ranging wildlife populations that have direct and regular contact with domestic dogs. The domestic dog is the most numerous of carnivores in the world with an estimated population of over 500 million worldwide.[112] Domestic dogs have been sources of many zoonotic viruses, bacteria, helminths, arthropods, protozoa, and fungi and have served as a link for exchange of pathogens among livestock, wildlife, and humans.[113–115] An International Expert Meeting on Dog Population Management was held in Banna, Italy, in March 2011 as a joint effort between the Food and Agricultural Organization of the United Nations and the World Society for the Protection of Animals with technical support from the World Health Organization, to address the challenges of domestic and stray dog population management throughout the world.[116] Regular domestic animal health care is not universally available in developing nations or even in remote areas of developed countries. This hinders development of effective disease detection and preventative veterinary medicine programs.[115] Lack of vaccination to achieve herd immunity, uncontrolled reproduction of domestic dogs, and free-roaming dogs, they are whether owned, abandoned, or feral, are major roadblocks to preventing further spread of CDV to all susceptible species.[72,73,117,118]

Studying the demographic characteristics of dog populations in urban and rural areas is critical for understanding the epidemiology of canine infectious diseases and to make decisions in planning and implementing dog population management schemes to control zoonotic diseases and diseases that are of conservation interest such as CDV.[72,117,118] Three recent prospective studies of large felids in Brazil, Iberian lynx in Andalusia, Spain, and wolves in the remote north coastal mainland and islands of British Columbia, Canada, suggest that unvaccinated dogs in towns and small settlements do pose a significant risk; seroprevalence for CDV exposure in these animals is high.[72,73,119] Additional prospective studies of disease in threatened and endangered species and dog populations that reside in transecting areas of urban populations, towns or settlements, and wilderness areas are needed to provide baseline health and serologic information. The heterogeneity of CDV genotypes that have been isolated in restricted geographical areas within the United States, Europe, and elsewhere are postulated as being the result of intense, legal, or uncontrolled trade and travel of domestic dogs and uncontrolled movement receptive wild species.[10,12,120] Recent reports of European Wildlife and EdoMex genotypes isolated from North American dogs that have not traveled outside the United States underscore the need to gather additional sequence information to elucidate the epidemiologic patterns of CDV on a local and global scale.[10] Characterization of circulating CVD genotypes in domestic dogs and wildlife within a discrete territory over a protracted timeline would also further our understanding of how the virus spreads and evolves within and between species. Reliable information about transmission of CDV among domestic and wild carnivores should enable more effective management of the disease.[76]

SUMMARY

Canine distemper is a highly contagious disease of domestic dogs that also infects multiple wildlife hosts, some that serve as secondary or amplifying reservoirs of the virus. Transmission of CDV among dogs and other susceptible hosts continues to present many challenges in the United States and worldwide. Control of distemper in dog populations requires a strong commitment by many constituencies. CDV is the most significant viral threat to the extinction of endangered carnivores, eclipsing rabies. Effective vaccines for distemper are available to control CDV in domestic dogs, although the vaccine strains that are used in commercial vaccines have not changed in the past 60 years. Client education about the serious consequences of CDV to both their pet dogs and to wildlife is the critical first step to curtail the spread of CDV, followed by reducing reproduction rates of dogs and abandonment of pets. It is important for veterinarians, dog owners, animal control officers, wildlife wardens, and quarantine officers to understand that canine distemper can cross continents during the transportation of dogs. A major challenge in diagnostic testing is differentiating infection due to attenuated vaccine virus from infection caused by wild-type virus so that recently CDV-vaccinated dogs are not unnecessarily euthanized where outbreaks of distemper occur, particularly in animal shelters. Because canine distemper is an RNA virus, a potential for emergence of antigenic variants exists, particularly in situations where wildlife that are infected with a strain of CDV that has adapted to that host spills back to domestic dogs. Introduction of novel canine distemper viruses in improperly vaccinated dog populations with insufficient immunity can cause new outbreaks of CDV. Increased surveillance of CDV in dog and wildlife populations to identify new genotypes and trace movement of strains within and between species will broaden our epidemiologic knowledge base and advise the veterinary profession and biologics industry as to the need for changes to vaccine strains to protect domestic dogs.

REFERENCES

1. Cleaveland S, Kaare M, Knobel D, et al. Canine vaccination—providing broader benefits for disease control. Vet Microbiol 2006;117(1):43–50.
2. Deem SL, Spelman LH, Yates RA, et al. Canine distemper in terrestrial carnivores: a review. J Zoo Wildl Med 2000;31(4):441–51.
3. Harder TC, Kenter M, Vos H, et al. Canine distemper virus from diseased large felids: biological properties and phylogenetic relationships. J Gen Virol 1996; 77(3):397–405.
4. Myers DL, Zurbriggen A, Lutz H, Pospischil A. Distemper: not a new disease in lions and tigers. Clin Diag Lab Immunol 1997;4(2):180–4.
5. Carpenter MA, Appel MJ, Roelke-Parker ME, et al. Genetic characterization of canine distemper virus in Serengeti carnivores. Vet Immunol Immunopathol 1998; 65(2-4):259–66.
6. Craft ME, Volz E, Packer C, Meyers LA. Disease transmission in territorial populations: the small-world network of Serengeti lions. J R Soc Interface 2011;8(59):776–86.
7. Mamaev LV, Denikina NN, Belikov SI, et al. Characterisation of morbilliviruses isolated from Lake Baikal seals (Phoca sibirica). Vet Microbiol 1995;44(2-4):251–9.
8. Osterhaus ADME, de Swart RL, Vos HW, et al. Morbillivirus infections of aquatic mammals: newly identified members of the genus. Vet Microbiol 1995;44(2-4): 219–27.
9. Jessup DA, Murray MJ, Casper DR, et al. Canine distemper vaccination is a safe and useful preventive procedure for southern sea otters (Enhydra lutra nereis). J Zoo Wildl Med 2009;40(4):705–10.
10. Kapil S, Allison RW, Johnston L, et al. Canine distemper virus strains circulating among North American dogs. Clin Vaccine Immunol 2008;15(4):707–12.
11. Program for Monitoring Emerging Diseases. ProMED Mail. International Society for Infectious Diseases. Available at: http://www.promedmail.org/pls/apex/f?p=2400: 1000. Accessed July 30, 2011.
12. Martella V, Elia G, Buonavoglia C. Canine distemper virus. Vet Clin North Am Small Anim Pract 2008;38:787–97.
13. von Messling V, Zimmer G, Herrler G, et al. The hemagglutinin of canine distemper virus determines tropism and cytopathogenicity. J Virol 2001;75(14):6418–27.
14. Ohishi K, Ando A, Suzuki R, et al. Host-virus specificity of morbilliviruses predicted by structural modeling of the marine mammal SLAM, a receptor. Comp Immunol Microbiol Infect Dis 2010;33(3):227–41.

15. Harder TC, Osterhaus ADME. Canine distemper virus—A morbillivirus in search of new hosts? Trends Microbiol 1997;5(3):120–4.
16. von Messling V, Oezguen N, Zheng Q, et al. Nearby clusters of hemagglutinin residues sustain slam-dependent canine distemper virus entry in peripheral blood mononuclear cells. J Virol 2005;79(9):5857–62.
17. Zipperle L, Langedijk JP, Orvell C, et al. Identification of key residues in virulent canine distemper virus hemagglutinin that control CD150/SLAM-binding activity. J Virol 2010;84(18):9618–24.
18. Suter SE, Chein MB, von Messling V, et al. In vitro canine distemper virus infection of canine lymphoid cells: a prelude to oncolytic therapy for lymphoma. Clin Cancer Res 2005;11(4):1579–87.
19. Fujita K, Miura K, Yoneda M, et al. Host range and receptor utilization of canine distemper virus analyzed by recombinant viruses: Involvement of heparin-like molecule in CDV infection. Virology 2007;359(2):324–35.
20. Appel MJ, Shek WR, Summers BA. Lymphocyte-mediated immune cytotoxicity in dogs infected with virulent canine distemper virus. Infect Immun 1982;37(2): 592–600.
21. Beineke A, Puff C, Seehusen F, et al. Pathogenesis and immunopathology of systemic and nervous canine distemper. Vet Immunol Immunopathol 2009; 127(1-2):1–18.
22. Tatsuo H, Ono N, Yanagi Y. Morbilliviruses use signaling lymphocyte activation molecules (CD150) as cellular receptors. J Virol 2001;75(13);5842–50.
23. Seki, F, Ono N, Yamaguchi R, et al. Efficient isolation of wild strains of canine distemper viruses in Vero cell expressing canine SLAM (CD150) and their adaptability to marmoset B95a cells. J Virol 2003;77(18): 9943–50.
24. Örvell C, Sheshberadaran H, Norrby E. Preparation and characterization of monoclonal antibodies directed against four structural components of canine distemper virus. J Gen Virol 1985;66(3):443–56.
25. Iwatsuki K, I okiyoshi S, Hirayama N. Antigenic differences in the H proteins of canine distemper viruses. Vet Microbiol 2000;71(3-4):281–6.
26. USDA Center for Veterinary Biologics. Veterinary Biological Products. Licensees and Permittees. Prepared July 7, 2011. Available at: http://www.aphis.usda.gov/animal_health/vet_biologics/vb_licensed_products.shtml. Accessed July 30, 2011.
27. Demeter Z, Palade EA, Hornyák A, et al. Controversial results of the genetic analysis of a canine distemper vaccine strain. Vet Microbiol 2010;142(3-4):420–6.
28. Zhao JJ, Yan XJ, Chai XL, et al. Phylogenetic analysis of the haemagglutinin gene of canine distemper virus strains detected from breeding foxes, raccoon dogs and minks in China. Vet Microbiol 2010;140(1-2):34–42.
29. Wang F, Yan X, Chai X, et al. Differentiation of canine distemper virus isolates in fur animals from various vaccine strains by reverse transcription-polymerase chain reaction-restriction fragment length polymorphism according to phylogenetic relations in China. Virology J 2011;8:85–92.
30. Si W, Zhou S, Wang Z, Cui SJ. A multiplex reverse transcription-nested polymerase chain reaction for detection and differentiation of wild-type and vaccine strains of canine distemper virus. Virol J 2010;7:86–91.
31. Chulakasian S, Lee MS, Wang CY, et al. Multiplex amplification refractory mutation system polymerase chain reaction (ARMS-PCR) for diagnosis of natural infection with canine distemper virus. Virol J 2010;7:122–30.
32. Martella V, Elia G, Lucente MS, et al. Genotyping canine distemper virus (CDV) by a hemi-nested multiplex PCR provides a rapid approach for investigation of CDV outbreaks. Vet Microbiol 2007;122(1-2):32–42.

33. Green RG, Swale FS. Vaccination of dogs with modified distemper virus. J AmVet Med Assoc 1939;95:469–70.

34. Schatzberg SJ, Li Q, Porter BF, et al. Broadly reactive pan-paramyxovirus reverse transcription polymerase chain reaction and sequence analysis for the detection of canine distemper virus in a case of canine meningoencephalitis of unknown etiology. J Vet Diagn Invest 2009;21(6):844–9.

35. American Animal Hospital Association Canine Vaccine Task Force. 2006 AAHA Canine Vaccine Guidelines, Revised. Available at: http://www.aahanet.org. Accessed July 30, 2011.

36. Povey RC. Distempter vaccination of dogs: factors which could cause vaccine failure. Can Vet J 1986;27(9):321–3.

37. Schultz RD, Thiel B, Mukhtar E, et al. Age and long-term protective immunity in dogs and cats. J Comp Pathol 2010(Suppl 1);142:S102–8.

38. Larson LJ, Schultz RD. Three-year duration of immunity in dogs vaccinated with a canarypox-vectored recombinant canine distemper virus vaccine. Vet Ther 2007; 8(2):101–6.

39. Larson LJ, Schultz RD. Three-year duration of immunity in dogs vaccinated with a canarypox-vectored recombinant canine distemper virus vaccine. Vet Ther 2007: 8(2):101–106 [Erratum in: Vet Ther 2008;9(3):248].

40. Larson LJ, Schultz RD. Effect of vaccination with recombinant canine distemper virus vaccine immediately before exposure under shelter-like conditions. Vet Ther 2006;7(2):113–8.

41. American Ferret Association. Ferret Vaccination Policy. Revised August 2006. Available at: http://www.ferret.org/read/vaccinations.html. Accessed July 30, 2011.

42. Krakowka S, Olsen RG, Axthelm MK, et al. Canine parvovirus potentiates canine distemper encephalitis attributable to modified live-virus vaccine. J Am Vet Med Assoc 1982;180(2):137–9.

43. Chappuis G. Control of canine distemper. Vet Microbiol 1995;44(2-4):351–8.

44. Lan NT, Yamaguchi R, Inomata A, et al. Comparative analyses of canine distemper viral isolates from clinical cases of canine distemper in vaccinated dogs. Vet Microbiol 2006;115(1-3):32–42.

45. Martella V, Cirone F, Elia G, et al. Heterogeneity within the hemagglutinin genes of canine distemper virus (CDV) strains detected in Italy. Vet Microbiol 2006;116(4): 301–9.

46. Gemma T, Watar T, Akiyama K, et al. Epidemiological observations on recent outbreaks of canine distemper in Tokyo area. J Vet Med Sci 1996;58(6):547–50.

47. Lan NT, Yamaguchi R, Furuya Y, et al. Pathogenesis and phylogenetic analyses of canine distemper virus strain 007Lm, a new isolate in dogs. Vet Microbiol 2005; 110(3-4):197–207.

48. Simon-Martínez J, Ulloa-Arvizu R, Soriano VE, et al. Identification of a genetic variant of canine distemper virus from clinical cases in two vaccinated dogs in Mexico. Vet J 2008;175(3):423–6.

49. Pardo ID, Johnson GC, Kleiboeker SB. Phylogenetic characterization of canine distemper viruses detected in naturally infected dogs in North America. J Clin Microbiol 2005;43(10):5009–17.

50. Lee MS, Tsai KJ, Chen LH, et al. The identification of frequent variations in the fusion protein of canine distemper virus. Vet J 2010;183(2):184–90.

51. Sawatsky B, von Messling V. Canine distemper viruses expressing a hemagglutinin without N-glycans lose virulence but retain immunosuppression. J Virol 2010;84(6): 2753–61.

52. Armstrong JA, Froelich EJ. Inactivation of viruses by benzalkonium chloride. Appl Microbiol 1964;12(2):132–7.
53. Watanabe Y, Miyata H, Sato H. Inactivation of laboratory animal RNA-viruses by physicochemical treatment. Jikken Dobutsu 1989;38:305–11.
54. Pratelli A. Canine distemper virus: the emergence of new variants. Vet J 2011;187(3): 290–1.
55. Gámiz C, Martella V, Ulloa R, et al. Identification of a new genotype of canine distemper virus circulating in America. Vet Res Commun 2011;35(6):381–90.
56. Woma TY, van Vuuren M, Bosman AM. Phylogenetic analysis of the haemagglutinin gene of current wild-type canine distemper viruses from South Africa: lineage Africa. Vet Microbiol 2010;143(2-4):126–32.
57. Calderon MG, Remorini P, Periolo O, et al. Detection by RT-PCR and genetic characterization of canine distemper virus from vaccinated and non-vaccinated dogs in Argentina. Vet Microbiol 2007;125(3-4):341–9.
58. Blancou J. Dog distemper: imported into Europe from South America? Hist Med Vet 2004;29(2):35–41.
59. McCarthy AJ, Shaw MA, Goodman SJ. Pathogen evolution and disease emergence in carnivores. Proc Biol Sci 2007;274(1629):3165–74.
60. Han GZ, Liu XP, Li SS. Cross-species recombination in the haemagglutinin gene of canine distemper virus. Virus Res 2008;136(1-2):198–201.
61. Monne I, Fusaro A, Valastro V, et al. A distinct CDV genotype causing a major epidemic in Alpine wildlife. Vet Microbiol 2011;150(1-2):63–9.
62. Sekulin K, Hafner-Marx A, Kolodziejek J, et al. Emergence of canine distemper in Bavarian wildlife associated with a specific amino acid exchange in the haemagglutinin protein. Vet J 2011;187(3):399–401.
63. Pomeroy LW, Bjørnstad ON, Holmes EC. The evolutionary and epidemiological dynamics of the paramyxoviridae. J Mol Evol 2008;66(2):98–106.
64. Lednicky JA, Dubach J, Kinsel MJ, et al. Genetically distant American canine distemper virus lineages have recently caused epizootics with somewhat different characteristics in raccoons living around a large suburban zoo in the USA. Virol J 2004;1:2–15.
65. Qui W, Zhen Y, Zhang S, et al. Canine distemper outbreak in Rhesus monkeys, China. EID 2011;17(8):1541–3.
66. Yoshikawa Y, Ochikubo F, Matsubara Y, et al. Natural infection with canine distemper virus in a Japanese monkey (Macaca fuscata). Vet Microbiol 1989;20(3):193–205.
67. Appel MJ, Yates RA, Foley GL, et al. Canine distemper epizootic in lions, tigers, and leopards in North America. J Vet Diagn Invest 1994;6(3):277–88.
68. Ramanathan A, Malik PK, Prasad G. Seroepizootiological survey for selected viral infections in captive Asiatic lions (Panthera leo persica) from western India. J Zoo Wildl Med 2007;38(3):400–8.
69. Roelke-Parker ME, Munson L, Packer C, et al. A canine distemper virus epidemic in Serengeti lions (Panthera leo). Nature 1996;379(6564):441–5.
70. Riley SP, Foley J, Chomel B. Exposure to feline and canine pathogens in bobcats and gray foxes in urban and rural zones of a national park in California. J Wildl Dis 2004;40(1):11–22.
71. Biek R, Ruth TK, Murphy KM, et al. Factors associated with pathogen seroprevalence and infection in Rocky Mountain cougars. J Wildl Dis 2006;42(3):606–15.
72. Nava AF, Cullen L, Sana DA, et al. First evidence of canine distemper in Brazilian free-ranging felids. Ecohealth 2008;5(4):513–8.

73. Millán J, Candela MG, Palomares F, et al. Disease threats to the endangered Iberian lynx (*Lynx pardinus*). Vet J 2009;182(1):114–24.

74. Quigley KS, Evermann JF, Leathers CW, et al. Morbillivirus infection in a wild Siberian tiger in the Russian Far East. J Wildl Dis 2010 Oct;46(4):1252–6.

75. Acosta-Jamett G, Chalmers WS, Cunningham AA, et al. Urban domestic dog populations as a source of canine distemper virus for wild carnivores in the Coquimbo region of Chile. Vet Microbiol 2011 May 13. Epub ahead of print.

76. Craft ME, Volz E, Packer C, et al. Distinguishing epidemic waves from disease spillover in a wildlife population. Proc Biol Sci 2009;276(1663):1777–85.

77. Craft ME, Hawthorne PL, Packer C, et al. Dynamics of a multihost pathogen in a carnivore community. J Anim Ecol 2008;77(6):1257–64.

78. Rikula U, Nuotio L, Sihvonen L. Vaccine coverage, herd immunity and occurrence of canine distemper from 1990-1996 in Finland. Vaccine 2007;25(47):7994–8.

79. Montali RJ, Bartz CR, Teare JA, et al. Clinical trials with canine distemper vaccines in exotic carnivores. J Am Vet Med Assoc 1983;183(11):1163–7.

80. Wimsatt J, Biggins DE, Williams ES, et al. The quest for a safe and effective canine distemper virus vaccine for black-footed ferrets. In: Roelle JE, editor. Recovery of the black-footed ferret: progress and continuing challenges. Proceedings of the Symposium on the Status of the Black-footed Ferret and Its Habitat. Fort Collins (CO): USGS; 2004. p. 248–66.

81. Bush M, Montali RJ, Brownstein D, et al. Vaccine-induced canine distemper in a lesser panda. J Am Vet Med Assoc 1976;169(9):959–60.

82. Philippa J. Chapter 12. Vaccination of non-domestic carnivores: a review. In: Kaandorp J, editor. Transmissible Diseases Handbook. 4th edition. Compiled by the Infectious Diseases Working Group (IDWG) of the European Association of Zoo and Wildlife Veterinarians (EAZWV). Amsterdam: European Association of Zoos and Aquaria; 2010. Available at: http://www.eaza.net/activities/Pages/Activities.aspx. Accessed July 30, 2011.

83. Bronson E, Emmons LH, Murray S, et al. Serosurvey of pathogens in domestic dogs on the border of Noël Kempff Mercado National Park, Bolivia. J Zoo Wildl Med 2008;39(1):28–36.

84. Lamberski N. Updated vaccination recommendations for carnivores. In: Miller RE, Fowler M, editors. Fowler's zoo and wild animal medicine, vol. 7. St. Louis (MO): Elsevier Saunders; 2011. p. 442–50.

85. Carpenter JW, Appel MJ, Erickson RC, et al. Fatal vaccine-induced canine distemper virus infection in black-footed ferrets. J Am Vet Med Assoc 1976;169(9):961–4.

86. Thorne ET, Williams ES. Disease and endangered species: the black-footed ferret as a recent example. Conserv Biol 1988;2(1):66–74.

87. Black-footed Ferret Recovery Program. 2011. Available at: http://www.blackfootedferret.org/disease. Accessed July 30, 2011.

88. Timm SF, Munson L, Summers BA, et al. A suspected canine distemper epidemic as the cause of a catastrophic decline in Santa Catalina Island foxes (*Urocyon littoralis catalinae*). J Wildl Dis 2009;45(2):333–43.

89. Clifford D L, Mazet JA, Dubovi EJ, et al. 2006. Pathogen exposure in endangered island fox (*Urocyon littoralis*) populations: Implications for conservation management. Biol Conserv 2006;131(2):230–43.

90. Institute for Wildlife Studies. Santa Catalina Island Fox. 2011. Available at: http://www.iws.org/island_fox_studies_Santa_Catalina_Island.htm. Accessed July 30, 2011.

91. The International Union for Conservation of Nature (IUCN) Red List of Threatened Species. *Lycaon pictus*. 2011. Available at: http://www.iucnredlist.org/apps/redlist/details/12436/0. Accessed July 30, 2011.

92. van de Bildt MW, Kuiken T, Visee AM, et al. Distemper outbreak and its effect on African wild dog conservation. Emerg Infect Dis 2002;8(2):211–3.

93. Welter J, Taylor J, Tartaglia J, et al. Mucosal vaccination with recombinant poxvirus vaccines protects ferrets against symptomatic CDV infection. Vaccine 1999;17(4):30–8.

94. Welter J, Taylor J, Tartaglia J, et al. Vaccination against canine distemper virus infection in infant ferrets with and without maternal antibody protection, using recombinant attenuated poxvirus vaccines. J Virol 2000;74(14):6358–67.

95. Wimsatt J, Biggins D, Innes K, et al. Evaluation of oral and subcutaneous delivery of an experimental canarypox recombinant canine distemper vaccine in the Siberian polecat (*Mustela eversmanni*). J Zoo Wildl Med 2003;34(1):25–35.

96. National Wildlife Disease Program. 2011. Available at: http://www.aphis.usda.gov/wildlife_damage/nwdp/index.shtml. Accessed July 30, 2011.

97. DeLiberto TJ, Beach RH. USDA APHIS Wildlife Services' National Wildlife Disease Surveillance and Emergency Response System (SERS). In: Proceedings of the 22nd Vertebrate Pest Conference. Davis (CA), 2006. p. 329–33.

98. National Wildlife Disease Program. State Highlights—Eastern Region; Minnesota. In: The Carrier 2010;2(4):7. Available at: http://www.aphis.usda.gov/wildlife_damage/nwdp/pdf/The%20Carrier%20Vol%202%20Iss%204.pdf. Accessed July 30, 2011.

99. Innovative Solutions to Human–Wildlife Conflicts. NWRC Accomplishments 2005, p. 59. Available at: http://www.aphis.usda.gov/publications/wildlife_damage/content/printable_version/wildlife-report508.pdf. Accessed July 30, 2011.

100. Scott J. Wildlife Services: Partnering in Africa. Inside APHIS Quarterly Employee Newsletter, 2009 Summer Issue. Available at: http://www.aphis.usda.gov/inside_aphis/downloads/InsideAPHIS_2009_Summer.pdf. Accessed July 30, 2011.

101. NWRC Spotlight Archives. Scientists Help Save Wild Dogs and African Lions. January 5, 2010. Available at: http://www.aphis.usda.gov/wildlife_damage/nwrc/spotlight/african_Jan10.shtml. Accessed July 30, 2011.

102. U.S. Department of the Interior. 2011. Available at: http://www.doi.gov/index.cfm. Accessed July 30, 2011.

103. Marinari PE, Kreeger JS. 2006. An adaptive management approach for black-footed ferrets in captivity. In: Roelle JE, editor. Recovery of the black-footed ferret: progress and continuing challenges. Proceedings of the Symposium on the Status of the Black-footed Ferret and Its Habitat. Fort Collins, CO: USGS; 2004, p. 23–7.

104. NPS. Endangered Island Fox: On the Cusp of Biological Recovery. June 10, 2010. Available at: http://www.nps.gov/chis/parknews/island-fox-2010-update.htm. Accessed July 30, 2011.

105. Catalina Island Conservancy. Fox Rescue. 2011. Available at: http://www.catalinaconservancy.org. Accessed July 30, 2011.

106. Yellowstone National Park News Release. Yellowstone Wolf Population in Transition. February 16, 2010. Available at: http://www.nps.gov/yell/parknews/1006.htm.

107. Manitoba Veterinary Medical Association. Canine distemper outbreak reported in raccoons along the Seine River in South Winnipeg. December 22, 2010. Available at: http://www.mvma.ca. Accessed July 30, 2011.

108. Cleaveland S, Laurenson MK, Taylor LH. Diseases of humans and their domestic mammals: pathogen characteristics, host range and the risk of emergence. Phil Trans R Soc Lond B 2001;356:991–9.

109. Dobson A, Foufopoulos J. Emerging infectious pathogens of wildlife. Phil Trans R Soc Lond B 2001:356:1001–12.
110. Almberg ES, Cross PC, Smith DW. Persistence of canine distemper virus in the Greater Yellowstone ecosystem's carnivore community. Ecol Appl 2010;20(7):2058–74.
111. Almberg ES, Mech LD, Smith DW, et al. A serological survey of infectious disease in Yellowstone National Park's canid community. PLoS One 2009;16;4(9):e7042.
112. Food and Animal Organization of the United Nations. Animal Production and Health Division News Archives. 2011. Available at: http://www.fao.org/ag/againfo/home/en/news.htm. Accessed July 30, 2011.
113. MacPherson CN. Human behaviour and the epidemiology of parasitic zoonoses. Int J Parasitol 2005;35(11-12):1319–31.
114. Pedersen AB, Jones KE, Nunn CL, et al. Infectious diseases and extinction risk in wild mammals. Conserv Biol 2007;21(5):1269–79.
115. Salb AL, Barkema HW, Elkin BT. Dogs as sources and sentinels of parasites in humans and wildlife, northern Canada. EID 2008;14(1):60–3.
116. World Society for the Protection of Animals. WSPA and the FAO call for global dog population body. April 4, 2011. Available at: http://www.wspa-international.org/latestnews/2011/FAO-global-dog-population-body.aspx. Accessed July 30, 2011.
117. Acosta-Jamett G, Cleaveland S, Cunningham AA, et al. Demography of domestic dogs in rural and urban areas of the Coquimbo region of Chile and implications for disease transmission. Prev Vet Med 2010;94(3-4):272–81.
118. Acosta-Jamett G, Chalmers WS, Cunningham AA, et al. Urban domestic dog populations as a source of canine distemper virus for wild carnivores in the Coquimbo region of Chile. Vet Microbiol 2011. doi:10.1016/j.vetmic.2011.05.008.
119. Bryan HM, Darimont CT, Paquet PC, et al. Exposure to infectious agents in dogs in remote coastal British Columbia: Possible sentinels of diseases in wildlife and humans. Can J Vet Res 2011;75(1):11–7.
120. Demeter Z, Rusvai M. Canine distemper: still a major concern in Central Europe. Lucrari Stiintifice Universitatea de Stiinte Agricole a Banatului Timisoara, Medicina Veterinara 2009;42(1):136–50.

Astroviruses in Dogs

Vito Martella, DVM*, Paschalina Moschidou, DVM,
Canio Buonavoglia, DVM

KEYWORDS

- Astrovirus • Dog • Enteritis • Small rounded viruses

Astroviruses (AstVs) are small nonenveloped icosahedral viruses. Their genome is composed of plus-sense, single-stranded RNA with a 3′ polyadenylated [poly(A)] tail. AstVs have been identified from numerous animal species, including humans, and mainly associated with enteric disease.[1] Nonenteric disease has been also described in avian species.[2] Even more interestingly, AstVs have been detected in the central nervous system tissue of mink with neurologic disease[3] and of an immunocompromised patient with encephalitis.[4] Canine AstVs were first identified in the early 1980s,[5] but they have been recently "rediscovered" and characterized at the molecular level as a distinct species within the *Mamastrovirus* genus.[6–8]

CAUSES

AstVs (family Astroviridae) are small-rounded viruses (SRVs) with a peculiar starlike shape when observed on electron microscopy (EM), although this conformation is not always readily recognizable. AstV genome is composed of a plus-sense single-stranded RNA of 6.4 of 7.3 kb in size, containing 3 open reading frames (ORFs) and with a 3′ poly(A) tail.[1] Two ORFs, located at the 5′ end of the genome (ORF1a and ORF1b), encode nonstructural proteins, while ORF2, located at the 3′ end, encodes the capsid protein.[1] AstVs were first identified by EM in 1975 in Scotland in the stools of infants hospitalized with diarrhea.[9] Subsequently, similar SRVs have been identified from several mammalian and avian species,[10–18] including bats,[19] rats,[20] and aquatic mammals.[21] AstV infection is associated with gastroenteritis in most animal species, and human AstVs are regarded as the second or third most common cause of viral diarrhea in children.[1] AstVs have also been associated with extraintestinal diseases, such as nephritis in chicken,[2] hepatitis in ducks,[16] and shaking syndrome in mink.[3]

Based on the species of origin of the virus, the genome structure and genetic homology, 2 genera have been defined within the family Astroviridae: *Mamastrovirus*,

---

This work was granted by the project from the Italian Ministry of Health, Ricerca corrente 2009, project IZS VE 21/09 RC "Definizione di una procedura validata per la selezione di cani per programmi di Interventi Assistiti dagli Animali (IAA)".
The authors have nothing to disclose.
Dipartimento di Sanità Pubblica e Zootecnia, Università degli Studi Aldo Moro di Bari, S.p. per Casamassima Km 3, 70010 Valenzano, Bari, Italy
* Corresponding author.
E-mail address: v.martella@veterinaria.uniba.it

which infect mammals, and *Avastrovirus*, which include viruses detected from avian species. As viruses genetically highly diverse can circulate in a given host species,[22] a novel classification system based on comparison of the full length ORF2, the capsid precursor, has been proposed (http://talk.ictvonline.org/files/proposals/taxonomy_proposals_vertebrate1/m/vert01/2287.aspx). In this classification, 2 genogroups (GI and II) have been defined in *Mamastrovirus* genus. AstV strains within the same species display a p-distance lower than 0.312 and species are assigned consecutive letters. In this system, human AstVs type 1 to type 8 are GI.A, feline AstV is GI.B, and canine AstVs are GI.E.

Novel AstVs have been recently detected in humans, although only in a sporadic fashion. These novel human AstVs are distantly related to "classic" human AstV types 1 to 8, and more similar genetically to some animal AstVs.[23-25] Antibodies to one such novel AstV, strain MAstV/GII.B/Hu/THA/2001/NE-3010, have been detected in 20% to 36% of the sera of children.[26] These findings suggest recent interspecies transmission events of AstVs from animals to humans and, more importantly, widespread exposure of humans to these viruses.

ASTROVIRUSES IN DOGS

AstV-like particles have been detected only occasionally in dogs on EM. In some cases, due to their morphologic similarities (about 25 to 35 nm, rounded, absence of envelope) with caliciviruses and picornaviruses, they have generically been referred to as SRVs. AstV-like particles were first detected on EM in beagle pups with diarrheal disease in the United States in 1980, in mixed infection with canine parvovirus type-2 (CPV2) and canine coronaviruses (CCoV).[5] AstV-like particles were also detected on EM in 3 of 157 normal fecal samples (but not in 29 diarrheal samples) in a survey in Australia in 1984.[27] In a large EM-based survey in Germany, SRVs were identified in 41 of 4044 (about 1%) feces of dogs with diarrhea.[28] More recently, AstVs have been identified in dogs with enteric signs and characterized molecularly, suggesting that the detected viruses may represent a distinct AstV species.[6-8]

While early evidence suggested that AstV infection in dogs is rare or occasional, recent investigations based on sensitive and specific assays indicate that AstVs are indeed widespread in the canine population. By screening on RT-PCR with canine AstV-specific primers 625F-1 and 626R-1 (**Table 1**) in a collection of fecal samples obtained from 1- to 6-month-old pups with gastroenteric signs in Italy in 2007, AstV RNA was detected in 27 of 110 samples (24.5%), either alone (10 of 110, 9.0%) or in mixed infections with canine parvovirus type 2 (5 of 110, 4.5%) and canine coronavirus (8 of 110, 7.3%) or both (4 of 110, 3.6%). Also, AstV RNA was detected in 7 of 75 swabs (9.3%) obtained from asymptomatic young dogs.[7]

In a survey in Shangai, China, in 2008, using canine AstV-specific primers L5 and R5 (**Table 1**), AstVs have been detected on RT-PCR in 22 of 183 (12.02%) dogs with enteric signs but in 0 of 138 asymptomatic dogs (0%). The 3' end portion of the genome of a Chinese virus was sequenced and found to be distantly related (76.9% to 78.3% nucleotide [nt] identity in the full-length ORF2) to other canine AstVs, providing evidence for genetic heterogeneity in canine AstVs.[8]

Antibodies specific for canine AstV (virus Bari/08/ITA) have been detected by an indirect immunofluorescence assay in 32 of 54 (59.0%) serum samples. The majority (14 of 22, 63.6%) of the serum samples testing negative were from pups aged less than 3 months, while only 3 of 32 (9.4%) of the positive sera were from dogs aged less than 3 months.[7] This age-related pattern would be consistent with the fact that by 2 to 3 months of age, pups is susceptible to infectious agents as maternally derived immunity tends to wane.[29]

Table 1
List of primers used for diagnostic of canine AstVs

Primer	Sequence (5' to 3')	Sense	Target	Reference	Assay
CaAstV2Pb	6FAM-ATATGTACTTTTGCCATCAGGAGAG-BHQ1	+	ORF1b	Unpublished	qRT-PCR
CaAstV2-F	ATTACCACGATGTTGYTCTGTR	+	ORF1b	Unpublished	qRT-PCR
CaAstV2-R	CATCATTGGTATGTTGAAAAYYTG	–	ORF1b	Unpublished	qRT-PCR
CaAstV1Pb	6FAM-TACTGTGCTACTTCCATCTGGCGAG-BHQ1	+	ORF1b	Unpublished	qRT-PCR
CaAstV1-F	ATTACCACGATGTTGTTCTGTA	+	ORF1b	Unpublished	qRT-PCR
CaAstV1-R	CATGATTGGTATGTTGAAAATCTG	–	ORF1b	Unpublished	qRT-PCR
panAstVFor1	GARTTYGATTGGRCKCGKTAYGA	+	ORF1b	[19]	RT-PCR
panAstVFor2	GARTTYGATTGGRCKAGGTAYGA	+	ORF1b	[19]	RT-PCR
panAstVRev	GGYTTKACCCACATNCCRAA	–	ORF1b	[19]	RT-PCR
625F-1	GTACTATACCRTCTGATTTAATT	+	ORF1b	[7]	RT-PCR
626R-1	AGACCAARGTGTCATAGTTCAG	–	ORF1b	[7]	RT-PCR
L5	CAANTCACAACCCAAAACAAA	+	ORF2	[8]	RT-PCR
R5	TTTTNACNATCACTGCTAGNG	–	ORF2	[8]	RT-PCR

Unpublished data by Martella and colleagues, 2011.

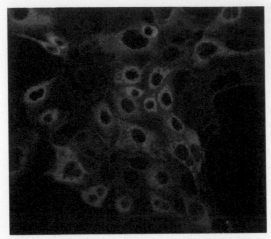

Fig. 1. Indirect immunofluorescence on 24-hour infected MDCK cells.

CULTIVATION IN VITRO

A canine AstV, strain Bari/08/ITA, has been isolated in a canine kidney cell line (Madin-Darby canine kidney [MDCK]). Likewise other mammalian AstVs, cultivation required supplementation with trypsin.[7] Virus replication in MDCK cells triggered a clear cytopathic effect consisting in enlargement and/or detaching of cells and appearance of fine granules in the cytoplasm. Viral antigens were observed in immunefluorescence in the cells as fine granules dispersed in the cytoplasm, aggregating in perinuclear position (**Fig. 1**). No significant mutation was mapped in the ORF2 and 3′ noncoding region (3′ -UTR) between the field virus and the tissue-adapted (third serial passage) isolate Bari/08/ITA.

GENOME ORGANIZATION OF CANINE ASTROVIRUSES

The full-length genome sequence of canine AstVs has not been determined yet, while the sequence of the 3′ end of the genome (the 3′ end of ORF1b, the full-length ORF2, and the 3′-UTR) is available for the isolate ITA/2008/Bari and for strain ITA/2010/Zoid. In addition, the full-length ORF2 sequences of an additional 6 canine strains from Italy and China are available in the databases. In these strains, ORF2 ranges from 765 to 774 amino acids in length, while the 3′-UTR ranges from 77 to 87 nt. There is an 8-nt overlap between the termination codon of ORF1b and the initiation codon of ORF2. The highly conserved nucleotide stretch upstream of ORF2, 5′-ATTTGGAGNGGNG-GACCNAAN$_{5-8}$ATGNC-3′,[30] believed to be part of a promoter region for synthesis of subgenomic RNA, is nearly completely conserved in the sequence of strains ITA/2008/Bari and ITA/2010/Zoid. Overall, these features mirror those observed in other mammalian AstVs.[1]

By comparison of the capsid protein, the canine AstV strains exhibit more than 70.% amino acid identity to each other and less than 33% amino acid identity to noncanine AstVs, thus constituting a genetically well-defined group (**Fig. 2**). The range of variation among canine AstVs is similar to those defined for human GI.A AstV types 1 to 8.[31] By analyzing the capsid protein of human AstVs, a high degree of conservation can be observed in the N-terminal portion (amino acids 1 to 415) of the capsid protein, while downstream the conserved 415 residues, considerable variability is seen among

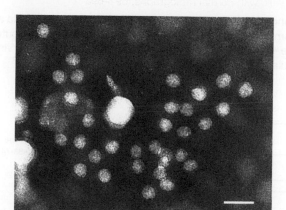

Fig. 2. EM observation of negatively stained AstV particles, aggregated by an AstV-specific antiserum. Scale bar 50 nm. (*Courtesy of* Dr Antonio Lavazza, Istituto Zooprofilattico Sperimentale di Lombardia ed Emilia Romagna, Sezione di Brescia, Italy.)

strains of different serotypes.[1] Likewise, among the canine AstV strains, a high degree of variation occurs between aa 422 and 668 (<50% aa identity), whilst the capsid sequence is more conserved at the NH_3- and COOH-ends. The hypervariable region is believed to form the spikes of the virion and to interact with the cell receptors[32] as neutralizing monoclonal antibodies have been mapped to this variable domain.[33,34] These findings may be predictive of marked antigenic differences among the various canine strains.

PATHOGENESIS

Using specific primers in RT-PCR, canine AstVs RNA has been detected exclusively in the stool and in the intestinal content of pups and no evidence for extraintestinal localization has been obtained thus far screening the tissues of animals dead from severe gastroenteritis.

AstV shedding was detectable in RT-PCR for at least 10 days in a 3-month-old pup hospitalized with watery diarrhea and severe dehydration. Clinical signs in the pup lasted 4 days, with viral shedding continuing for 8 days after the pup recovered from the disease. The pup tested negative to all other canine pathogens, suggesting that AstV was actually the causative agent of the disease.[7] By quantification of viral load in real time RT-PCR (qRT-PCR), a positive correlation between the clinical signs and the virus titers was observed with the highest viral loads occurring during the acute symptomatic phase. Also, specific IgGs were not detected in the serum sample collected at the time of hospitalization, but they were detectable 2 weeks after hospitalization, indicating seroconversion.[7] Interesting pieces of information have been gathered by monitoring an outbreak of gastroenteric disease associated with canine AstV, affecting 2 household dogs (aged 2 years and 2 months, respectively). The AstV strain, ITA/2010/Zoid, displayed limited amino acid identity (70.3% to 73.9%) to other canine AstV strains in the full-length capsid protein. Antibodies specific for the prototype canine astrovirus isolate ITA/2008/Bari were not detected in the convalescent sera of the animals, suggesting limited antigenic relatedness. In the 2 animals, virus shedding (up to 10^7 to 10^8 copies of genome equivalents/gr of feces) was correlated with clinical signs, with the disease being severer and virus shedding being more prolonged (more than 1 month) in the young pup (Martella and colleagues, unpublished information, 2011). Prolonged virus shedding after acute infection and resistance in the environments[35,36] could be factors facilitating virus diffusion in susceptible population.

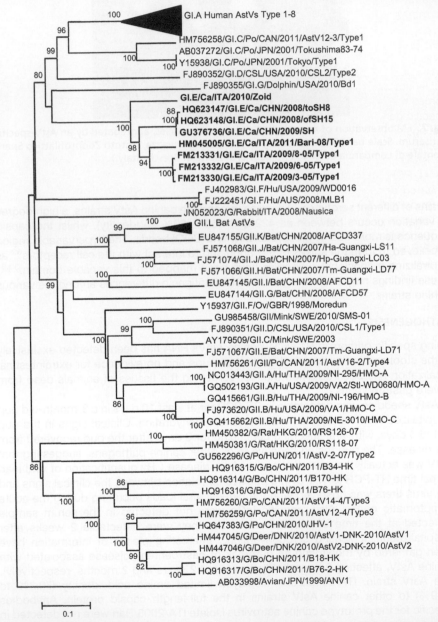

Fig. 3. Phylogenetic tree based on the full-length amino acid sequence of the capsid protein of AstVs of avian and mammalian origin. The tree was elaborated with the neighbor-joining method without any distance correction.

DIAGNOSTICS

EM observation has long been the only assay able to reveal the presence of SRVs in the stools of dogs (**Fig. 3**). The low prevalence rates on EM, compared to the high rates revealed in molecular assays, suggest AstV titers in the feces are above the EM detection limits for a restricted time period.[7] Also, EM is not always able to characterize firmly SRVs, as the peculiar morphology of AstVs is often lost during sample conservation and/or processing.[9] Several primer sets have been developed to recognize effectively canine AstVs in RT-PCR (**Table 1**). The primers have been designed in highly conserved regions of the ORF1b (RdRp) and ORF2 (capsid protein). Also, a quantitative RT-PCR (qRT-PCR) has been set up (**Table 1**). The qRT-PCR assay was able to detect AstV strains that markedly differed in the capsid gene and proved to be highly sensitive (Martella and colleagues, unpublished data, 2011). Using the strain Bari/08/ITA has antigen, an indirect immunofluorescence assay has been developed to identify canine AstV-specific IgGs.[7]

SUMMARY

Based on the present, yet limited, literature, canine AstVs appear to be widespread in different geographical areas. AstV prevalence seems to be significantly higher in pups with gastroenteric disease than in asymptomatic animals. In some cases AstVs can be detected alone (not in coinfection with other enteric pathogens) from animals with enteric disease and virus shedding can be correlated with the onset of gastroenteric signs. Interestingly, canine AstVs appear to be genetically heterogeneous. Animal experiments will be pivotal to investigate the pathogenic role of canine AstVs and understand whether prophylaxis tools are required. Also, the canine homologous model could offer valuable information for the study of human AstVs.

REFERENCES

1. Mendez E, Arias CF. Astroviruses. In: Fields Virology, Knipe DM, Howley PM, editors. 5th ed. Philadelphia: Lippincott Williams & Wilkins; 2007. p. 981–1000.
2. Imada T, Yamaguchi S, Mase M, et al. Avian nephritis virus (ANV) as a new member of the family Astroviridae and construction of infectious ANV cDNA. J Virol 2000;74: 8487–93.
3. Blomström A-L, Widén F, Hammer A-S, et al. Detection of a novel astrovirus in brain tissue of mink suffering from shaking mink syndrome by use of viral metagenomics. J Clin Microbiol 2010;48:4392–6.
4. Quan PL, Wagner TA, Briese T, et al. Astrovirus encephalitis in boy with X-linked agammaglobulinemia. Emerging Infect Dis 2010;16:918–25.
5. Williams FP Jr. Astrovirus-like, coronavirus-like, and parvovirus-like particles detected in the diarrheal stools of beagle pups. Arch Virol 1980;66:215–26.
6. Toffan A, Jonassen CM, De Battisti C, et al. Genetic characterization of a new astrovirus detected in dogs suffering from diarrhoea. Vet Microbiol 2009;139: 147–52.
7. Martella V, Moschidou P, Lorusso E, et al. Detection and characterization of astroviruses in dogs. J Gen Virol 2011;92(Pt 8):1880–7.
8. Zhu AL, Zhao W, Yin H, et al. Isolation and characterization of canine astrovirus in China. Arch Virol 2011;156(9):1671–5.
9. Madeley CR, Cosgrove BP. Letter: 28 nm particles in faeces in infantile gastroenteritis. Lancet 1975;2:451–2.

10. Bridger JC. Detection by electron microscopy of caliciviruses, astroviruses and rotavirus-like particles in the faeces of piglets with diarrhoea. Vet Rec 1980;107: 532–3.

11. Englund L, Chriél M, Dietz HH, et al. Astrovirus epidemiologically linked to pre-weaning diarrhoea in mink. Vet Microbiol 2002;85:1–11.

12. Hoshino Y, Zimmer JF, Moise NS, et al. Detection of astroviruses in feces of a cat with diarrhea. Brief report. Arch Virol 1981;70:373–6.

13. Kjeldsberg E, Hem A. Detection of astroviruses in gut contents of nude and normal mice. Brief report. Arch Virol 1985;84:135–40.

14. McNulty MS, Curran WL, McFerran JB. Detection of astroviruses in turkey faeces by direct electron microscopy. Vet Rec 1980;106:561.

15. Snodgrass DR, Gray EW. Detection and transmission of 30 nm virus particles (astroviruses) in faeces of lambs with diarrhoea. Arch Virol 1977;55:287–91.

16. Todd D, Smyth VJ, Ball NW, et al. Identification of chicken enterovirus-like viruses, duck hepatitis virus type 2 and duck hepatitis virus type 3 as astroviruses. Avian Pathol 2009;38(1):21–30.

17. Tzipori S, Menzies JD, Gray EW. Detection of astrovirus in the faeces of red deer. Vet Rec 1981;108(13):286.

18. Woode GN, Bridger JC. Isolation of small viruses resembling astroviruses and caliciviruses from acute enteritis of calves. J Med Microbiol 1978;11(4):441–52.

19. Chu DKW, Poon LLM, Guan Y, et al. Novel astroviruses in insectivorous bats. J Virol 2008;82(18):9107–14.

20. Chu DKW, Chin AWH, Smith GJ, et al. Detection of novel astroviruses in urban brown rats and previously known astroviruses in humans. J Gen Virol 2010; 91(Pt 10):2457–62.

21. Rivera R, Nollens HH, Venn-Watson S, et al. Characterization of phylogenetically diverse astroviruses of marine mammals. J Gen Virol 2010;91(Pt 1):166–73.

22. Finkbeiner SR, Holtz LR, Jiang Y, et al. Human stool contains a previously unrecognized diversity of novel astroviruses. Virol J 2009;6:161.

23. Bányai K, Meleg E, Moschidou P, et al. Detection of newly described astrovirus MLB1 in stool samples from children. Emerg Infect Dis 2010;16(1):169; author reply 169–70.

24. Finkbeiner SR, Le BM, Holtz LR, et al. Detection of newly described astrovirus MLB1 in stool samples from children. Emerg Infect Dis 2009;15(3):441–4.

25. Kapoor A, Li L, Victoria J, et al. Multiple novel astrovirus species in human stool. J Gen Virol 2009;90(Pt 12):2965–72.

26. Burbelo PD, Ching KH, Esper F, et al. Serological studies confirm the novel astrovirus HMOAstV-C as a highly prevalent human infectious agent. PLoS ONE 2011;6(8): e22576.

27. Marshall JA, Healey DS, Studdert MJ, et al. Viruses and virus-like particles in the faeces of dogs with and without diarrhoea. Aust Vet J 1984;61(2):33–8.

28. Vieler E, Herbst W. [Electron microscopic demonstration of viruses in feces of dogs with diarrhea]. Tierarztl Prax 1995;23(1):66–9.

29. Pollock RV, Carmichael LE. Maternally derived immunity to canine parvovirus infection: transfer, decline, and interference with vaccination. J Am Vet Med Assoc 1982;180(1):37–42.

30. Walter JE, Briggs J, Guerrero ML, et al. Molecular characterization of a novel recombinant strain of human astrovirus associated with gastroenteritis in children. Arch Virol 2001;146(12):2357–67.

31. Méndez-Toss M, Romero-Guido P, Munguía ME, et al. Molecular analysis of a serotype 8 human astrovirus genome. J Gen Virol 2000;81(Pt 12):2891–7.

32. Krishna NK. Identification of structural domains involved in astrovirus capsid biology. Viral Immunol 2005;18(1):17–26.
33. Bass DM, Upadhyayula U. Characterization of human serotype 1 astrovirus-neutralizing epitopes. J Virol 1997;71(11):8666–71.
34. Sanchez-Fauquier A, Carrascosa AL, Carrascosa JL, et al. Characterization of a human astrovirus serotype 2 structural protein (VP26) that contains an epitope involved in virus neutralization. Virology 1994;201(2):312–20.
35. Abad FX, Villena C, Guix S, et al. Potential role of fomites in the vehicular transmission of human astroviruses. Appl Environ Microbiol 2001;67(9):3904–7.
36. Abad FX, Pintó RM, Villena C, et al. Astrovirus survival in drinking water. Appl Environ Microbiol 1997;63(8):3119–22.

Canine Reproductive, Respiratory, and Ocular Diseases due to Canine Herpesvirus

James F. Evermann, PhD[a],*, Eric C. Ledbetter, DVM[b],
Roger K. Maes, DVM, PhD[c]

KEYWORDS

- Canine Herpesvirus • Reproductive • Respiratory • Ocular
- Diseases • Detection

Although canine herpesvirus (CHV) (also referred to as canine herpesvirus 1, canid herpesvirus 1, neonatal herpes, genital herpes, ocular herpes, and CHV-1) infections and related diseases have been recognized since the early 1960s,[1–5] there has been a resurgence of interest in the various clinical manifestations of the virus, which makes this review very timely.[6–11] The various forms of CHV-associated infections are listed in **Table 1**. In some cases these infections were directly related to clinical symptoms, such as acute neonatal viremia resulting in puppy mortality; systemic viremia in naive pregnant females resulting in fetal death, abortion, and mummification; and ocular-respiratory disease in dogs of various age ranges.[12]

What has changed within the past decade has been the ability to detect the virus in its subclinical state, which allows for a much clearer understanding of the importance of 2 subpopulations of dogs: carrier-shedder adult dogs, and CHV–latently infected dogs in the animal populations with which we work.[13–17] The increased sensitivity of both antibody-based serology assays and nucleic acid–based polymerase chain reaction (PCR) assays have increased our level of clinical inquiry regarding CHV, as well as the other canine infectious microorganisms.[18–22] In addition to recognizing CHV adult carriers in the general population, this new momentum has allowed for clinicians to screen dogs that are undergoing

The authors have nothing to disclose.
[a] Department of Veterinary Clinical Sciences and Washington Animal Disease Diagnostic Laboratory, College of Veterinary Medicine, Washington State University, Pullman, WA 99164, USA
[b] Department of Clinical Sciences, College of Veterinary Medicine, Cornell University, Ithaca, NY 14853, USA
[c] Diagnostic Center for Population and Animal Health, Michigan State University, 4125 Beaumont Road, Lansing, MI 48910, USA
* Corresponding author.
E-mail address: jfe@vetmed.wsu.edu

Vet Clin Small Anim 41 (2011) 1097–1120
doi:10.1016/j.cvsm.2011.08.007
0195-5616/11/$ – see front matter © 2011 Elsevier Inc. All rights reserved.

Table 1
Clinical features of canine herpesvirus infection and disease

Infection/Disease	Age Groups at Risk	Outcome/Comments
1. Mucosal form (respiratory/vaginal)	Older puppies (>3 weeks) and adults	Mild, often inapparent infection, active shedding, with establishment of latency
2. Latent infection	Older puppies, adults, and survivors of neonatal and mucosal forms	Lifelong infection, may show recrudescence at pregnancy and stress
3. Acute neonatal viremia	Puppies from birth to 3 weeks	Fatal systemic disease, active shedding, poor prognosis
4. Systemic infection of naïve pregnant females	Breeding dams	Fetal death, abortion, mummification, source of virus for acute neonatal viremia
5. Ocular form	Older puppies (> 3 wks) and adults	Mild conjunctivitis to severe ocular disease, with active shedding

Data from Anvik JO. Clinical considerations of canine herpesvirus infection. Vet Med 1991;82:394–403.

immunosuppressive regimens of therapy for various dermatologic conditions, as well as dogs being treated for various cancers. This review will provide a brief overview of the reproductive aspects of CHV disease and will then bring together the current literature, documenting the involvement of CHV in adult dog respiratory and ocular diseases.

CONTEMPORARY CLINICAL OBSERVATIONS
Reproductive Disorders

Consistent with the other alpha herpesviruses, CHV has a predilection for pregnant dogs and neonatal puppies.[23–26] Early reports focused on the effects of CHV on various reproductive parameters in the dog, in part due to the severity of the clinical symptoms and the profound pathologic effects. In the review by Anvik,[12] acute neonatal viremia and systemic infection of naïve pregnant females were regarded as 2 of the most important disease outcomes of CHV infection. The emphasis at that time was on the recognition of clinical symptoms for a rapid diagnosis. Since there are no commercial vaccines currently available for the prevention of CHV-induced disease, it has become paramount to understand the clinical features of CHV infections (see **Table 1**) and to incorporate this knowledge with sound management practices to minimize the effects on reproductive efficiency and puppy survival.[27]

As was mentioned previously, this has been the primary focus of the earlier literature on CHV infections. Infection may occur during pregnancy or may be acquired by puppies during the first few weeks of life. The key feature during both of these phases is that the pregnant female and puppies are *immunologically naïve* to CHV and therefore highly susceptible to disease. Puppies may acquire the infection in utero, from passage through the birth canal, from contact with oronasal secretions of the dam, or contact shedders. Humans may serve as fomites of the virus if attending to an adult carrier-shedder dog, and then proceeding to a nursery setting without proper disinfection. Naïve neonatal puppies, younger than 1 week, are at highest risk of fatal systemic disease, while naïve dogs older than 3 weeks are relatively resistant to disease but can still become infected.[27–29] Virus infection in naïve older dogs is generally acquired via aerosol, so that replication occurs in the nasopharynx tonsils and retropharyngeal and bronchial lymph nodes.[2,30–32] This respiratory site will become an important aspect of the ecology of the virus when both respiratory and ocular clinical outcomes are covered in subsequent sections.

Although neonatal infections are regarded as the most common, in utero infection with CHV may occur. Infertility and abortion of stillborn or of weak pups has been reported. While the mortality rate usually approaches 100% for the fetal puppy, there may be no further clinical manifestations reported in the dam.[1,5,26]

Passive immunity acquired from the dam appears to be of primary biological importance in the survival of infected pups.[12,27,33–35] Puppies that are nursing from CHV-seronegative dams usually develop the fatal multisystemic disease, while puppies that suckle from CHV-seropositive dams remain asymptomatic but still become infected. The CHV is usually recovered from the oropharyngeal region in these disease-resistant pups. It is generally accepted that maternal antibody and/or immune lymphocytes acquired through the milk explain why naturally infected dams that have a diseased litter will usually give birth to normal litters on subsequent pregnancies.

Since CHV is one of the few canine viral infections that can proceed to fatal disease and there is no commercial vaccine routinely available, it has become necessary for *infection management* to prevent reproductive disease. The literature has focused on 3 aspects of the virus and its relationship with host immunity and its carrier-spread dynamics within a population of susceptible dogs.

Infection management—understanding the risk factors

The risk factors associated with CHV infection and reproductive disease has been intensively studied over the past 5 years.[36,37] The studies have used various diagnostic assays including serology, virus isolation, and polymerase chain reaction (PCR). These studies have provided valuable information on controlling CHV-associated reproductive diseases (ie, infertility, abortion, stillbirths, and neonatal mortality). **Table 2** lists the 12 risk factors that were studied and whether there was an association with reproductive disease. Of the 12 factors, 8 were identified as having a positive correlation with disease: breeding kennel, age, mating experience, cycle (stage), concurrent kennel cough, kennel size, breeding management, and hygiene.

The underlying risks in the aforementioned factors are CHV infection and an immune susceptible dog. This has led to strategies to naturally immunize (via contact with adult dogs) susceptible female dogs prebreeding, to screen female dogs for CHV infection (by serology and/or PCR) prior to breeding, and to use a defined quarantine period for pregnant dogs with an unknown CHV infection status. An age-risk, immunologically naïve-risk strategy has been used by clinicians and clients to focus on the most susceptible time periods for disease. This time encompasses the pregnant female during the last 3 weeks prior to whelping, and her puppies up to 3 weeks post whelping.[12,27,33] This understanding has constituted the rationale for the "6-week danger period."[12,27]

The primary contributing risk factors that allow for CHV infection and disease are kennel size, hygiene, and kennel cough. All 3 of these are important in the spread and retention of CHV in high-risk dog populations. While the controversy over CHV being a significant contributor to the kennel cough syndrome has been an ongoing debate (see subsequent section on respiratory–ocular infections), it should be noted that CHV was initially reported as a respiratory pathogen as early as it was a reproductive pathogen.[2] The data from Ronsse and coworkers[22] support the contention that CHV

Table 2
Risk factors studied to determine the association between CHV infection and reproductive diseases in dogs

Risk Factors	Risk Criteria	Disease Correlation
Breeding Kennel	77 kennels sampled	Yes
Sex	Male (n = 137); female (n =4 09)	No
Shows	Attended or not	No
Breed	41 different breeds	No
Age	14 different age ranges	Yes
Mating experience	Males mated or not	Yes
Cycle (stages)	Five different stages	Yes
Number of litters	Zero to >1	No
Kennel cough	History of respiratory disease	Yes
Kennel size	Ranged from <6 to >20 dogs	Yes
Breeding management	Use of nonresident males	Yes
Hygiene–biosecurity	Ranged from very good to insufficient	Yes

Data from Evermann JF. Canine herpesvirus infection: Update on risk factors and control measures. Vet Forum 2005;69:32–7; and Ronsse V, Verstegen J, Onclin K, et al. Risk factors and reproductive disorders associated with canine herpesvirus-1 (CHV-1). Theriogenology 2004;61:619–36.

is primarily maintained and spread among dogs in a multidog environment as a respiratory infection.

Respiratory Disorders

The disease outcomes of CHV infections are age dependent. In naive puppies that are less than 1 month of age, natural and experimental infection with CHV may be highly fatal. Natural exposure of pups occurs by ingestion or inhalation of virus containing material. The primary replication sites are nasal mucosa, pharynx, and tonsil. Systemic spread of the virus is enhanced by a cell-associated viremia.[29–32] The pathology induced by CHV in the lungs of newborn pups is depicted in **Figs. 1** and **2**.

Experimental infection of older dogs (3 months or older) with CHV has resulted in a mild rhinitis and pharyngitis. Symptoms of tracheobronchitis were produced following experimental inoculation with CHV isolated from naturally infected dogs.[38,39] Experimental infection of 5- to 12-week-old pups induced mild rhinitis and pharyngitis and virus replication was demonstrated in the upper respiratory tract. Although CHV has been isolated from dogs with upper respiratory disease, reproduction of "kennel cough" has only been rarely reported. Thompson and coworkers[32] reported that aerosol exposure of 12-week-old dogs caused a necrotizing rhinitis, broncheointerstitial pneumonia, and multifocal alveolar necrosis. More severe disease can occur when CHV infects dogs that are immunosuppressed.[9] A case of generalized CHV infection in a 9-year-old dog with a normal immune system was documented recently (Gadsden BJ, Langohr IM, Maes R. Fatal herpesviral infection in an adult dog. Submitted for publication, 2011). The most severe lesions were seen in the liver. The histologic lesions observed in the lung of this dog are presented in **Fig. 3**.

Infection rates, based on serologic studies, are high enough to explain entry of CHV into multidog environments, either as an active infection or as the result of reactivation of latent virus in environments associated with natural, or pharmacologically induced immunosuppression. In Belgium the seroprevalence in adult dogs was found to be

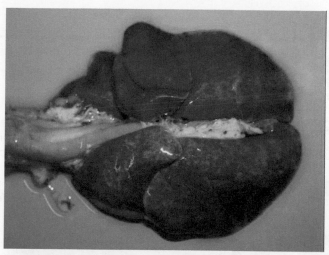

Fig. 1. Dog, puppy, canine herpesvirus 1 infection. The lung is diffusely non-collapsed and has numerous small coalescing pale foci suggestive of a necrotizing interstitial pneumonia. (*Courtesy of* Dr David Driemeier, Universidade Federal do Rio Grande do Sul, Porto Alegre, RS, Brazil.)

45.8%.[22] Rijsewijk and colleagues[21] reported a seroprevalence of 39% in the Netherlands. Reading and Field,[20] using an antibody detection ELISA, found a seroprevalence of 88% in the United Kingdom. In Japan, the seroprevalence was recently reported to be 21.7%.[6] Since CHV is regarded as a weak immunogen, these antibody-based surveys are probably an underrepresentation of the true infection rate in the dog populations.[33]

Canine infectious respiratory disease (CIRD) is most commonly seen in rescue centers, boarding kennels, and veterinary hospitals. Most of the affected dogs have a dry cough of limited duration. In complicated cases, bronchopneumonia is seen and can be fatal. Multiple infectious agents can play a role in the induction of CIRD. Canine parainfluenza virus and *Bordetella bronchiseptica* are frequently involved. Canine distemper and canine adenovirus type 2 (CAV-2) have been associated with CIRD but are not routinely detected due in part to effective vaccines, and the population immunity is fairly high. Canine influenza, canine respiratory coronavirus, and, most recently, canine pneumovirus, are emerging components of CIRD, which have added to the complexity of this disease syndrome.[18,19,40]

Although CHV infections have been documented in multidog environments, its etiologic role in CIRD is still being assessed. During a 2-year longitudinal study of viruses associated with CIRD at a rescue center in the United Kingdom, CHV was found in 12.8% of the tracheal samples examined and in 0.0% of the lung samples. Infections with CHV were seen 3 to 4 weeks after entry and were associated with more severe respiratory signs.[18] The delay in detection of the virus by PCR was corroborated by the serologic data, which also indicated that CHV infections occurred at a later time point. A possible explanation offered for its detection in more severe cases was the possibility that latent CHV could have been reactivated as a result of the stress induced by a primary CIRD episode that was triggered by other viral or bacterial agents. The virus source was not determined. The authors speculated that genetically different CHV strains would have been detected if the source of virus was the result of reactivation of latent virus from different dogs. It has been reported, however, that CHV strains show very low sequence variability.[41]

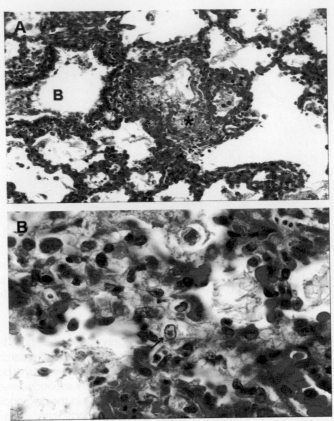

Fig. 2. (*A*) Dog, puppy (2 weeks of age), canine herpesvirus 1 infection. The pulmonary parenchyma is focally effaced by fibrin exudate and necrotic cell debris (*). Similar exudate also fills part of the bronchiolar lumen (B). The alveolar septa in the remaining lung are mildly expanded by inflammatory cell infiltrate (fibrinonecrotizing bronchointerstitial pneumonia) (hematoxylin-eosin, original magnification ×20). (*B*) Dog, puppy (2 weeks of age), canine herpesvirus 1 infection. High magnification of the previous figure. An epithelial cell contains a round, eosinophilic, intranuclear inclusion body surrounded by a clear halo and marginated chromatin within an area of lymphohistiocytic inflammation of the pulmonary parenchyma (hematoxylin-eosin, original magnification ×60). (*Courtesy of* Dr Ingeborg Langohr, Michigan State University, East Lansing, MI.)

Erles and Brownlie[19] monitored dogs in 2 training centers in the United Kingdom for 1 year. All dogs were vaccinated against CAV-2, CPV-2, and *Leptospira interrogans*. Tonsillar swabs and serum samples were collected at entry and every 3 months thereafter. Blood samples were collected at entry and every 4 weeks thereafter. Most CIRD cases were observed in autumn and winter. Most dogs were healthy at arrival and were in the kennel for at least 2 weeks before developing clinical signs. Seroconversion to CHV was detected throughout the year. The most logical explanation for the seroconversion pattern would be continuous introduction in the kennel by acutely infected dogs or reactivation of latent virus in the resident population. The authors concluded that while CHV contributed to the CIRD, it was not an obligate pathogen in that environment, since some asymptomatic dogs also seroconverted.

Kawakami and colleagues[6] described an outbreak of infectious tracheobronchitis in Japan accompanied by death in adult dogs. The only pathogen identified during the outbreak was CHV. Molecular testing led to the conclusion that a single strain was involved, with virulence characteristics that were only slightly higher than those of previously tested CHV strains. As was the case in the study reported by Erles and colleagues,[18] it was not clear whether the virus was introduced into the center in the form of acute infections or was the result of reactivation of latent infections in the resident population. Regardless, the authors emphasized that there was sufficient amounts of immunosuppression in shelter populations to allow for CHV to be a significant primary pathogen in that environment.

Ocular Disorders

Ocular manifestations of CHV infection may develop during both primary and recurrent infection and are dependent upon host age and immune status. In fetal and neonatal dogs with primary CHV infection, severe intraocular lesions are frequently present concurrent with systemic viral disease. Subclinical or mild recurrent ocular surface disease is typically observed in immunocompetent mature dogs. In immuno-suppressed mature dogs, ocular lesions associated with CHV infected are often more severe, persist for a longer duration, and may be refractory to treatment.

Primary CHV infection in fetal and neonatal dogs

Primary CHV infection occurring after in utero or early neonatal CHV transmission (ie, first 2 to 3 weeks of life) is associated with a cell-associated viremia. Hematogeneous dissemination of virus results in CHV infection of intraocular tissues with severe clinical ocular manifestations. Ocular disease is typically bilateral and becomes evident within a short period after the development of systemic disease in many, but not all, dogs.[1,3] Panuveitis, retinitis, and optic neuritis with extensive monocular and neutrophilic infiltrates, edema, hemorrhage, and necrosis are observed histopathologically within the iris, ciliary body, choroid, retina, and optic nerve.[42] Intranuclear viral inclusions are frequently detected during the acute inflammatory phase in uveal and retinal tissues. As the palpebral fissures do not open until 10 to 14 days postpartum in dogs, ocular changes may not be externally visible in young animals. In dogs with open eyelids, most clinically detectable ocular lesions are sequelae to panuveitis and include keratitis, corneal edema, aqueous flare, anterior synechiae, cataracts, and chorioretinitis (**Fig. 4**).[42] Reduced vision or blindness may result from various combinations of the ocular lesions.

Following the acute inflammatory stage of infection, developmentally mature tissues (eg, cornea, uvea) undergo varying degrees of necrosis, fibrosis, gliosis, and atrophy.[42] The canine retina is incompletely developed at birth and responds by a combination of necrosis, disorganization, and reorganization. Retinal dysplasia, characterized by formation of retinal folds with rosette-like structures, and retinal degeneration are the final result. In dogs surviving neonatal CHV infection, blindness, cataracts, optic nerve atrophy, retinal degeneration, and retinal dysplasia are frequent residual sequelae.[43]

Primary and recurrent ocular CHV infections in mature dogs

In contrast to fetal and neonatal dogs, ocular lesions associated with CHV infection in mature dogs are typically restricted to the ocular surface with a variety of corneal, conjunctival, and eyelid lesions.[44] In immunocompetent dogs these lesions are frequently mild and self-limiting; however, they are a source of discomfort and their recurrent nature may be frustrating to clients. Nonspecific clinical signs associated

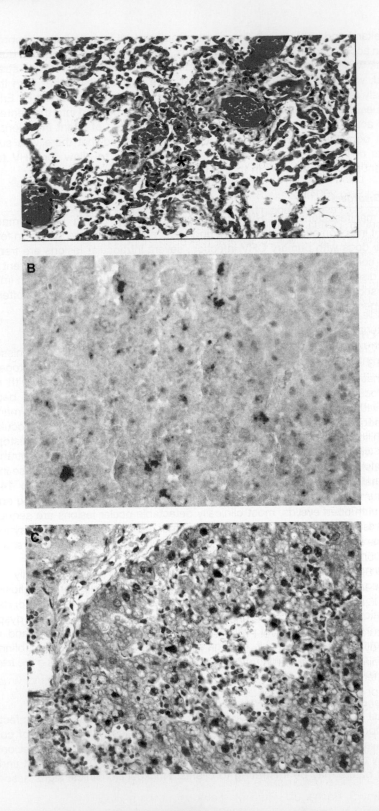

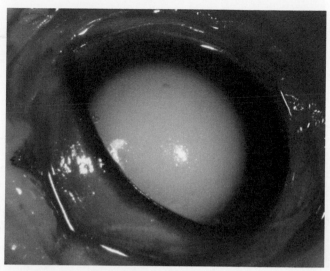

Fig. 4. Canine herpesvirus disease in puppy (12 days old). Diffuse corneal edema, marked aqueous flare, and a mature cataract are evident.

with CHV ocular infection in mature dogs include blepharospasm, photophobia, and ocular discharge. Blepharospasm and ocular pain are often disproportionally severe compared to that expected from the extent of ocular lesions. Ocular discharge is initially restricted to epiphora, but becomes mucoid, mucopurulent, or serosanguineous with progression of infection.[7,44]

Primary and recurrent ocular CHV infection may be subclinical or associated with various combinations of blepharitis, conjunctivitis, keratitis, and corneal ulceration.[7,44-46] In all published descriptions of naturally-acquired primary ocular CHV infection, clinical lesions were bilateral; however, the severity and specific manifestations of CHV infection were not always symmetrical between eyes of individual dogs. In most cases, primary ocular CHV infection resolves spontaneously and without permanent ocular lesions; however, recovered dogs are at risk for developing recrudescent ocular disease associated with reactivation of latent CHV. Recrudescent CHV ocular disease may present with either unilateral or bilateral lesions. Recurrent CHV ocular infection may occur in dogs with no identifiable risk factors; however, an immunocompromise state is present in most dogs.[7,44] Naturally acquired recurrent CHV ocular infection is reported in dogs with a variety of immunomodulating

Fig. 3. (A) Dog, adult dog (9 years of age), canine herpesvirus 1 infection. The pulmonary architecture is focally mildly disrupted by fibrin, cell debris, and hemorrhage (*). Vessels are acutely congested and alveoli are flooded with macrophages and proteinaceous material indicative of diffuse pulmonary edema (hematoxylin-eosin, original magnification ×20). (*Courtesy of* Dr Ingeborg Langohr, Michigan State University, East Lansing, MI.) (B) Liver; dog. Canid herpesviral 1 protein is detected within areas of hepatic necrosis (immunohistochemistry). (*Courtesy of* Dr Matti Kiupel, Michigan State University, East Lansing, MI.) (C) Liver; dog. Canid herpesviral 1 nucleic acid is present in the areas of hepatic necrosis. In situ hybridization. (*Courtesy of* Dr Matti Kiupel, Michigan State University, East Lansing, MI.)

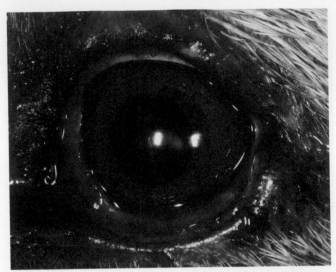

Fig. 5. Canine herpesvirus disease in adult dog (8 years old). Recurrent blepharoconjunctivitis following administration of chemotherapy for lymphoma. Eyelid erythema, mucopurulent ocular discharge, conjunctival hyperemia, chemosis, and conjunctival petechiae are present.

systemic conditions and receiving a variety of immunosuppressive therapeutics. Systemic conditions included diabetes mellitus, immune-mediated thrombocytopenia, and lymphoma. Immunosuppressive therapeutics included topical ocular corticosteroids, topical ocular cyclosporine, systemic corticosteroids, and a variety of antineoplastic chemotherapeutics (eg, cyclophosphamide, doxorubicin, vincristine). In many reported dogs, potentially immunosuppressive conditions were concurrently present with the administration of multiple topical and systemic immunosuppressive medications.

Blepharitis is occasionally present with ocular CHV and may appear as focal or generalized eyelid erythema, edema, exudates, and crusting. Regions of alopecia may be present. The blepharitis may represent self-trauma resulting from discomfort associated with conjunctival or corneal disease, or active viral infection of eyelid cutaneous epithelium as described for other dermal regions in dogs with CHV infection.[46] Conjunctivitis is the most frequently reported ocular lesion associated with both primary and recurrent CHV infection[44,47] and can be presented with conjunctival hyperemia, chemosis, and ocular discharge. Ulceration of the conjunctival epithelium may occur and appears as flat, irregular, pale or pink regions on the conjunctival surface surrounded by regions of hyperemia. Conjunctival ulcerations are readily detected with application of sodium fluorescein, rose Bengal, or lissamine green stains. Although the clinical features of CHV conjunctivitis are often indistinguishable from other etiologies, conjunctival petechiae are frequently reported in dogs with CHV infection (**Fig. 5**).[9,44,47] Although not specific to CHV infection, this clinical finding is uncommon with most other etiologies of conjunctivitis and should be considered suggestive of CHV.

Ulcerative keratitis and nonulcerative keratitis are frequent lesions associated with primary and recurrent ocular CHV infection.[7,8,47] A variety of clinical manifestations are observed in the cornea associated with CHV infection and these likely represent

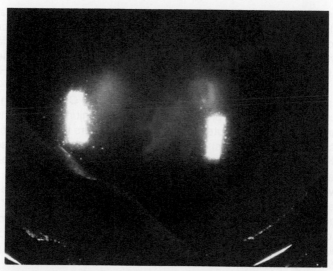

Fig. 6. Canine herpesvirus disease in adult dog (10 years old). Dendritic corneal ulcerations developed during topical ocular corticosteroid treatment. Fluorescein-stained linear, branching, superficial corneal ulcerations with prominent terminal end bulbs are detected in the central cornea.

a continuum along the progression of active corneal epithelial infection. Punctate keratitis is the earliest detectable CHV corneal ulceration and appears clinically as a fine stippling of epithelial loss. This subtle lesion is often clinically overlooked when examination is performed without the aid of magnification, but application of corneal vital stains (particularly rose Bengal or lissamine green) facilitate detection.[47] As punctate ulcerations progress, they form the classic alphaherpesvirus corneal lesion of dendritic corneal ulcers. Dendritic corneal ulcerations are strongly suggestive of CHV infection in the dog. These linear, branching ulcers stain brightly with sodium fluorescein, rose Bengal, and lissamine green (**Fig. 6**).[7,47] Prominent terminal end bulbs are a consistent feature of CHV dendritic ulcers in the dog and can be used to differentiate CHV corneal lesions from other potential causes of linear corneal ulcers that might appear clinically similar (eg, external trauma, cilia abnormalities, entropion). Terminal end bulbs are club-shaped, rounded ends to the CHV dendritic ulcer branches, and are not seen with other causes of linear corneal ulcers. Coalescence of dendritic ulcerations may result in the formation of geographic corneal ulcers.[47] These appear as larger, irregular-shaped areas of corneal epithelial loss. In dogs with CHV ulcerative keratitis, corneal ulcers are commonly located in discrete groups or linear arrangements on the corneal surface. Unless complicated by secondary bacterial infection, CHV corneal ulcers remain superficial and corneal stromal loss is not appreciable. Nonulcerative keratitis is a less frequent lesion reported with CHV ocular infection.[47] Clinically, nonulcerative keratitis appears as a circumferential ring of cornea stromal neovascularization with epithelial and subepithelial leukocyte infiltrates in the peripheral cornea. Nonulcerative keratitis may represent a resolution stage of active corneal epithelial disease.

The largest published case series of primary CHV ocular disease described an outbreak of CHV infection a closed colony of young adult laboratory beagles.[47] In this group of 27 dogs, conjunctivitis was detected in 100% of dogs, ulcerative keratitis in

26% of dogs, and nonulcerative keratitis in 19% of dogs. Corneal ulcerations were further subclassified by clinical appearance as punctate (7% of dogs), dendritic (19% of dogs), and geographic (4% of dogs). This report confirmed CHV-associated ocular disease in group housed susceptible dogs, and provides an overview of the spectrum and relative frequency of ocular lesions associated with primary ocular CHV infection in dogs.

Under experimental conditions, acquisition of primary CHV infection by ocular surface inoculation consistently produces self-limiting conjunctivitis in immunocompetent mature dogs.[29,46] This route of infection likely occurs frequently under natural conditions and has direct clinical relevance.[47] Viral inoculation by other anatomic routes, such as the genital tract, is associated with inconsistent development of ocular disease.[48] Clinical signs were manifested in both eyes, even when viral inoculation was unilateral, but the magnitude of conjunctivitis may not be symmetric between eyes. The clinical severity of ocular lesions peak approximately 7 to 10 days after infection and lesions slowly resolve over the following 2 weeks. Histopathologic findings in dogs with acute experimental CHV conjunctivitis include conjunctival epithelial necrosis, subepithelial lymphocyte and macrophage infiltration, and edema of the substantia propria.[28,29]

Experimental induction of recurrent ocular CHV infection was demonstrated by administering immunosuppressive dosages of systemic corticosteroids to latently infected dogs recovered from primary CHV ocular infection.[8] Recrudescent CHV ocular disease was detected in 83% of immunosuppressed dogs in one study.[8] Bilateral conjunctivitis or linear corneal ulcers developed as early as 3 days after initiating corticosteroid administration. The mean duration of detectable ocular disease was 8.6 days and was shorter than the experimental primary ocular CHV infection in the dogs. Cellular lesions observed by in vivo confocal microscopy in the dogs included conjunctival leukocyte infiltrates, corneal leukocyte infiltrates, abnormal corneal epithelial cell morphologies, and corneal Langerhans cell infiltrates. Subsequent research determined topical ocular corticosteroid administration does not result in recurrent CHV ocular disease in latently infected dogs under experimental conditions.[15] In this study, topical ophthalmic prednisolone acetate (1.0% suspension) was administered 4 times daily for 28 days to both eyes of dogs with experimentally induced latent CHV infection. Viral shedding and recurrent CHV ocular disease were not detected; however, crystalline corneal opacities developed in some dogs. These bilateral corneal lesions appeared clinically as subepithelial and anterior stromal punctate, white, refractile opacities within the central cornea. It was unclear if the crystalline corneal opacities were a nonspecific result of corticosteroid administration or influenced by prior CHV corneal disease.

In immunocompromised dogs, such as lymphoma who are receiving chemotherapy or dogs with autoimmune systemic disorders receiving long-term immunosuppressive therapy, relatively severe ocular lesions may develop during recurrent CHV infection.[7,9] These lesions include severe ulcerative conjunctivitis and extensive corneal ulceration that is refractory to treatment. Development of viremia, systemic CHV dissemination, and visceral hemorrhagic necrosis, similar to what is typically observed in fetal and neonatal dogs, has been reported in a mature dog with ocular CHV infection while receiving chemotherapy for lymphoma.[9] In the reported dog, it was speculated that viremia and systemic CHV disease developed secondary to localized ocular CHV reactivation with an insufficient immune response to contain virus to the anatomic site of recurrent disease.

Recent evidence suggests CHV ocular diseases in mature dogs are clinically underappreciated. A survey of dogs with idiopathic conjunctivitis determined CHV was the most common viral etiology of conjunctivitis in mature, vaccinated dogs and was detected in ocular samples from approximately 17% of study dogs.[44] Conjunctivitis is among the most common ocular diseases in dogs presented to veterinarians and, if these results are extrapolated to the general canine population, it implies CHV ocular diseases occur commonly.[49]

VIRUS DETECTION
Latency Sites

To determine the sites of latency of CHV, Miyoshi and colleagues[16] experimentally inoculated adult seronegative dogs via the intranasal (n = 2), intranasal and intravenous (n = 3), or intravaginal (n = 3) routes with a strain of CHV. Although clinical signs were not observed, infectious virus was isolated from swabs until 4 to 6 days postinoculation. Tissues were collected 2 to 4 months postinoculation and examined for the presence of latent viral DNA. It was determined that the trigeminal ganglion (TG) was an important latency site for CHV, regardless of the inoculation route. Latency was detected also in lumbosacral ganglia of 2 of 3 dogs inoculated intravaginally, 1 of 2 dogs inoculated intranasally, and 1 of 3 dogs inoculated both intranasally and intravenously. Abortion and stillbirths could also be associated with reactivation of latent CHV, but the mechanism by which this takes place has not been investigated. Retropharyngeal lymph nodes were another important latency site, since latency was detected in this tissue in 7 of 8 dogs. Conversely, all attempts to demonstrate latency in peripheral blood lymphoid cells were negative.

In humans, herpesviruses have been detected in the inner ear and are considered to play a role in vestibular dysfunction. Parzefall and colleagues[50] reported on the prevalence of canine herpesvirus DNA in the vestibular ganglia (VG) and vestibular labyrinth (VL) of 52 dogs that were included in their study. CHV DNA was detected in the VL of 17% of the dogs and in the VG of 19% of the dogs. Although no attempt was made to differentiate between acute and latent infection, it is very likely that the PCR was detecting latent virus. Interestingly, infection of the VG or VL was not always associated with infection of TG. Since the VG, in contrast to the trigeminal and geniculate ganglia, do not have direct connection with sensory nerve endings on body surfaces, it remains most probable that there was primary infection of the TG or geniculate ganglia, with subsequent spread to the VG.

Spontaneous Reactivation

Burr and colleagues[13] examined tissues from 12 adult dogs that had been euthanized for various reasons. From each dog 12 tissues that have been associated with latency in other herpesvirus infections were examined. Viral DNA was detected in the organs of 9 of the 12 dogs. The tissues most commonly found to be positive were lumbosacral ganglia, tonsil, parotid salivary gland, and liver. Based on the data, lumbosacral ganglia are an important site of latency and potential source of reactivated virus for venereal infections and infection of pups as they pass through the birth canal. Finding of latent virus in tonsils and salivary glands points to the role of oronasal spread in the transmission of CHV. It was noted that viral DNA was detected in the trigeminal ganglia extracts of only 2 of the dogs. None of the 12 blood samples tested were found to be positive, indicting a lack of detectable viremia. The authors commented that CHV is either totally absent from peripheral blood or that the level of infection is limited to 1 genomic copy per 2000 mononuclear cells. They also pointed out that basing the incidence of CHV infection on serology only may lead to an underestimation of the true infection rate.

The difficulty in detecting circulating CHV in a kennel situation is highlighted in a study by Ronsse and colleagues.[11] Dogs in a breeding facility were followed for the duration of 1 reproductive cycle. A number of dogs seroconverted (negative to positive) to CHV during this period. Conversely, antibody-positive dogs became seronegative. The serologic data clearly indicate that CHV was circulating in this kennel in the form of acute and/or reactivated form, primary infections. However, despite the fact that samples were taken at regular intervals, the results of PCR testing with a previously validated assay were uniformly negative both on all nasal and vaginal swabs and buffy coat samples. A possible explanation is that the shedding interval after reactivation is very short. Even during acute infection, shedding of CHV is limited to 2 to 6 days.

Reactivation Following Corticosteroid Administration

Latent CHV has been reactivated by treatment with corticosteroids. Okuda and colleagues[51] treated dams with a history of CHV infection with 600 mg of prednisolone for 5 consecutive days. Reactivation of latent CHV infection was confirmed in 4 of 5 dams. Infectious CHV was recovered from nasal, oral, vaginal, and ocular secretions on the 5th to 21st days after initiation of treatment and also from nasal mucosa and tonsil tissues. These results indicate that latent CHV infections develop frequently and that the latent virus may be reactivated, without clinical signs, in dogs with a history of CHV infection.

Ledbetter and colleagues[8] investigated whether systemic administration of an immunosuppressive regimen of corticosteroids (3 mg/kg/day for 7 consecutive days) to experimental adult dogs would lead to reactivation and recrudescence. Group 1 dogs were latently infected and received corticosteroid treatment. Group 2 dogs were latently infected and received a placebo. Group 3 dogs were control dogs and received corticosteroid treatment. Bilateral ocular disease, consisting of conjunctivitis and keratitis, was seen in 83% of the group 1 dogs between days 3 and 18 of the experiment. Ocular shedding was detected in 50% of the group 1 dogs, and a 4-fold rise in antibody titer was detected in all dogs in group 1. None of the dogs in the control groups showed ocular disease, shed virus, or seroconverted. Corticosteroid-induced reactivation is likely the result of enhanced expression of both viral and cellular genes. Corticosteroid also lead to host immune response suppression, As discussed by the authors, the immunosuppression could be involved directly in the reactivation event, or indirectly in facilitating the spread of reactivated virus to peripheral tissues, leading to renewed replication at peripheral mucosal sites and potential transmission to susceptible animals that are in contact with the animal in which reactivation takes place.

Ledbetter and colleagues[15] also administered topical ocular prednisolone acetate or a placebo to mature dogs experimentally inoculated with CHV via the ocular route and previously tested for reactivatable latency by systemic administration of an immunosuppressive dose of corticosteroids. The dogs were treated 4 times daily for a total of 28 days. The results of this study showed that topical ocular prednisolone at the concentration and treatment regimen used did not result in detectable reactivation of CHV latency, based on a combination of recrudescent clinical signs, confocal microscopy findings, ocular infectious virus shedding, real-time PCR findings, and serologic response. A potential explanation for the data is that the concentration of topically administered corticosteroid that is absorbed systemically is insufficient to induce reactivation.

Malone and colleagues described a disseminated CHV infection, which led to euthanasia, in an adult dog.[9] The dog had undergone chemotherapy for the treatment of generalized lymphoma. It was not clear whether generalized infection in this case was the result of enhanced susceptibility to CHV as a result of immunosuppression or whether it was due to reactivation of a preexisting latent CHV infection in this dog.

Molecular Methods to Detect CHV

Amplification of target sequences by PCR method is currently the most common and most sensitive molecular diagnostic approach to the detection of CHV in natural or experimentally infected animals. The PCR assays described initially were gel based, implying that the amplified products are visualized by UV illumination of ethidium bromide–stained agarose gels. Miyoshi and colleagues[16] combined a nested PCR with Southern blotting and showed that the detection limit of this combination was equivalent to 1 $TCID_{50}$.

Schultze and Baumgärtner[17] described nested gel-based PCR and in situ hybridization assays to diagnose acute CHV infection in formalin-fixed paraffin-embedded tissues of 1- to 3-week-old puppies that were naturally infected. The specificity of the PCR products was confirmed by restriction endonuclease digestion. Viral DNA was detected in a variety of cell types, such as bronchiolar and alveolar epithelial cells, hepatocytes, renal tubular epithelial cells, neurons, fibrocytes, cardiac myocytes, and endothelial cells. This is in accordance with the previously described "pantropism" of CHV. When paraffin-embedded tissues are used for PCR, it has to be kept in mind that the quality of the DNA can be affected by several factors, such as the length of time between tissue removal and fixation, the presence of nucleases in the tissue, and the length of storage of the paraffin blocks.

Burr and colleagues[13] developed a gel-based PCR for CHV and used it in conjunction with Southern blotting to confirm the authenticity of the amplicons. They also assessed the PCR compatibility of each sample for CHV PCR by first verifying that primers specific for a portion of the canine pancreatic lipase gene-amplified their target in each of the tissue extracts. The assay was capable of detecting approximately 14 genomic copies spiked into 1 μg of placental DNA and approximately 3500 copies when spiked into 0.2 ml of blood.

Erles and colleagues[18] described a gel-based PCR targeting a 494–base pair region of a gene homologous to HSV-1 UL 37. Reubel and colleagues[52] described a nested PCR that had a sensitivity that was 100 times higher than virus isolation. Ronsse and colleagues[22] described the use of 2 PCR assays for CHV. One of these assays had a sensitivity of 0.01 $CCID_{50}$.

The most sensitive and specific method currently available to detect CHV DNA is probe-based real-time PCR. A fluorogenic real-time PCR assay was described by Reubel and colleagues[52] and reported to have a detection limit of 10 copies of viral DNA. The first probe-based multiplex real-time PCR for CHV was reported by Ledbetter and colleagues.[8] Very recently, Dooaro and colleagues[11] reported the development and complete validation of a probe-based real-time quantitative PCR for the detection and quantitation of CHV DNA in clinical samples. The assay was found to be very sensitive, since it could detect as few as 10 copies of the target per sample. In comparison with the gel-based PCR assay described by Schulze and Baumgärtner,[17] which was used in parallel, this assay has a 10-fold lower detection limit. Specificity for CHV was very high, as determined by lack of amplification of other canine viruses. The dynamic range was validated by successful amplification of a number of CHV-positive samples from different geographic locations. Reproducibility of the assay was determined by determining both intra-assay and interassay variability between the results obtained with samples containing variable amounts of target DNA. Both intra-assay and interassay variability, expressed as a coefficient of variation, were fairly low, were dependent on the target concentration, and were found to increase with decreasing target copy numbers. A potential pitfall of PCR assays is that the sample contains substances that are inhibiting the reaction, thus potentially leading to false-negative results. To control for this possibility, an internal control construct was spiked into each sample at known quantity and co-amplified. This way, any inhibition would be readily detectable from a decrease in the expected signal resulting from the amplification of this internal control. A relatively simple way to avoid inhibition was to prepare a 10-fold dilution of the sample.

Since it allows absolute quantitation, the assay was used to determine viral loads in tissues of pups that had died from acute infection and a vaginal swab collected from the dam. The viral load in the vaginal swab was 1.57×10^3 copies/10 μl. The highest viral load in tissues was 5.76×10^9 copies/10 μl, present in kidney homogenates. The authors concluded that, since it quantitates copy numbers over a wide range, this assay will be very useful not only for diagnostic purposed, but also for future pathogenesis studies and for the testing of the effect of antivirals on the replication of CHV.

CARRIER STATES AND SHEDDING PATTERNS
Carriers

The phrase "carrier animal" has been used extensively to describe an animal that harbors an infectious agent *beyond* the usual time allowed for the incubation phase of the infection and the acute and convalescent phases of clinical disease.[53] When it comes to the herpesviruses this is problematic since there are at least 2 phases that exceed those previously mentioned and are characterized by latency and exacerbation of clinical symptoms from latency. According to Povey, a carrier animal may or may not shed virus in excretions or secretions, and shedding may occur continuously or intermittently.[53] As was noted in the preceding section, latency in its strict definition is the lack of viral transcription and translation, so no mature virus is being produced. A latently infected dog with CHV would be defined as a carrier dog that is not shedding virus and would not be contagious to in-contact, susceptible dogs. Exacerbation of the latent state to a replicative state would result in virus replication and shedding. The dog may have mild to severe clinical symptoms during this exacerbation phase.

Shedding Patterns

Primary, systemic neonatal CHV infection is associated with extensive viral shedding from numerous anatomic sites. High CHV viral titers are detected in respiratory secretions, ocular discharge, saliva, and urine and on many mucosal surfaces (eg, genital, nasal, ocular, oral, pharyngeal, rectal, tracheal[4,28]). Viral shedding may persist for up to 3 weeks in dogs that survive neonatal infection. Viral shedding from infected neonates may serve to spread CHV, either through direct contact or fomites, to littermates and other dogs.

Primary and recurrent CHV infection in mature dogs is associated with mucosal viral shedding that it detectable by PCR assay or virus isolation. The duration and anatomic site of shedding vary markedly between dogs and infection episodes in individual animals. Canine herpesvirus-1 shedding often occurs from multiple mucosal surfaces simultaneously and may be detected at sites anatomically distant to regions of overt clinical disease. Reports of experimentally induced primary and recurrent CHV infection suggest viral shedding during primary infection is prolonged and associated with higher viral titers than recurrent infection.[8,45,51,54] There is an individual dog susceptibility to CHV reactivation and shedding. Latent CHV infection can be reactivated, with induction of viral shedding, by short durations of corticosteroid administration in some dogs; however, other dogs are resistant to corticosteroid-induced viral reactivation.[8,51,54]

When naturally infected mature bitches that previously aborted CHV-infected pups where experimentally immunosuppressed by a 5-day course of systemic corticosteroid administration, CHV was shed from the nasal, oral, ocular, and vaginal mucosa.[51] Viral shedding could not be induced in all dogs. Viral shedding was detected by virus isolation as early as 5 days, and as late as 20 days, after initiating corticosteroid administration. The duration of detected CHV shedding ranged from 1 to 7 days in individual dogs. In a similar study[54] using 3-month- and 2-year-old dogs experimentally infected with CHV by nasal and intravenous routes, CHV reactivation and mucosal viral shedding were repeatedly induced by systemic corticosteroid administration. Primary oronasal infection was associated with nasal CHV shedding of approximately 2 weeks' duration. Following recovery from primary infection, systemic corticosteroid administration induced viral shedding from the nasal, oropharyngeal, and genital mucosa. The onset of detectable shedding was between 5 and 9 days after initiating corticosteroid treatment and persisted for up to 32 days with marked variation between individual dogs. A second round of corticosteroid administration was administered 3 months later and again resulted in viral shedding in some, but not all, dogs. The duration of viral shedding was shorter in all dogs during the second experimental reactivation and was associated with a tendency for lower viral titers.

In studies examining ocular CHV infection, a similar pattern of viral shedding is reported. Experimental primary ocular CHV infection in mature dogs produced by direct ocular surface inoculation resulted in conjunctival viral shedding that persisted for 10 days after inoculation.[46] Virus was detected in conjunctival samples by virus isolation and CHV PCR, and viral titers peaked 5 days postinoculation. CHV was inoculated into a single eye, but viral shedding was detected bilaterally in some dogs. Following recovery from primary ocular infection, viral shedding was not detected over the subsequent 8 months. Experimental recurrent ocular CHV infection induced by systemic corticosteroid administration to dogs recovered from primary ocular infection again resulted in viral shedding.[8] Ocular CHV shedding was detected by PCR assay in 50% of dogs between 10 and 13 days after administering the first dose of corticosteroid. In comparison to primary ocular CHV infection, ocular viral shedding associated with recurrent infection was briefer and viral titers in samples were lower.

Experimental primary CHV genital mucositis in mature dogs, produced by intravaginal and intrapreputial CHV inoculation, resulted in genital viral shedding that was detected by virus isolation for up to 20 days.[46] Several dogs also developed nasal, pharyngeal, and conjunctival viral shedding during this period. Canine herpesvirus tracheobronchitis induced by intranasal viral inoculation was associated with viral shedding for up to 18 days.[2] In the dogs with CHV upper respiratory tract infection, viral shedding from the nasal mucosa was detected by virus isolation in all dogs and a some had concurrent tracheal and rectal viral shedding.

CLINICAL ECOLOGY AND EPIDEMIOLOGY
Five Key Questions

The clinical ecology and epidemiology of CHV can be summarized in **Table 3**. It basically starts with a series of questions that inquire into the status of the virus, the host, and the environment with which both are localized.[55] The critical question is whether CHV infection and disease are of economic concern? As was mentioned earlier, the reproductive diseases associated with CHV were the initial driving force

Table 3	
Clinical ecology and epidemiology of canine herpesvirus infection and disease	
1. Is the infection/disease of economic concern?	Yes, may result in high mortality of litters, increased respiratory and ocular disease in susceptible dogs.
2. Is the infection/disease a public health risk? (zoonosis)	No, restricted host range to the canids.
3. Where is the agent when not causing disease? (ecology)	Subclinical carrier animals, latency. Readily inactivated outside dog's body.
4. What are the key contributing factors to the infection/disease process? (epidemiology)	Naïve susceptible puppies, naïve pregnant dams, and susceptible (stressed) adult dogs.
5. What factors can we control to minimize or eliminate the infection/disease process?	Shedding to susceptible dogs/puppies during critical 6 week danger period; maintain good kennel biosecurity. No vaccine available.

Data from Evermann JF, Eriks ES. Diagnostic medicine: The challenge of differentiating infection from disease and making sense for the veterinary clinician. Adv Vet Med 1999;41:25–38.

behind the recognition of the economic and emotional effects upon dog owners. While the costs of CHV-associated reproductive diseases have not been reported, it would be conceivable that a dam that loses an entire litter to CHV would result in a loss of $10,000, since multiple puppies are involved. In cases of respiratory disease and ocular disease, the costs of treatment and long-term care of recurrent infections may exceed $1000 per case.

The second question pertains to the zoonotic or public health risks associated with CHV infections. The virus is species specific and there is no evidence to support its involvement in human disease.[26]

The third question is the key to the persistence of CHV in the canine population—Where is the virus when *not* causing disease? This has been a key factor in understanding the virus and controlling it. The virus maintains itself in subclinical carrier dogs by way of latency. It may be exacerbated throughout life by stress, which results in mild to severe clinical symptoms that most commonly affect the respiratory and ocular systems. Concurrent with these clinical episodes there is shedding from excretions and secretions to susceptible dogs. The 2 most susceptible age groups are pregnant CHV naïve dogs and puppies of these dams (in utero, postnatal).

The fourth question revolves around the epidemiology of CHV once its infection occurs in the susceptible dog. The course of the infection to disease is variable and has been reviewed earlier under the contemporary clinical observations. One important aspect to reiterate here is the importance of immunity in controlling the infection–disease process in pregnant dams and their offspring during the postnatal period. Early postnatal infection (3 weeks or less) results in high morbidity accompanied by high mortality.[34] Later infection (3 weeks or later) results in low morbidity and very low mortality. However, it is usually the later postnatal infection that establishes the lifelong carrier state via latency.

The fifth question is a natural extension of the sequence of clinical inquiry and addresses the control of CHV, so that infection is minimized during disease-susceptible periods and maximized during disease-resistant periods. As noted previously, shedding states are important in maintaining the virus infection on the population to attain a certain degree of population immunity. Knowing when dogs are potentially contagious, and maintaining the 6-week barrier to infection, allows for maximum protection during this susceptible period. Since there is no reliable vaccine available, kennel hygiene and biosecurity are essential.[34]

THERAPEUTICS

Therapy for neonatal CHV infection is largely supportive and carries a poor prognosis for survival once clinical disease is manifested.[23] In instances where dogs survive neonatal CHV infection, cardiac, neurologic, and ocular lesions may be permanent. Elevating the environmental temperature of dogs in a litter after CHV infection is diagnosed may provide some protection to uninfected pups. Viral replication is reduced at elevated body temperatures and there are lower morbidity and mortality rates in dogs that are subsequently infected; however, this is ineffective for individual dogs if implemented after viral infection.[23] Intraperitoneal injection of immune sera obtained from CHV-seropositive dogs is described as a method to reduce mortality in an exposed litter, but it must be administered prior to infection to be most effective.[26] Lactoferrin possesses in vitro antiviral activity against CHV and inhibits cellular infection.[56] Administration of lactoferrin to dogs at risk for infection could theoretically provide protection; however, this is not demonstrated in vivo. Isolated reports of apparently successful therapy of neonatal CHV infection with the antivirals vidarabine and acyclovir are described. Acyclovir was administered orally as a 10-mg total dose per dog at 6-hour intervals until 3.5 weeks of age.[26]

The pharmacokinetics and tissue distribution of intravenous, subcutaneous, and oral acyclovir were investigated in dogs.[57,58] Additionally, a sustained release buccal tablet form of acyclovir was evaluated in the dog.[59] Acyclovir is bioavailable when administered orally to dogs and is widely distributed within tissues; however, target plasma concentrations and effective dosages for CHV infection are currently unknown.[57–59] Acyclovir toxicosis resultant from accidental ingestion is reported in dogs with dosages as low as 40 mg/kg and the routine clinical use of this, and other systemic antiviral medications, in dogs for CHV infection requires further investigation of safety and efficacy.[60] The canine pharmacokinetics of newer-generation anti-herpesviral drugs, including famciclovir, are reported. Similar to acyclovir, safe and effective doses for dogs with CHV infection are undetermined.[61]

Treatment of respiratory and genital CHV infection is primarily symptomatic. Unless complicated by secondary bacterial infection, these conditions are typically self-limiting and specific antiviral therapy is not reported. In contrast to respiratory and genital infection, there are detailed reports of the successful clinical management of ocular CHV infection. In addition to nonspecific treatments to prevent secondary bacterial infection (topical ocular antimicrobials) and improve comfort (topical ocular atropine), antiviral therapy with 0.1% idoxuridine or 1% trifluridine ophthalmic solution was used. Idoxuridine and trifluridine are nucleoside analogues, possess good anti-herpesvirus activity, and are well tolerated by dogs when applied topically as ocular formulations. Trifluridine is available under the trade name Viroptic, and idoxuridine can be acquired from compounding pharmacies. Both antivirals are administered 6 to 8 times daily for the first 48 hours and then 4 times daily until resolution of clinical signs of active infection. Cidofovir 0.5% ophthalmic solution is an alternative ophthalmic antiviral for CHV ocular disease that is effective with twice daily administration (E.C. Ledbetter, unpublished data, 2011).

SUMMARY

This review has documented well that our level of clinical inquiry expands as our knowledge base about CHV increases. While earlier studies focused on the

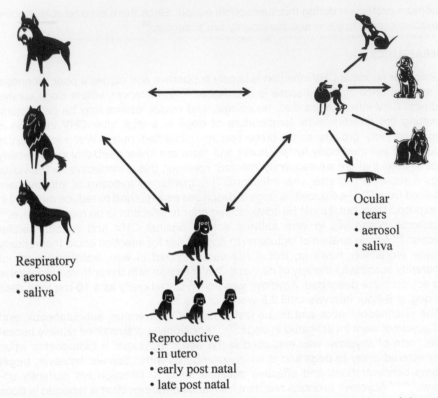

Respiratory
• aerosol
• saliva

Ocular
• tears
• aerosol
• saliva

Reproductive
• in utero
• early post natal
• late post natal

Fig. 7. Schematic of the potential interactions amongst three subpopulations of dogs and the infection-disease cycles of CHV.

reproductive effects of CHV in susceptible pregnant dogs and neonatal puppies, it has become apparent that in order to control CHV-related diseases that we must understand the various forms of CHV infection that may occur in the dog population (**Fig. 7**). This has prompted the veterinary community to develop more sensitive diagnostic assays, such as PCR, in order to answer the questions, where is the virus when not causing disease, and what is its relationship with respiratory and ocular diseases in adolescent and adult dogs (1 year or older)?

Molecular and serologic studies have clearly demonstrated that we are dealing with an infection that is more common than we considered a decade ago. Reports have indicated that up to 70% of some high-risk dog populations have been infected with and are latent carriers of CHV. This is important for veterinarians to know as we confer with clients on the best management steps we can take to protect our at-risk populations. While pregnant CHV-naïve dams and neonatal puppies born from a CHV-naïve dam are considered at high risk for disease, we must also take into consideration dogs in kennels and rescue centers. It is these dogs that are at risk for either exposure-infection or stress-induced exacerbation of latent CHV, which had been acquired at an earlier age.

The manifestations of CHV in adolescent and mature dogs may range from subclinical to severe respiratory and/or ocular diseases. The reports by Malone and colleagues,[9] Gadsden and colleagues (submitted, 2011), and Ledbetter and colleagues[7,47] all indicate that CHV can cause disease in older dogs and that it is not just a "puppy disease."

Recognition of the various forms of CHV-induced disease, availability of diagnostic assays with increased sensitivity, and the formation of reliable biosecurity measures will allow for better control steps to be taken in dogs at-risk for infection and disease.

ACKNOWLEDGMENTS

The authors would like to acknowledge those clinicians and veterinary researchers who provided insights and recommendations for our understanding of CHV pathogenesis and the management of CHV; these include Dr L. Carmichael, Dr M. Appel, Dr J. Gorham, Dr R. Ott, Dr A. Hashimoto, Dr A. Sears, and Dr M. Spector. The technical support of A. McKeirnan and L. Tanaka is greatly appreciated. The assistance of T. Pfaff in preparing the Word document was essential. This manuscript is dedicated to all the men and women who serve as dog handlers in roles of community protection, rescue operations, guide dogs, and national defense.

REFERENCES

1. Carmichael LE, Squire RA, Krook L. Clinical and pathologic features of a fatal viral disease of newborn pups. Am J Vet Res 1965;26:803–14.
2. Karpas A, Garcia FG, Calvo F, et al. Experimental production of canine tracheobronchitis (kennel cough) with canine herpesvirus isolated from naturally infected dogs. Am J Vet Res 1968;29:1251–7.
3. Percy DH, Olander HJ, Carmichael LE. Encephalitis in the new born pup due to canine herpesvirus. Vet Pathol 1968;5:135–45.
4. Huxsoll DL, Hemelt IE. Clinical observations of canine herpesvirus. J Am Vet Med Asso 1970;156:1706–13.
5. Hashimoto A, Hirai K, Yamaguchi T, et al. Experimental transplacental infection of pregnant dogs with canine herpesvirus. Am J Vet Res 1982;43:844–50.
6. Kawakami K, Ogawa H, Maeda K, et al. Nosocomial outbreak of serious infectious tracheobroncitis (kennel cough) caused by canine herpesvirus infection. J Clin Micro 2010;48:1176–81.
7. Ledbetter EC, Riis RC, Kern TJ, et al. Corneal ulceration associated with naturally occurring canine herpesvirus-1 infection in two adult dogs. J Am Vet Med Assoc 2006;229:376–84.
8. Ledbetter E, Kim SG, Dubovi EJ, et al. Experimental reactivation of latent canine herpesvirus-1 and induction of recurrent ocular disease in adult dogs. Vet Micro 2009;138:98–105.
9. Malone EK, Ledbetter EC, Rassnick KM, et al. Disseminated canine herpesvirus-infection in an immunocompromised adult dog. J Vet Intern Med 2010;24.965–8.
10. Ronsse V, Verstegen J, Onclin K, et al. Risk factors and reproductive disorders associated with canine herpesvirus-1 (CHV-1). Theriogenology 2004;61:619–36.
11. Ronsse V, Verstegehn J, Thiry E, et al. Canine herpesvirus-1 (CHV-1): clinical, serological and virological patterns in breeding colonies. Theriogenology 2005;64:61–74.
12. Anvik JO. Clinical considerations of canine herpesvirus infection. Vet Med 1991;82:394–403.
13. Burr PD, Campbell EME, Nicholson L, et al. Detection of canine herpesvirus-1 in a wide range of tissues using the polymerase chain reaction. Vet Micro 1996;53:227–37.

14. Decaro N, Amorisco F, Desario C, et al. Development and validation of a real-time PCR assay for specific and sensitive detection of canid herpesvirus-1. J Virol Meth 2010;169:176–80.

15. Ledbetter EC, Kice NC, Matusow RB, et al. The effect of topical ocular corticosteroid administration in dogs with experimentally induced latent canine herpesvirus-1 infection. Exp Eye Res 2010;90:711–7.

16. Miyoshi M, Ishii Y, Takiguchi M, et al. Detection of canine herpesvirus DNA in the ganglionic neurons and the lymph node lymphocytes of latently infected dogs. J Vet Med Sci 1999;61:375–9.

17. Schulze C, Baumgärtner W. Nested polymerase chain reaction and in situ hybridization for diagnosis of canine herpesvirus infection in puppies. Vet Pathol 1998; 35:209–17.

18. Erles K, Dubovi EJ, Brooks HW, Brownlie J. Longitudinal study of viruses associated with canine infectious respiratory disease. J Clin Micro 2004;42:4524–9.

19. Erles K, Brownlie J. Investigation into the causes of canine infectious respiratory disease: antibody responses to canine respiratory coronavirus and canine herpesvirus in two kenneled dog populations. Arch Virol 2005;150:1493–504.

20. Reading MJ, Field HJ. A serological study of canine herpesvirus-1 infection in the English dog population. Arch Virol 1998;143:1477–88.

21. Rijsewijk FA, Luiten EJ, Daus FJ, et al. Prevalence of antibodies against canine herpesvirus-1 in dogs in the Netherlands in 1997–1998. Vet Micro 1999;65:1–7.

22. Ronsse V, Verstegen J, Onclin K, et al. Seroprevalence of canine herpesvirus-1 in the Belgian dog population in 2000. Reprod Domest Anim 2002;37:299–304.

23. Carmichael LE. Herpesvirus canis: aspects of pathogenesis and immune response. J Am Vet Med Assoc 1970;156:1714–21.

24. Casal M. Clinical approach to neonatal conditions. In: England GE, editor. BSAVA manual of canine and feline reproduction and neonatology. Gloucester (UK): British Small Animal Veterinary Association; 2011. p. 147–54.

25. Evermann JF, Kennedy MA. Viral infections. In: Peterson ME, Kutzler MA, editors. Small animal pediatrics. The first 12 months of life. St Louis (MO): Elsevier-Saunders; 2011. p. 79–129.

26. Greene CE, Carmichael LE. Canine herpesvirus infection. In: Greene CE, editor. Infectious diseases of the dog and cat. 3rd edition. St Louis (MO): Saunders Elsevier; 2006. p. 47–53.

27. Kraft S, Evermann JF, McKiernan AJ, et al. The role of neonatal canine herpesvirus infection in mixed infections in older dogs. Compend Cont Educ Prac Vet 1986;8: 688–96.

28. Appel MJ, Menegus M, Parsonson IM, et al. Pathogenesis of canine herpesvirus in specific-pathogen-free dogs; 5-to 12-week-old pups. Am J Vet Res 1969;30: 2067–73.

29. Wright NG, Cornwell JC. The susceptibility of six-week of puppies to canine herpes virus. J Small Anim Pract 1970;10:699–74.

30. Buonavoglia C, Martella V. Canine respiratory viruses. Vet Res 2007;38:355–73.

31. Ford RB. Canine infectious tracheobronchitis. In: Greene CE, editor. Diseases of the dog and cat. 3rd edition. St Louis (MO): Elsevier; 2006. p. 54–61.

32. Thompson H, Wright NG, Cornwell HJ. Canine herpesvirus respiratory infection. Res Vet Sci 1972;13:123–6.

33. Evermann JF. Canine herpesvirus infection: update on risk factors and control measures. Vet Forum 2005;69:32–7.

34. Evermann JF, Wills TB. Immunologic development and immunization. In: Peterson ME, Kutzler MA, editors. Small animal pediatrics. The first 12 months of life. St Louis (MO): Elsevier-Saunders; 2011. p. 104–12.

35. Poulet HI, Guigal PM, Soulier M, et al. Protection of puppies against canine herpesvirus by vaccination of the dams. Vet Rec 2001; 148:691–5.

36. Morresey PR. Reproductive effects of canine herpesvirus. Comp Cont Educ Prac Vet 2004;26:804–11.

37. Decaro N, Martella V, Bounavoglia C. Canine adenoviruses and herpesvirus. Vet Clin Small Anim 2008;38:799–814.

38. Gaskell R, Willoughby K. Herpesviruses of carnivores. Vet Micro 1999; 69:73–88.

39. Appel M. Canine herpesvirus. In Virus infections of carnivores. Philadelphia: Elsevier; 1987. p. 5–15.

40. Renshaw R, Laverack M, Zylich N, et al. Genomic analysis of a pneumovirus isolated from dogs with acute respiratory disease. Vet Micro 2011;150:88–95.

41. Reubel GH, Pekin J, Webb-Wagg K, et al. Nucleotide sequence of glycoprotein genes B,C,D,G,H and I, the thymidine kinase and protein kinases and gene homologue UL24 of an Australian isolate of canine herpesvirus. Virus Genes 2002;25:195–200.

42. Albert DM, Lahav M, Carmichael LE, et al. Canine herpes-induced retinal dysplasia and associated ocular anomalies. Invest Ophthalmol 1976;15:267–78.

43. Percy DH, Carmichael LE, Albert DM, et al. Lesions in puppies surviving infection with canine herpesvirus. Vet Pathol 1971;8:37–53.

44. Ledbetter EC, Hornbuckle WE, Dubovi EJ. Virologic survey of dogs with naturally acquired idiopathic conjunctivitis. J Am Vet Med Assoc 2009;235:954–9.

45. De Palma VE, Ayala MA, Gobello C, et al. An atypical presentation for the first isolation of canid herpesvirus-1 in Argentina. Arq Braz Med Vet Zootec 2010;62:1267–70.

46. Ledbetter EC, Dubovi EJ, Kim SG, et al. Experimental primary ocular canine herpesvirus-1 infection in adult dogs. Am J Vet Res 2009;70:513–21.

47. Ledbetter EC, Kim SG, Dubovi EJ. Outbreak of ocular disease associated with naturally-acquired canine herpesvirus-1 infection in a closed domestic dog colony. Vet Ophthalmol 2009;12:242–7.

48. Hill H, Mare CJ. Genital disease in dogs caused by canine herpesvirus. Am J Vet Res 1974;35:669–72.

49. Lund EM, Armstrong PJ, Kirk CA, et al. Health status and population characteristics of dogs and cats examined at private veterinary practices in the United States. J Am Vet Med Assoc 1999;214:1337–41.

50. Parzefall B, Fischer A, Blutke A, et al. Naturally-occurring canine herpesvirus-1 infection of the vestibular labyrinth and ganglion of dogs. Vet J 2011;189:100–2.

51. Okuda Y, Hashimoto A, Yamaguchi T, et al. Virus reactivation in bitches with a medical history of herpesvirus infection. Am J Vet Res 1993;54:551–4.

52. Rubel GH, Pekin J, Venables D, et al. Experimental infection of European red foxes (Vulpes vulpes) with canine herpesvirus. Vet Micro 2001;83:217–33.

53. Povey RC. Persistent viral infection. The carrier state. Vet Clin N Am Small Anim Pract 1986;16:1075–95.

54. Okuda Y, Hashimoto A, Yamaguchi T, et al. Repeated canine herpesvirus (CHV) reactivation in dogs by an immunosuppressive drug. Cornell Vet 1993;83:291–302.

55. Evermann JF, Eriks ES. Diagnostic medicine: The challenge of differentiating infection from disease and making sense for the veterinary clinician. Adv Vet Med 1999;41:25–38.

56. Tanaka T, Nakatani S, Xuan X, et al. Antiviral activity of lactoferrin against canine herpesvirus. Antiviral Res 2003;60:193–9.

57. Krasny HC, de Miranda P, Blum MR, et al. Pharmacokinetics and bioavailability of acyclovir in the dog. J Pharmacol Exp Ther 1981;216:281–8.

58. de Miranda P, Krasny HC, Page DA, et al. The disposition of acyclovir in different species. J Pharmacol Exp Ther 1981;219:309–15.

59. Degim T, Elgen B, Ocak O. A sustained release dosage form of acyclovir for buccal application: an experimental study in dogs. J Drug Target 2006;14:35–44.

60. Richardson JA. Accidental ingestion of acyclovir in dogs: 105 reports. Vet Hum Toxico 2000;42:370-37–1.

61. Filer CW, Ramji JV, Allen GD, et al. Metabolic and pharmacokinetic studies following oral administration of famciclovir to the rat and dog. Xenobiotica 1995;25:477–90.

Canine Coronavirus: Not Only an Enteric Pathogen

Nicola Decaro, DVM, PhD*, Canio Buonavoglia, DVM

KEYWORDS

- Canine coronavirus • *Alphacoronavirus-1* • Pantropic CCoV
- Experimental infection • Molecular virology

Canine coronavirus (CCoV) is strictly related to coronaviruses of cats and pigs, with which it is now included in a unique viral species.[1] To date, two different canine coronavirus genotypes are known, which have been designated types I and II,[2] and canine/porcine recombinant strains have been also identified in recent years.[3,4] CCoV is generally recognized as the etiologic agent of self-limiting infections of the small intestine, which can lead to mild gastroenteritis.[5] However, a few years ago a highly virulent strain (pantropic CCoV) was isolated that was responsible for an outbreak of fatal, systemic disease in pups.[6] Such a strain displayed some genetic changes with respect to extant strains circulating in the dog population. The disease induced by the strain isolated from the natural outbreak was reproduced under experimental conditions.[7–9] This article reviews the currently available literature on pantropic CCoV, providing a meaningful update on the virologic, epidemiologic, clinical, diagnostic, and prophylactic aspects of the infections caused by this emerging pathogen of dogs.

AN OVERVIEW OF CANINE CORONAVIRUSES
Coronavirus Structure, Genome, and Taxonomy

Coronaviruses (family Coronaviridae, order Nidovirales) are enveloped viruses associated mainly with enteric and respiratory diseases in mammals and birds. The round and sometimes pleomorphic coronavirion, 80 to 120 nm in diameter, contains a linear, positive-strand RNA molecule, which is complexed with the highly basic nucleocapsid phosphoprotein (N) to form a helical capsid found within the viral envelope. The coronavirus membranes contain at least three viral proteins: the spike (S), envelope (E), and membrane (M) proteins. The S glycoprotein mediates viral attachment to specific cell receptors and fusion between the envelope and plasma membrane and it is the main inducer of virus-neutralizing antibodies. The E protein plays an important role in viral envelope assembly, but it is not essential for virus propagation. The M protein, the most abundant structural component, is a type III glycoprotein consisting of a short amino-terminal ectodomain, a triple-spanning transmembrane domain, and

Department of Veterinary Public Health, Faculty of Veterinary Medicine of Bari, Strada per Casamassima Km 3, 70010 Valenzano, Bari, Italy
* Corresponding author.
E-mail address: n.decaro@veterinaria.uniba.it

Vet Clin Small Anim 41 (2011) 1121–1132
doi:10.1016/j.cvsm.2011.07.005
0195-5616/11/$ – see front matter © 2011 Elsevier Inc. All rights reserved.

a long carboxyl-terminal inner domain. Some coronaviruses possess an additional structural protein, the hemagglutinin-esterase (HE), closely related to the hemagglutinin-esterase fusion protein of influenza C virus.[10]

Among RNA viruses, coronaviruses possess the largest genome, 27.6 to 31 kb in size. The 5'-most two thirds of the genome comprise the replicase gene, which consists of two overlapping open reading frames, ORF 1a and 1b. Located downstream of ORF1b are up to 11 ORFs that code for the 4 common structural proteins and a variable set of accessory proteins. Number, nucleotide sequence, and order of these additional genes can vary remarkably among different coronaviruses. The function of the accessory proteins is in most cases unknown. Albeit not essential for virus replication, they play an important role in virus–host interactions because they are generally maintained during natural infection, and their loss—either through spontaneous mutation or reversed genetics—results in reduced virulence.[10]

Until a few years ago, three major coronavirus groups were distinguished based on phylogenetic and antigenic analyses. CCoV was included in phylogroup 1, together with feline coronaviruses (FCoVs) type I and type II, transmissible gastroenteritis virus (TGEV) of swine, porcine respiratory coronavirus (PRCoV), porcine epidemic diarrhea virus (PEDV), and human coronaviruses 229E (HCoV-229E) and NL63 (HCoV-NL63).[10] Subsequently, a ferret coronavirus[11] and viruses identified in bats[12] were proposed as tentative members of this group. Recently, the International Committee of Taxonomy of Viruses accepted the proposal of the Coronavirus Study Group to revise the family Coronaviridae to include the corona- and toroviruses as subfamilies (Corona- and Torovirinae) and to convert the coronavirus phylogroups 1, 2, and 3 into genera (*Alpha-*, *Beta-*, and *Gammacoronavirus*, respectively).[1] The new taxonomy is based upon rooted phylogeny and quantitative pairwise sequence comparison and includes a clear definition of coronavirus species demarcation in accordance with that used in other virus families. Given their close genetic relatedness (>96% amino acid identity in the key replicase 1ab domains), TGEV, CCoV, and FCoV are now considered not as separate viruses but rather as host range variants of the same species, *Alphacoronavirus-1*.

Apart from the enterotropic virus CCoV, dogs harbor a genetically and antigenically unrelated coronavirus, canine respiratory coronavirus (CRCoV).[13] This virus displays high sequence identity to bovine coronavirus (BCoV)[14,15] and is now recognized as a host variant of the unique species *Betacoronavirus-1* of the genus *Betacoronavirus*,[1] together with BCoV and BCoV-related viruses.[16,17]

Origin and Evolution of CCoV

The first report on CCoV infection appeared in 1971, when Binn and colleagues isolated a coronavirus (strain 1-71) from dogs with acute enteritis in a canine military unit in Germany.[18] The disease could be reproduced in young dogs by experimental infection with the purified virus, thus fulfilling Koch's postulates.[19] Since then, several CCoV outbreaks have been reported worldwide, showing that CCoV is an important enteropathogen of dogs. Serologic and virologic investigations demonstrated that CCoV is widespread in the dog population, and the virus is highly prevalent in kennels and animal shelters.[5] Enteric CCoV infection is characterized by high morbidity and low mortality. The virus is shed at high titers in the feces and transmitted via the fecal–oral route. CCoV infection is generally restricted to the alimentary tract, leading to the onset of clinical signs typical of gastroenteritis including loss of appetite, vomiting, fluid diarrhea, dehydration, and, only very rarely, death.[5] Although, in general, CCoV does not cause systemic disease, the virus has been isolated from several tissues (tonsils, lungs, and liver) of experimentally infected pups.[20] Fatal disease commonly occurs as a consequence of mixed infections of CCoV with canine parvovirus type 2 (CPV-2),[21,22] with canine adenovirus type 1 (CAdV-1)[23] or with canine distemper virus (CDV).[24]

Currently, two genotypes of CCoV are known, which have been designated CCoV types I (CCoV-I) and II (CCoV-II).[25–32] These genotypes differ mainly in their spike proteins that share only 54% identity.[25] Moreover, CCoV-I strains possess a unique ORF, 624 nt in length, that is completely absent in FCoV-I strains and of which only remnants remain in the genomes of CCoV-II and TGEV.[33] In addition, CCoVs with a recombinant origin between CCoV-II and TGEV have been identified in the feces of dogs with diarrhea and have been found to be widespread in dog populations. Accordingly, CCoV-II has been further classified into two subtypes, CCoV-IIa and CCoV-IIb, including "classic" CCoVs and TGEV-like strains, respectively.[3] Subtype CCoV-IIb has been reported in several European countries,[4,34] as well as in Japan.[31]

PANTROPIC CCoV
Virus Emergence and Clinical Outbreaks

Similar to other coronaviruses, CCoV can mutate, resulting in more virulent strains and corresponding increased severity of enteric illness.[35–38]

On May 2005, a severe outbreak of fatal, systemic disease affected seven dogs housed in a pet shop in Apulia region, Italy. Clinical signs were first observed in three miniature pinschers and a cocker spaniel, 45 and 53 days of age, respectively, and were highly suggestive of canine parvovirus infection, consisting of fever (39.5°–40°C), lethargy, anorexia, vomiting, hemorrhagic diarrhea, and neurologic signs (ataxia, seizures) followed by death within 2 days after the onset of the symptoms. Veterinarians also reported a marked leukopenia, with total WBC counts below 50% of the baseline values. After a few days, the same signs were observed in two other 45-day-old miniature pinschers and in one 56-day-old Pekinese dog, which underwent a rapid fatal outcome.[6]

Necropsy on the carcasses of these three pups revealed severe lesions in the alimentary tract, tonsils, lungs, liver, spleen, and kidneys. The most prominent lesion was hemorrhagic gastroenteritis. Tonsils were enlarged and contained multifocal hemorrhages. Lobar subacute bronchopneumonia was evident both in the cranial and caudal lobes (**Fig. 1**), and accompanied effusions in the thoracic cavity. Spleens were

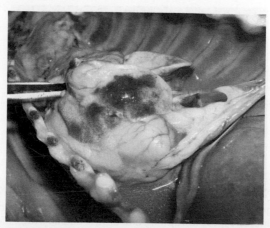

Fig. 1. Lung of a dog with pantropic CCoV infection. Pneumonia in the caudal lobe.

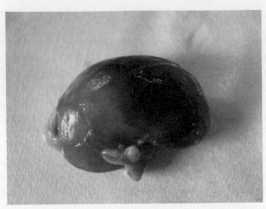

Fig. 2. Kidney of a dog with pantropic CCoV infection. Extensive hemorrhagic areas in the cortex.

enlarged and exhibited subcapsular hemorrhages. Necrosis and lipidosis with hemorrhages was evident in the livers. Infarction and hemorrhages were detected in the cortex and medulla of kidneys (**Fig. 2**; Ref.[6] and Buonavoglia and colleagues, unpublished data, 2006).

Histopathology in the mucosa of the small intestine consisted of atrophy and flattening of most villi, with denudating of the lining epithelium, mononuclear infiltration of the lamina propria, and cell depletion of the centers of lymphoid follicles. Severe coalescing bronchoalveolar lesions in the lungs consisted of a densely cellular fibrinopurulent exudate (**Fig. 3**). Diffuse hepatocyte degeneration was present with moderate microvacuolar fatty change and minimal random necrosis (**Fig. 4**). Splenic lesions were characterized by a diffuse fibrinoid degeneration with arteriolar necrosis. There was leukocytolysis within residual follicles and many macrophages infiltrated the hemorrhagic and hyperemic parenchyma. Diffuse lymphoid depletion was noted in the spleens. Diffuse deep and superficial areas of the renal

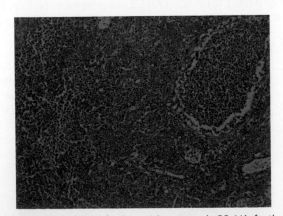

Fig. 3. Photomicrograph of the lung of a dog with pantropic CCoV infection. Densely cellular fibrinopurulent exudates, septae disruption, and diffuse edema (H&E). (*Courtesy of* Prof. M. Castagnaro, University of Padua.)

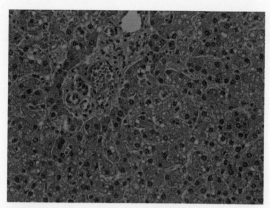

Fig. 4. Photomicrograph of the liver of a dog with pantropic CCoV infection. Diffuse hepatocyte degeneration and microvacuolar fatty change (H&E). (*Courtesy of* Prof. M. Castagnaro, University of Padua.)

cortex exhibited coagulative necrosis with peripheral hyperemia (**Fig. 5**) and degeneration of arteriolar walls.[39]

Virologic and bacteriologic investigations on the parenchymatous organs failed to detect common canine pathogens, whereas CCoV-I and CCoV-II were identified in the intestinal content of all pups by genotype-specific real-time reverse transcriptase-polymerase chain reaction (RT-PCR) assays. Unexpectedly, CCoV-II RNA was also detected at high titers in lungs, spleen, liver, kidney, and brain. A coronavirus strain (CB/05) was isolated on A-72 cells from all the examined tissues but brain. Immuno-histochemistry using an *Alphacoronavirus-1* monoclonal antibody detected viral antigen in all tissues, including lungs (**Fig. 6**).

Other outbreaks of pantropic CCoV infection occurred in France, Belgium,[40] and Belgium. J Small Anim Pract. Submitted for publication), and Greece (V. Ntafis and E. Xylouri-Fragkiadaki, personal communication, 2009). Between March 2008 and

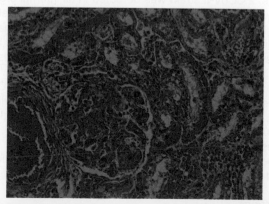

Fig. 5. Photomicrograph of the kidney of a dog with pantropic CCoV infection. Coagulative necrosis associated with marked hyperemia (H&E). (*Courtesy of* Prof. M. Castagnaro, University of Padua.)

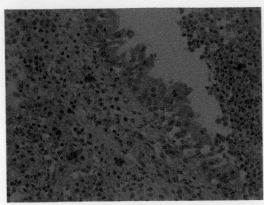

Fig. 6. Immunohistochemical staining with monoclonal anti-CCoV antibody of a lung section from a dog with pantropic CCoV infection. CCoV-infected cells are brown stained. (*Courtesy of* Prof. M. Castagnaro, University of Padua.)

August 2009, five outbreaks of a fatal systemic disease occurred in breeding kennels or pet shops of the north of France and Belgium, involving a total of 21 pure-bred pups, 20 of which died. Clinical signs were the same in all outbreaks and consisted of lethargy, vomiting, anorexia, diarrhea, and convulsions.

Post mortem examination revealed minimal to severe changes in the intestines and major organs. Lesions of discrete to moderate enteritis were generally confined to the small intestine, the serosa of which was often rough and pitted, and pale to old-pink. Loco-regional lymph nodes were enlarged and occasionally congested. Many puppies presented light to severe hepatic degeneration, with a yellow-brown discoloration. The spleen was slightly thickened and congestive and lungs were congested.

Histopathologically, apart from the changes in the intestinal mucosa (denudation and atrophy of the intestinal villi and necrosis of the crypts), edema and depletion of lymphoid tissues were evident. Other peculiar changes included discrete to severe hepatocyte degenerative changes with cytoplasm microvacuolization and extensive subacute interstitial pneumonia with intense vascular congestion.

In four outbreaks, a CCoV-II strain was detected in all internal organs, although in three cases there was a coinfection with CPV-2c. In one outbreak, lethal disease was associated to single pantropic CCoV infection in all examined organs (gut, spleen, liver, lung, brain). In the remaining case, a coinfection with CPV-2c and CCoV-I was identified, but the systemic spread of CCoV-I was associated to a possible synergistic effect of the CPV-induced enteritis.[40]

To date, limited information is available about the Greek pantropic CCoV outbreak, but preliminary data seem to confirm the same clinical and pathologic findings observed in the Italian, French, and Belgian cases (V. Ntafis and E. Xylouri-Fragkiadaki, personal communication, 2009).

Additional cases of pantropic CCoV disease, with or without concurrent CPV infection, have been observed in recent years, but these outbreaks are still under study (Decaro and colleagues, unpublished data, 2011).

Experimental Infections

Experimental infection of five CCoV-seronegative pups with strain CB/05 reproduced the disease with occurrence of severe clinical signs, including pyrexia, anorexia, depression, vomiting, diarrhea, and leucopenia.[7] A different clinical course was observed according to the age of the infected pups. The older dogs, 6 months of age, slowly recovered from the disease, whereas two out of three 2.5-month-old dogs were euthanized due to the severity of the CB/05-induced disease. The pantropism of the virus was confirmed by the presence of gross lesions in the internal organs of the dead dogs, as well as by the detection of viral RNA in those tissues, including brains, albeit at lower titers with respect to those detected in dogs that succumbed to natural infection. Traces of viral RNA were detected in the blood of a single dog, although further unpublished studies have demonstrated that detectable viremia can occur easily during CB/05 experimental infection (Decaro and colleagues, unpublished data, 2010).

Subsequently, strain CB/05 was proven to be able to infect even dogs recovered from a recent infection caused by enteric CCoV, inducing the occurrence of mild clinical signs.[8] Although the dogs used in that study had a strong humoral immunity to enteric CCoV at the time of challenge, experimental infection with strain CB/05 was successful in all pups irrespective of the viral dose administered. Exposure to even low amounts of virus would have a similar pattern of infection on seropositive animals, as dogs inoculated with different viral loads displayed the same duration of the viral shedding and not so very different viral titers in the feces. The duration of viral shedding was shorter and the clinical signs milder with respect to previous observations in seronegative dogs,[7] attributed mainly to the cross-protection induced by antibodies against enteric CCoV. Lymphotropism of strain CB/05 was clearly demonstrated by the occurrence of moderate lymphopenia in several infected pups. However, despite the moderate lymphopenia and the presence of the virus in the lymphoid tissues, the viral RNA was not detected in the blood at any time.

A further experiment aimed to evaluate the effects of pantropic CCoV infection on circulating monocytes and lymphocyte populations.[9] Infection of 11-week-old pups with strain CB/05 resulted in a profound depletion of T cells and a slight loss of B cells in the first week postinfection. In particular, while the CD8$^+$ and the B lymphocytes returned to baseline levels by day 7 postinfection, the CD4$^+$ T cells remained significantly low for 1 month and recovered completely after only 2 months. Monocytosis was also observed after CB/05 infection with a peak at day 5 postinfection. In this study, the polyclonal production of serum IgG or IgM against CCoV was not altered. However, the prolonged depletion of circulating CD4$^+$ T cells may affect humoral as well as cell-mediated immunity, thus compromising the ability to generate or maintain an effective immune response.

In contrast with findings observed in natural outbreaks, most recent experimental studies demonstrated that the outcome of pantropic CCoV infection is not invariably fatal. Indeed, the main effect of this new pathogen is the long-term lymphopenia, which could determine a severe impairment of the dog immune response against concurrent pathogens or vaccinal antigens. In fact, in environmental conditions of kennels and animal shelters, pups are exposed to multiple pathogens and a concurrent infection with pantropic CCoV may exacerbate the clinical course of other viruses, thus leading to a rapid death of the affected pups. In addition, routine vaccinations are usually carried out in pups at the age of 40 to 60 days, when CCoV infection reaches the maximal frequency.

Molecular Virology

Sequence analysis of the 3′ genome end, including ORFs 2 (S gene), 3a, 3b, 3c, 4 (E gene), 5 (M gene), 6 (N gene), 7a and 7b, showed that strain CB/05 had a high degree of amino acid identity to the cognate ORFs of CCoV-II, although the S protein displayed the highest identity to FCoV-II strain 79-1683. A genetic marker was identified in the CB/05 genome, consisting of a 38-nt deletion in ORF3b, which was responsible for a predicted truncated nonstructural protein 3b.[41]

The further pantropic CCoV strains identified so far have not been extensively analyzed at the genetic level. However, preliminary data seem to indicate that those strains are highly similar to prototype virus CB/05, but most of them lack the ORF3b deletion that was proposed as a genetic marker for pantropic CCoV.

At present, the genetic changes associated to the pantropism of the virus are far to be determined, representing a challenge for the future, analogously to what described for the strictly related feline infectious peritonitis virus (FIPV).[42] Therefore, there is the need to develop a reverse genetics system similar to that established for FIPV,[43] which could be useful to understand the molecular basis of the change of virulence and tropism.

Diagnosis

Diagnosis of pantropic CCoV infection cannot be made on the basis of clinical and post mortem findings, considering that the course of infections caused by other canine pathogens, such as CPV and CAdV, may be undistinguishable. Thus, making a definitive diagnosis of pantropic CCoV-induced disease is difficult. In the absence of a clear genetic marker, that should be common to all pantropic strains identified so far, the detection of a CCoV-II strain in the internal organs is the essential condition required for a definitive diagnosis.

Considering the widespread circulation of enteric CCoV and the cross reactions existing between this virus and the pantropic strains, serologic tests such as enzyme-linked immunosorbent assay, virus neutralization,[44] and Western blotting[45] are not suitable to diagnose a pantropic CCoV infection. In contrast, virologic methods developed for detection of enteric CCoV are also employed for diagnosis of systemic infections.

Viral isolation on cell lines of canine (A-72) or feline (Crandel feline kidney) origin using tissue homogenates is usually followed by detection of viral antigens by immunofluorescence assay. However, CCoV is quite unstable in the environment, so that virus isolation succeeds only if samples contain high viral titers and are stored and transported in the cold chain. In contrast, methods based on nucleic acid amplification are highly sensitive, even in the presence of low amounts of viral RNA. Several RT-PCR assays have been developed to detect CCoV in fecal specimens,[46–48] the majority of which can be easily conducted on RNA extract from internal organs.

Quantitative PCR using TaqMan chemistry has allowed for sensitive detection of strain and amount of virus[49] and for rapid discrimination between the CCoV genotypes.[27]

Pantropic CCoV antigens can be also detected in tissue sections by immunochemical staining within macrophages in inflammatory sites and within arterial walls.[6,39]

Treatment and Prevention

There is no specific treatment for infections caused by pantropic CCoV. As for other viral diseases of dogs, management must emphasize supportive treatment to maintain fluid and electrolyte balance. Although rarely indicated, broad-spectrum antimicrobial agents can be given to treat secondary bacterial infections.

To date, no homologous vaccines against pantropic CCoV are available on the market. Inactivated vaccines that are currently used against enteric CCoV were shown to be poorly effective, as they induced high serum antibody levels but no protection after experimental infection with enteric CCoV.[50] Analogously, a killed, MF59-adjuvanted vaccine recently developed against TGEV-like strains (CCoV-IIb) was not able to prevent fecal shedding of the challenge virus.[51] Only an experimental modified-live virus vaccine administered oronasally has been able to induce complete protection from disease as well as from infection.[52] Considering that the immunity induced by natural infection with enteric CCoV is not able to protect pups from challenge with strain CB/05, the efficacy of currently used vaccines prepared with enteric CCoV strains may be poorer against pantropic CB/05-like viruses. According to this scenario, dogs vaccinated with enteric CCoV may acquire subclinical infections with pantropic CCoV resulting in lymphopenia that may represent a predisposing factor for opportunistic pathogens and for a more severe disease induced by "true" pathogens (CPV, CAdV, CDV, and others).

Extensive epidemiologic surveys would assess whether the pantropic CCoV infection is widespread in dog populations. Systematic vaccination programs using homologous live vaccines would seem important in environments such as kennels, shelters, and pet shops that are at high risk of exposure to this newly identified virus.

SUMMARY

Canine coronavirus (CCoV) is an enteric pathogen, which is currently included in the new species *Alphacornavirus-1* of the *Alphacoronavirus* genus. To date, two genotypes of CCoV have been described, CCoV-I and CCoV-II, with the latter including two different subtypes, CCoV-IIa and CCoV-IIb. Usually, CCoV causes mild to severe diarrhea in pups, whereas fatal infections have been associated mainly with concurrent infections by other canine pathogens. However, a few years ago, an outbreak of fatal, systemic disease caused by a highly virulent CCoV-II strain (CB/05) was reported. To date, pantropic CCoV outbreaks have occurred in different parts of Europe, with clinical presentations and post mortem findings similar to those observed in the first outbreak. The pantropic CCoV-induced disease was also reproduced under experimental conditions, although the most prominent finding was a severe, long-lasting lymphopenia (mainly associated to a dramatic reduction of $CD4^+$ cells), rather than the death of the infected pups. Lacking any specific vaccine against this emerging pathogen of dogs, further studies should carefully evaluate (1) the worldwide distribution of the virus in dog populations and (2) the efficacy of existing vaccines, based on enteric CCoV, against pantropic viruses.

REFERENCES

1. Carstens EB. Ratification vote on taxonomic proposals to the International Committee on Taxonomy of Viruses (2009). Arch Virol 2010;155:133–46.
2. Pratelli A, Decaro N, Tinelli A, et al. Two genotypes of canine coronavirus simultaneously detected in the fecal samples of dogs with diarrhea. J Clin Microbiol 2004;42: 1797–9.
3. Decaro N, Mari V, Campolo M, et al. Recombinant canine coronaviruses related to transmissible gastroenteritis virus of swine are circulating in dogs. J Virol 2009;83: 1532–7.
4. Decaro N, Mari V, Elia G, et al. Recombinant canine coronaviruses in dogs, Europe. Emerg Infect Dis 2010;16:41–7.
5. Decaro N, Buonavoglia C. An update on canine coronaviruses: viral evolution and pathobiology. Vet Microbiol 2008;132:221–34.
6. Buonavoglia C, Decaro N, Martella V, et al. Canine coronavirus highly pathogenic for dogs. Emerg Infect Dis 2006;12:492–4.

7. Decaro N, Campolo M, Lorusso A, et al. Experimental infection of dogs with a novel strain of canine coronavirus causing systemic disease and lymphopenia. Vet Microbiol 2008;128:253–60.
8. Decaro N, Elia G, Martella V, et al. Immunity after natural exposure to enteric canine coronavirus does not provide complete protection against infection with the new pantropic CB/05 strain. Vaccine 2010;28:724–9.
9. Marinaro M, Mari V, Bellacicco AL, et al. Prolonged depletion of circulating CD4+ T lymphocytes and acute monocytosis after pantropic canine coronavirus infection in dogs. Virus Res 2010;152:73–8.
10. Enjuanes L, Brian D, Cavanagh D, et al. Family *Coronaviridae*. In: van Regenmortel MHV, Fauquet CM, Bishop DHL, et al, editors. Virus taxonomy, classification and nomenclature of viruses. New York: Academic Press; 2000. p. 835–49.
11. Wise AG, Kiupel M, Maes RK. Molecular characterization of a novel coronavirus associated with epizootic catarrhal enteritis (ECE) in ferrets. Virology 2006;349: 164–74.
12. de Groot RJ, Ziebuhr J, Poon LL, et al. Revision of the family Coronaviridae. Taxonomic proposal of the Coronavirus Study Group to the ICTV Executive Committee. Available at: http://talk.ictvonline.org/media/p/1230.aspx. Accessed October 20, 2009.
13. Erles K, Toomey C, Brooks HW, et al. Detection of a group 2 coronavirus in dogs with canine infectious respiratory disease. Virology 2003;310:216–23.
14. Decaro N, Desario C, Elia G, et al. Serological and molecular evidence that canine respiratory coronavirus is circulating in Italy. Vet Microbiol 2007;121:225–30.
15. Lorusso A, Desario C, Mari V, et al. Molecular characterization of a canine respiratory coronavirus strain detected in Italy. Virus Res 2009;41:96–100.
16. Decaro N, Martella V, Elia G, et al. Biological and genetic analysis of a bovine-like coronavirus isolated from water buffalo (*Bubalus bubalis*) calves. Virology 2008;370: 213–22.
17. Decaro N, Cirone F, Mari V, et al. Characterisation of bubaline coronavirus strains associated with gastroenteritis in water buffalo (*Bubalus bubalis*) calves. Vet Microbiol 2010;145:245–51.
18. Binn LN, Lazar EC, Keenan KP, et al. Recovery and characterization of a coronavirus from military dogs with diarrhea. Proc Annu Meet US Anim Health Assoc 1974;78: 359–66.
19. Keenan KP, Jervis HR, Marchwicki RH, et al. Intestinal infection of neonatal dogs with canine coronavirus 1-71: studies by virologic, histologic, histochemical, and immunofluorescent techniques. Am J Vet Res 1976;37:247–56.
20. Tennant BJ, Gaskell RM, Kelly DF, et al. Canine coronavirus infection in the dog following oronasal inoculation. Res Vet Sci 1991;51:11–8.
21. Decaro N, Martella V, Desario C, et al. First detection of canine parvovirus type 2c in pups with haemorrhagic enteritis in Spain. J Vet Med B Infect Dis Vet Public Health 2006;53:468–72.
22. Decaro N, Desario C, Elia G, et al. Occurrence of severe gastroenteritis in pups after canine parvovirus vaccine administration: a clinical and laboratory diagnostic dilemma. Vaccine 2007;25:1161–6.
23. Decaro N, Campolo M, Elia G, et al. Infectious canine hepatitis: an "old" disease reemerging in Italy. Res Vet Sci 2007;83:269–73.
24. Decaro N, Camero M, Greco G, et al. Canine distemper and related diseases: report of a severe outbreak in a kennel. New Microbiol 2004;27:177–81.
25. Pratelli A, Martella V, Decaro N, et al. Genetic diversity of a canine coronavirus detected in pups with diarrhoea in Italy. J Virol Methods 2003;110:9–17.

26. Yeşilbağ K, Yilmaz Z, Torun S, et al. Canine coronavirus infection in Turkish dog population. J Vet Med B Infect Dis Vet Public Health 2004;51:353–5.
27. Decaro N, Martella V, Ricci D, et al. Genotype-specific fluorogenic RT-PCR assays for the detection and quantitation of canine coronavirus type I and type II RNA in faecal samples of dogs. J Virol Methods 2005;130:72–8.
28. Benetka V, Kolodziejek J, Walk K, et al. M gene analysis of atypical strains of feline and canine coronavirus circulating in an Austrian animal shelter. Vet Rec 2006;159:170–4.
29. Wang Y, Ma G, Lu C, et al. Detection of canine coronaviruses genotype I and II in raised Canidae animals in China. Berl Munch Tierarztl Wochenschr 2006;19:35–9.
30. Decaro N, Desario C, Billi M, et al. Western European epidemiological survey for parvovirus and coronavirus infections in dogs. Vet J 2011;187:195–9.
31. Soma T, Ohinata T, Ishii H, et al. Detection and genotyping of canine coronavirus RNA in diarrheic dogs in Japan. Res Vet Sci 2010; 90:205–7.
32. McElligott S, Collins PJ, Sleator RD, et al. Detection and genetic characterization of canine parvoviruses and coronaviruses in southern Ireland. Arch Virol 2011; 156:495–503.
33. Lorusso A, Decaro N, Schellen P, et al. Gain, preservation and loss of a group 1a coronavirus accessory glycoprotein. J Virol 2008;82:10312–7.
34. Erles K, Brownlie J. Sequence analysis of divergent canine coronavirus strains present in a UK dog population. Virus Res 2009;141:21–5.
35. Naylor MJ, Walia CS, McOrist S, et al. Molecular characterization confirms the presence of a divergent strain of canine coronavirus (UWSMN-1) in Australia. J Clin Microbiol 2002;40:3518–22.
36. Sanchez-Morgado JM, Poynter S, Morris TH. Molecular characterization of a virulent canine coronavirus BGF strain. Virus Res 2004;104:27–31.
37. Evermann JF, Abbott JR, Han S. Canine coronavirus-associated puppy mortality without evidence of concurrent canine parvovirus infection. J Vet Diagn Invest 2005;17:610–4.
38. Escutenaire S, Isaksson M, Renström LH, et al. Characterization of divergent and atypical canine coronaviruses from Sweden. Arch Virol 2007;152:1507–14.
39. Zappulli V, Caliari D, Cavicchioli L, et al. Systemic fatal type II coronavirus infection in a dog: pathological findings and immunohistochemistry. Res Vet Sci 2008;84:278–82.
40. Zicola A, Jolly S, Mathijs E, et al. Fatal outbreaks in dogs with pantropic canine coronavirus in France and Belgium. J Small Anim Pract, in press.
41. Decaro N, Martella V, Elia G, et al. Molecular characterisation of the virulent canine coronavirus CB/05 strain. Virus Res 2007;125:54–60.
42. Haijema BJ, Rottier PJM, de Groot RJ. Feline coronaviruses: a tale of two-faced types. In Thiel V, editor. Coronaviruses. Molecular and cellular biology. Norfolk (UK): Caister Academic Press; 2007. p. 183–203.
43. Haijema BJ, Volders H, Rottier PJ. Switching species tropism: an effective way to manipulate the feline coronavirus genome. J Virol 2003;77:4528–38.
44. Pratelli A, Elia G, Martella V, et al. Prevalence of canine coronavirus antibodies by an enzyme-linked immunosorbent assay in dogs in the south of Italy. J Virol Methods 2002;102:67–71.
45. Elia G, Decaro N, Tinelli A, et al. Evaluation of antibody response to canine coronavirus infection in dogs by Western blotting analysis. New Microbiol 2002;25:275–80.
46. Bandai C, Ishiguro S, Masuya N, et al. Canine coronavirus infections in Japan: virological and epidemiological aspects. J Vet Med Sci 1999;61:731–6.

47. Pratelli A, Tempesta M, Greco G, et al. Development of a nested PCR assay for the detection of canine coronavirus. J Virol Methods 1999;80:11–15.

48. Naylor MJ, Harrison GA, Monckton RP, et al. Identification of canine coronavirus strains from faeces by S gene nested PCR and molecular characterization of a new Australian isolate. J Clin Microbiol 2001;39:1036–41.

49. Decaro N, Pratelli A, Campolo M, et al. Quantitation of canine coronavirus RNA in the faeces of dogs by TaqMan RT-PCR. J Virol Methods 2004;119:145–50.

50. Pratelli A, Tinelli A, Decaro N, et al. Efficacy of an inactivated canine coronavirus vaccine in pups. New Microbiol 2003;26:151–5.

51. Decaro N, Mari V, Sciarretta R, et al. Immunogenicity and protective efficacy in dogs of an MF59-adjuvanted vaccine against recombinant canine/porcine coronavirus. Vaccine 2011;29:2018–23.

52. Pratelli A, Tinelli A, Decaro N, et al. Safety and efficacy of a modified-live canine coronavirus vaccine in dogs. Vet Microbiol 2004;99:43–9.

Feline Coronavirus in Multicat Environments

Yvonne Drechsler, PhD[1], Ana Alcaraz, DVM, PhD,
Frank J. Bossong, DVM, Ellen W. Collisson, PhD,
Pedro Paulo V.P. Diniz, DVM, PhD*,[1]

KEYWORDS

- Cats • Feline infectious peritonitis • Diagnosis • Outbreak
- Prevention • Control

Feline coronavirus (FCoV) is a highly contagious virus that is ubiquitous in multicat environments. This virus commonly causes an asymptomatic infection, which can persist in certain individuals. Sporadically and unpredictably, FCoV infection leads to feline infectious peritonitis (FIP), a highly fatal systemic immune-mediated disease. The pathogenesis of FIP is not fully understood. Despite the low incidence of FIP among FCoV-infected cats, FIP is a major cause of mortality.[1,2] Since it can take weeks to months for FIP to develop after the initial infection with FCoV, the disease may only become apparent after a cat has been adopted or sold, resulting in devastating consequences for clients and adoption or breeding facilities. Currently, the development of FIP in a FCoV-infected cat is unpredictable, and once FIP develops, diagnosis confirmation is difficult. Historically, therapy has been limited to palliative treatment, although recent therapeutic protocols have improved survival time. This review provides interdisciplinary information about the virus, the pathophysiology of the disease, the available diagnostic methods, as well as the management and control of the virus and the disease in shelters and other multicat environments.

ETIOLOGY OF FELINE CORONAVIRUSES

FCoVs belong to a family of considerable importance in veterinary medicine. Viruses within the Coronaviridae family infect and often cause enteric and respiratory disease, especially in young animals.[3–9] In general, these viruses tend to be transmitted between and infectious for only closely related hosts.[10] However, with the discovery of the severe acute respiratory syndrome coronavirus (SARSCoV) that commonly

[1] These authors contributed equally to this work.

Disclosure: Pedro Diniz has received speaker honoraria from Boehringer Ingelheim Pharmaceuticals, Inc.

College of Veterinary Medicine, Western University of Health Sciences, 309 East Second Street, Pomona, CA 91766-1854, USA

* Corresponding author.

E-mail address: pdiniz@westernu.edu

Vet Clin Small Anim 41 (2011) 1133–1169
doi:10.1016/j.cvsm.2011.08.004
0195-5616/11/$ – see front matter © 2011 Elsevier Inc. All rights reserved.

infects bats and apparently "jumped" from civets and raccoon dogs to humans, the broader range of transmission and zoonotic potential of animal coronaviruses is a reality.[11]

Group 1 Coronaviruses

The coronaviruses can be classified into at least 4, if not 5, groups.[11,12] The mammalian viruses are represented in 3 or 4 of these groups with the feline viruses residing in group 1, along with the porcine, canine, rabbit, and ferret coronaviruses, and a human coronavirus, that is distinct from the virus associated with severe acute respiratory syndrome (SARS).[13–15] Within group 1 viruses, the feline, porcine, and canine members are closely related.[14,16–18] There are 2 distinct serotypes of FCoVs that are genetically related and, by definition, can be distinguished on the basis of specific antibodies.[19–24] Whereas serotype I FCoV shares genetics with the porcine virus, transmissible gastroenteritis virus (TGEV), type II FCoV shares homology with the canine coronavirus. The TGEV genomic sequences identified in the FCoV I and canine coronavirus sequences identified in FCoV II indicated these viruses likely originated in part by recombination events resulting in this exchange of genome regions.[19,25–27] Recombination is a common event for coronaviruses.[19,28–33] The FCoV I isolates have repeatedly been shown to more commonly infect cats worldwide than FCoV serotype II viruses.[34–38] However, the FCoV type II viruses are most commonly studied because of a greater propensity to replicate in vitro in cell culture. Unlike the type I FCoV, but similar to most of the group 1 coronaviruses, the FCoV type II viruses use their species-specific aminopeptidase N as the cell receptor for entry.[39–42]

Of considerable clinical interest is the manifestation of 2 FCoV biotypes, which are associated with distinct diseases or pathologies.[22,38,43] The feline enteric coronavirus (FECV) biotype is ubiquitous, commonly infecting the gut of cats and generally in the absence of disease, while the feline infectious peritonitis virus (FIPV) biotype is responsible for fatal, systemic disease. Because FECV and FIPV from the same cattery are nearly identical, both antigenically and genetically, while geographically separated isolates display greater sequence differences, it has been generally accepted that the FIPV arises from the FECV strains, within the same animal.[38,44–47] It is important to understand how the 2 biotypes relate to FCoV serotypes. Both FIPV and FECV are represented within both FCoV serotypes I and II.[37] Thus, the terms biotype and serotype are distinct and should not be confused.

Feline Coronavirus Genetics and Biotype Considerations

The infectious vehicle for transmission from cat to cat or from cell to cell is the coronavirus virion or viral particle (**Fig. 1**). The single-stranded RNA genome, lying within the core of the virion, is coated with nucleocapsid proteins.[13,24] A bilipid membrane, or envelope, originating from the host cell surrounds the nucleocapsid coated genome. Embedded within this membrane envelope are 3 major proteins that complete the repertoire of the virion particle. The membrane proteins are the glycosylated, envelope spike protein (S); the glycosylated, highly hydrophobic membrane protein (M); and a smaller hydrophobic envelope protein (E). The S protein can be cleaved into 2 parts resulting in the transmembrane S2, which anchors the protein in the cell derived envelope, and the more exterior S1. It is the S1 protein that houses the major determinants for virus attachment and thus antibody neutralization and serotype determination.[48,49]

The order of the genes encoded on the FCoV genome is similar to that of other coronaviruses. The information encoding the polymerase activity required for making

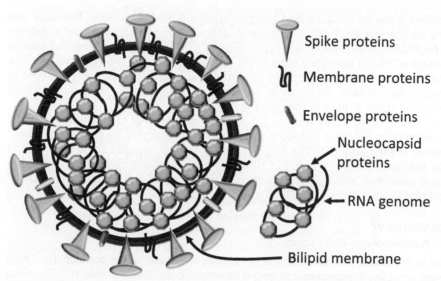

Spike proteins

Membrane proteins

Envelope proteins

Nucleocapsid proteins

RNA genome

Bilipid membrane

Fig. 1. Schematic of the FCoV virion (viral particle). Nucleocapsid proteins coat the RNA genome. The spike, membrane, and envelope proteins are anchored in the bilipid membrane of cell origin.

messenger RNA and genomic RNA is located in the 5′ two-thirds of the genome (**Fig. 2**).[24,50,51] The information encoded in the remaining third of the genome at the 3′ end encodes those proteins that make up the viral particle (see **Fig. 1**). These 3′ genes lie in an order of S, E, M, and N. Additional group I coronavirus ORFs encoding proteins of unknown function lie between the S and E genes (3a, 3b and 3c), and downstream of the N gene (7a, 7b).

The potential for mutations in the RNA genome of coronaviruses provides the background for variations that may result in changes in the nature of the viral antigens or disease resulting from viral infection. Whereas antigenic changes are responsible for vaccine failures in the case of the avian coronaviruses, mutations in the FCoV may also be responsible for the metamorphosis of the fairly benign enteric virus to a highly pathogenic relative, responsible for FIP.[28,30,44,46,52–54] The defining question is what

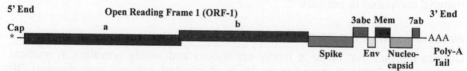

5′ End   Open Reading Frame 1 (ORF-1)   3abc Mem   7ab   3′ End

Cap   a   b

AAA

Spike   Env   Nucleo-   Poly-A
capsid   Tail

Fig. 2. Schematic of the gene organization on the FCoV genome. A cap structure at the 5′ end and the 3′ end poly-adenylated tail are typical structures on an RNA used as message for generating protein within a cell. The entire genome is approximately 29,000 nucleotide bases in length. The overlapping ORFs 1a and 1b encode proteins involved in RNA synthesis required for generating mRNA, the genome, and their negative sense templates. The spike refers to the gene encoding the highly glycosylated spike protein (S), Mem refers to the gene encoding the membrane protein (M), env refers to the gene encoding the envelope protein (E), and nucleocapsid refers to the gene encoding the nucleocapsid protein (N).

mutations in the enteric virus lead to a pathogenic, fatal viral progeny. The large size of the coronavirus RNA genome presents difficulties in identifying single mutations that might be instrumental in defining virulence.[51,55] Although differences can also be identified within the extremely large ORF1 (at the beginning of the genome), the size of this region has been an obstacle to pinpointing mutations potentially involved in biotype determination. Thus, gene comparisons have concentrated on selected genes lying in the 3′ third of the genome.[44,46,52–54]

An intact 3c region between the S and M genes has been associated with FECV replicating in the gut while mutations that prevent expression of the protein have been identified in FIPV strains.[44] The ORF 7b gene was also reported to be truncated in FECV but intact in FIPV strains.[56,57] However, such deletions may not be relevant to biotype since they also can occur with in vitro passage[53] and Lin and colleagues[58] found that small deletions in ORF7b could be found in both biotypes.

EPIDEMIOLOGY

FCoV Prevalence and Risk Factors

FCoV is distributed worldwide and is ubiquitous in virtually all cat populations. There is great variability in prevalence among different cat populations (**Table 1**).[59] The virus is transmitted via the fecal-oral route; therefore, the prevalence of FCoV infection is generally associated with the number and density of cats housed together. A serologic survey from Davis, California reported a seroprevalence of 20% in pet cats living in private households and 87% for purebred cats living in catteries.[60] Among 2,214 relinquished cats at 14 British shelters, the risk of being seropositive was 2.3-fold higher for cats originating from multicat households than for cats from single-cat households.[61] In other populations, more than 90% of the cats were seropositive, and certain cats could remain seropositive for 10 years or longer.[62] The length of time in multicat environments also increases the risk of exposure, which was estimated to be 5 times higher for cats living in shelters for longer than 60 days.[61] Although these environments are not the primary source of FCoV for many relinquished cats, factors intrinsic to the shelter environment amplify shedding and increase spread to susceptible individuals. One study demonstrated that FCoV-infected cats entering a shelter increased FECV shedding from 10- to 1 million-fold in 1 week.[63] Housing and husbandry practices that reduce exposure to feces and contaminated environments have a tremendous influence on the number of cats exposed to the virus.[62] As shown in **Table 1**, stray or feral cats generally have a lower prevalence of infection than pet cats, likely due to lower population densities and because burying feces outdoors results in less exposure to contaminated fecal material compared to pet cats.[64]

FIP Incidence and Risk Factors

Despite the fact that FCoV is highly contagious and widely prevalent in multicat environments (**Table 1**), only 5% to 12 % of infected cats will ever develop FIP syndrome.[60,65–68] However, depending on the population density, length of stay, and husbandry practices, the frequency rates in multicat environments can be as low as 0.6% to 0.8%.[69,70] The FIP incidence of 1 in every 200 new cases was determined based on 226,720 cats seen at 24 veterinary teaching hospitals in the United States over a period of 10 years (1986–1995).[1] Several risk factors for the development of FIP have been identified. Sexually intact male and young cats have the highest risk of developing FIP.[71] Over 40% of 1,182 cats with confirmed FIP seen in US teaching hospitals were from 6 months to 2 years of age.[1] In one study in Taiwan, 88% of 51

Table 1
Frequency of cats exposed to or infected with FCoV in selected populations

Sample Tested	Country	Population Type	Prevalence	No. Positive/Total	Diagnostic Method	Breed	Ref.
Serum	Australia	Multicat environment	44%	59/135	ELISA	Many	185
	Australia	Single cat household	24%	33/140	ELISA	Many	185
	Australia	Stray	0%	0/49	ELISA	Not disclosed	185
	Germany	Multicat environment	69%	29/42	IFA	Mixed-breed	68
	Italy	Multicat environment	82%	98/120	ELISA	Not disclosed	155
	Sweden	<5 cats in the environment	29%	a/129	IFA	Many	186
	Sweden	≥5 cats in the environment	71%	a/24	IFA	Many	186
	Turkey	Multicat environment	62%	18/29	VN	Not disclosed	187
	Turkey	Single cat households	4%	3/71	VN	Not disclosed	187
	UK	Multicat environment	23%	28/100	IFA	Many	98
	UK	Single cat household	16%	14/88	IFA	Many	98
	UK	Multicat environment	26%	432/1654	IFA	Many	61
	UK	Multicat environment	84%	110/131	IFA	Many	188
	UK	Stray	22%	111/506	IFA	Many	189
	USA, Florida	Stray	18%	101/553	IFA	Many	64
	USA, California	Single cat households	21%	7/33	IFA	Not disclosed	60
	USA, California	Multicat environment	87%	94/108	IFA	Not disclosed	60
Feces	Germany	Multicat environment	38%	16/42	Nested RT-PCR	Mixed-breed	68
	Malaysia	Multicat environment	96%	23/24	RT-PCR	Persian	190
	Malaysia	Multicat environment	70%	14/20	RT-PCR	Mixed-breed	190
	Sweden	Multicat environment	80%	12/15	Nested PCR	Persian	191
	Sweden	Single cat household	25%	24/98	Nested PCR	Many	191
Blood	Netherlands	Multicat environment	5%	23/424	mRNA RT-PCR	Many	170
	Malaysia	Multicat environment	15%	6/40	mRNA RT-PCR	Many	169
	Turkey	Stray	45%	10/22	mRNA RT-PCR	Many	168

Abbreviations: ELISA, enzyme-linked immunosorbent assay; IFA, immunofluorescent antibody assay; mRNA, messenger RNA; RT-PCR, reverse transcriptase polymerase chain reaction; VN, virus neutralization assay.
a Number of seropositives not provided.

FIP-confirmed cats were less than 2 years old.[72] The risk decreases to 4% when cats reach 36 months of age.[65] The disease is overrepresented in certain pure breeds, but the incidence of FIP can vary greatly between regions and countries. Abyssinian, Australian mist, Bengal, Birman, British shorthair, Burmese, Cornish rex, Himalayan, Persian, ragdoll, and rex breeds have been suggested as risk factors,[71–74] but FIP development is probably more related to bloodlines within a breed than to breeds themselves.[59] It has been demonstrated that the development of FIP in certain lineages occurs at higher frequencies than other lineages, independently of environment, antibody titers, or viral shedding patterns.[1,75] Cats with high FCoV titers or continuous exposure to persistent shedders also have a greater risk of developing FIP.[45,59,66]

Cats with immunosuppressive conditions, such as advanced FeLV or FIV infections, are more susceptible for developing FIP when exposed to FCoV.[66,76,77] It has been demonstrated that in FIV-infected cats the levels of FECV shedding are increased by 100-fold, with prolonged duration of fecal shedding.[45] In this study, it was demonstrated that 2 cats in the FIV-infected group later developed FIP. It is theorized that the immunosuppression from the chronic FIV infection may have enhanced the evolution and selection of FIPV mutants because of the increased rate of FECV replication in the bowel and the affected individuals' decreased ability to fight off mutant viruses that may occur.[45]

Stress also plays a very large factor as to whether an FCoV-infected cat develops FIP.[78] Stressors such as moving to a new environment, cat density, or surgery may increase the risk of an individual developing FIP. Virtually all cats in shelters and other multicat environments experience some level of stress and exposure to an array of pathogens; thus, higher incidence and outbreaks are expected in stressful environments.

Outbreaks

An outbreak is defined as a frequency of FIP-confirmed cases of greater than 10% in a multicat environment. However, rates lower than 10% may characterize an outbreak in shelters with low FIP prevalence. For example, in shelters with very low FIP frequency (<1%),[69,70] rates higher than 1% may be a cause of concern.[79] Outbreaks with prevalences of 3% to 49% have been described.[59,80] Several factors have been associated with outbreaks, including (1) *host-related factors*: age at exposure, sex, and lineage susceptibility; (2) *virus-related factors*: strain virulence, high replication rate in the intestine, and a tendency to mutate to FIPV; and (3) *environment-related factors:* frequency of exposure to FECV, infective dose, exposure to chronic shedders, and length of exposure.[79,81]

PATHOLOGY

FIP is classified as 2 forms: a noneffusive or dry and an effusive or wet form. Although the gross findings are different, the microscopic lesions are similar in both the dry and wet forms of FIP.[82,83] Furthermore, in most individual patients a mixture of both forms can be identified.

Gross Pathology

Both the wet and dry forms of FIP present with severe systemic disease and produce variable degrees of thoracic or abdominal effusions.[59] The effusive or wet form produces abundant clear, proteinaceous, straw-colored peritoneal effusions (**Fig. 3**A).[84] Large amounts of thick exudative fluid containing copious amounts of fibrin (see **Fig. 3**B)

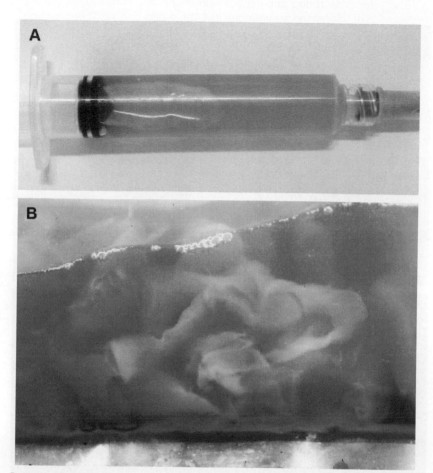

Fig. 3. Peritoneal effusion from a cat with classic wet (or effusive) form of FIP. (*A*) Characteristic color of peritoneal effusion collected by abdominocentesis. (*B*) Close view of a plastic bag containing 350 ml of abdominal effusion and large clumps of fibrin. The high viscosity of the effusion due to high protein content can be seen in Video 1. (*A, courtesy of* Daniel Gerardi, Universidade Federal do Rio Grande do Sul, Brazil.)

severely distend the abdomen. However, this is not the only lesion, as the exudate is accompanied by a perivascular inflammatory reaction (**Fig. 4**) The distinctive characteristic of FIP is a whitish, slightly granular, inflammatory exudate observed in the kidneys and the omentum and covering the hepatic or splenic capsule and extending into the parenchyma (**Fig. 5**). The soft, thin, granular, whitish layer or thin plaques are found in the liver or on the splenic capsule (**Fig. 6**). Other abdominal organs, such as the intestines, lymph nodes, pancreas, or urinary bladder, may be affected to variable degrees. Inflammatory exudates can also be seen in the lungs and heart, which are frequently affected by similar, small, slightly granular nodules to plaquelike lesions with subtle vascular orientation.[85]

In the noneffusive or dry form of FIP, where there is minimal to no effusion, the inflammatory reaction can be restricted to individual organs, such as kidneys, eyes, or brain. In these cases, the lesions still have the distinctive vascular orientation

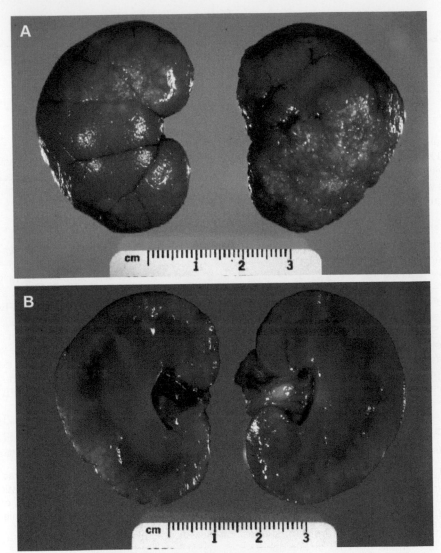

Fig. 4. Cat kidneys. (*A*) Multifocal to coalescing granulomatous inflammation (white, rough appearance) following the superficial blood vessels. (*B*) Cut section also shows the vascular-oriented distribution. (*Courtesy of* RN Fuji, VMD, Ithaca, NY.)

characteristic of the disease. The inflammatory response in the dry form is characterized by a perivascular oriented granulomatous to pyogranulomatous reaction with or without vasculitis.

FIPV and Hypersensitivity

The characteristic perivascular granulomatous lesions associated with FIPV infection have been attributed to type III and IV hypersensitivity reactions.[86-88] Type III hypersensitivity occurs when soluble antigen binds to antibody, forming immune complexes that can be deposited into the vessel walls, also leading to vasculitis.[89]

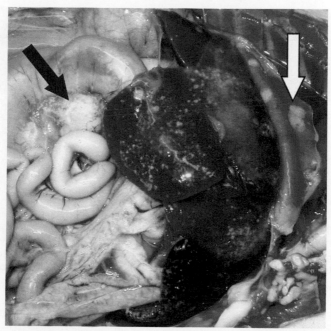

Fig. 5. Peritoneal cavity of a cat: intestine, liver, lymph node, spleen, and diaphragm. White-to-yellow soft plaques covering the parietal and visceral peritoneal surfaces (*white arrow*). The lymph nodes associated with large intestine are enlarged and yellow (*black arrow*).

Complement activation and deposition in tissues also occur during FIPV. This response triggers disseminated intravascular coagulation (DIC), vasculitis, and blood vessel necrosis. Type IV hypersensitivity is a delayed reaction due to excessive stimulation of T-cells and macrophages, which may also contribute to granuloma formation.[90] On the other hand, the pathology findings associated with hypersensitivity reactions might be secondary to monocyte activation in the development of vasculitis.[83] This is further supported by new findings that release of vascular endothelial growth factor (VEGF) by FIPV-infected monocytes induces vascular permeability and effusions.[91]

Shedding of FCoV

Following exposure to FCoV, the primary stage of infection lasts from 7 to 18 months, when the highest levels of viral shedding occur.[92] A dramatic decrease in shedding over 2 years has been reported in naturally infected cats.[68] Therefore, infected cats can be broadly divided into 3 categories: those that shed FECV relatively consistently over long periods of time (consistent shedders, about 10%–15%), intermittent shedders (about 70%–80%), and nonshedders (<5%).[92–94] In one study, 27% of adults shed FECV virus 75% of the time.[95] Apparently, these consistent shedders were persistently infected with the same strain of the virus,[68,96] but cats that recovered from the infection were susceptible to reinfection with the same strain or different strains of the virus.[96] It has been demonstrated that the colon is the major site of FECV persistence and a probable source for recurrent shedding.[97] It is

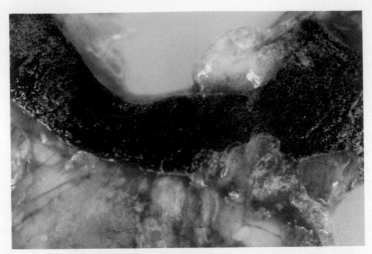

Fig. 6. Spleen from a cat. The capsular surface shows severe fibrinous inflammatory reaction that extends to the omentum. The inflammatory reaction is admixed with copious amounts of fibrin.

presumed that stress factors may contribute to persistent or intermittent shedding, especially in kittens,[59] where fecal shedding starts within in 1 week and remains at consistently high levels from 2 to 10 months after infection.[92] In addition, kittens shed higher levels of FECV than adult cats.[66,92] In one study, one-third of older cats and 90% of kittens and juveniles presented to shelters in Sacramento, California, USA, were shedding FECV at the time of entry.[63] Approximately one third of cats positive for antibodies specific for FCoV shed the virus in the feces.[98] It is of particular interest that cats shedding virus tended to have higher antibody titers (immunofluorescence assay [IFA] titers ≥100) than cats no longer shedding virus (titers ≥25).[92] Quantification of virus may not be an absolute indicator of the viral load, because of the presence of factors that inhibit reverse trasncription–polymerase chain reaction (RT-PCR) in feline feces.[50,92] Cats may be able to clear the infection within 6 to 8 months if there is no reinfection.[92] Virus clearance has been correlated with humoral[99] and cell-mediated immune responses to the virus.[100]

FIPV and Innate Immunity

Several studies have shown that FIPV replicates in monocytes/macrophages,[20,48,101,102] but there are few studies regarding the nature of the innate immune response to FIPV infection. Natural killer cells (NK) typically release type I interferons (IFNα and IFNβ) in response to viral infection inducing interferon-stimulated gene (ISG) transcription.[103–105] These results in an antiviral state, which coronaviruses such as SARSCoV have been shown to suppress.[106,107] In addition, monocytes and macrophages release proinflammatory cytokines such as tumor necrosis factor TNFα, interleukin (IL)-1, IL-6, and IL-12 in response to viral pathogens but also antiinflammatory IL-10 as an immune regulator that increases TNFα, which in turn has implications for the mostly cell-mediated adaptive immune response. Cats with FIP have been shown to express increased levels of these cytokines and monocytes or macrophages are suspected to play a role.[108,109]

FIPV and Humoral Immunity

In most viral infections, the humoral response results in the generation of viral neutralizing antibodies, which are pertinent in preventing infection. However, in the case of FIPV, there is evidence that the humoral antibody response contributes to pathogenesis by a mechanism called antibody-mediated enhancement.[87,110] Antibodies to the spike protein, which is responsible for viral attachment, facilitate the uptake of the virus through Fc receptors on macrophages.[111] Macrophages from FIPV-infected cats release increased levels of B-cell differentiation and survival cytokines, suggesting that enhanced B-cell activation plays a role in antibody-mediated enhancement of infection.[112] Vaccine development has been discouraged mainly because of concerns regarding vaccine-induced enhancement of infection.[113] However, antibody-mediated enhancement of FCoV infection has only been experimentally demonstrated with laboratory strains, and not with field strains.[65] In addition, clearance of FCoV infection in naturally infected cats was associated with the presence of antibodies against spike protein of FIPV.[99] The overall conclusions from experimentally infected cats indicate that humoral immunity does not play a large role in preventing FIPV infection and spread but might rather contribute to pathogenesis, at least in the laboratory setting.

FIPV and Cell-Mediated Immunity

In contrast to humoral immunity, it appears that the cell-mediated immune response plays an important role in fighting FIPV infection and several studies support this assumption. Pedersen and colleagues[59] hypothesized that differences in humoral and cellular immunity manifest in differences in pathogenesis in cats with FIP. They suggested that a strong humoral response and weak cellular immunity lead to the wet effusive form of FIP, while humoral immunity with an intermediate cellular immune response results in the dry form of FIP. It has been shown with other coronavirus infections that a strong cellular response will prevent the disease.[114,115] Additionally, infection with FeLV (feline leukemia virus), a strong suppressor of cellular immunity, is associated with a higher incidence of FIP.[76,77,116,117] FIP is characterized by depletion of T-lymphocytes,[118,119] with CD4$^+$ and CD8$^+$ T-lymphocyte counts remaining low.[100] It is not clear how this depletion occurs, as T cells do not appear to be susceptible to FIPV infection.[118] De Groot-Mijnes[100] theorized that this depletion leads to an acute immunodeficiency and that virus-induced T-cell responses face an uphill battle fighting the infection.

Recently, TNFα and interferon IFNγ have been shown to play a significant role in immunity and pathogenesis associated with FIPV infection. T-cells, B-cells, NK cells, and professional antigen-presenting cells (APCs) such as macrophages and dendritic cells secrete IFNγ,[120] which is important in further activation of immune cells, especially macrophages,[121,122] and is likely to be important in early host defenses.[121,123] Macrophage recognition of PAMPs (pathogen-associated molecular patterns) induces the release of IL-12 and chemokines, which attract NK cells to the site of inflammation, promoting IFNγ synthesis.[124,125] Negative regulators of IFNγ production include anti-inflammatory cytokines, as well as glucocorticoids.[126] IFNγ therefore, is crucial for the early innate response, as well as linking the innate to the adaptive immune response, especially cell-mediated adaptive immunity. Interestingly, clinically normal FCoV-infected cats living in catteries had higher serum IFNγ levels than cats with fulminant FIPV infection, suggesting it has an important role in suppressing the development of FIP.[127] The IFNγ response can be compromised by several factors, in FIPV-infected cats, including stress.

Elevated TNFα release are linked to apoptosis of CD4$^+$ and CD8$^+$ T-lymphocytes, as well as macrophage upregulation of the aminopeptidase N receptor (APN),[109,128] the receptor for FIPV type II. Significant changes were observed in cats after immunization with FIPV and subsequent challenge, regarding proinflammatory cytokine messenger RNA (mRNA) levels in blood leukocytes. Specifically, cats developing the disease expressed high levels of TNFα and low levels of IFNγ. In contrast, in cats that were immune and did not develop FIP, TNFα levels were low with IFNγ levels being elevated. In summary, these studies suggest that FIPV infection leads to reduced cell-mediated immunity, possibly through compromising IFNγ release from blood leukocytes, increased TNFα release from infected monocytes/macrophages, and subsequent T-cell depletion.

Immunity and Stress in Shelter Cats

Shelter cats live in environments that predispose them to increased chronic stress. Stress leads to elevated glucocorticoid release, which in turn negatively regulated IFNγ production, and impaired T-cell function[129,130] with negative effects on cell-mediated immunity. Considering that cell-mediated immunity is most likely responsible for clearance of FIPV infection, it becomes obvious that reducing stress in shelter cats potentially improves their odds of successfully combating infection. Additionally, the close contact of cats in shelters facilitates transmission of any virus, enabling an RNA virus such as FCoV to proliferate and evolve, eventually, to a virulent virus. To address the problem of widespread FECV infection in shelter cats, as well as their increased risk of FIPV infection and consequent disease, it is critical to increase efforts to elucidate the role of the host immune response to FCoV.

DISEASE PRESENTATION
Common Historical Findings

When cats are initially exposed to FCoV, they may be asymptomatic or have diarrhea and/or upper respiratory signs.[82] Cats with coronavirus-associated enteritis can have mild signs of vomiting and/or diarrhea, which can be of short duration or last for weeks or even months.[131] Gastrointestinal signs are generally mild or subclinical, and therapy is not required in most of the cases.

Physical Examination Findings

Although there is often a distinction made between the wet and dry forms of FIP, they are not mutually exclusive, and the progression of the disease may change from one form to the other. With both forms, an array of multiple clinical signs many be present, but none of them is pathognomonic for the disease. Patients may be asymptomatic or present with different levels of depression and anorexia. Other common findings include weight loss, pale mucous membranes, fever of unknown origin, and uveitis.[73,81]

In the wet (effusive) form (see Video 1 online [within this article at www.vetsmall.theclinics.com, November 2011 issue]), ascites with abdominal distention is the most common presentation (**Fig. 7**). A fluid wave on physical examination may be evident, but some cats will have less fluid accumulation, only detectable by abdominal ultrasound. Pleural effusion with secondary dyspnea, tachypnea, and muffled heart sounds may present (**Fig. 8**), whereas pericardial effusion is uncommon.[59,131] The wet form can also be associated with several clinical signs identified in the dry form, described later.

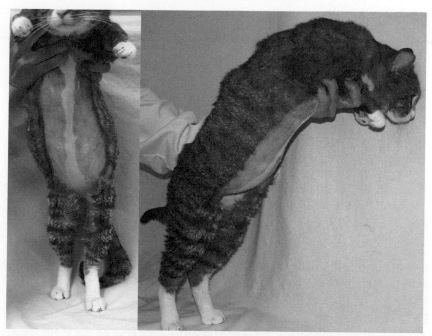

Fig. 7. Cat with wet (effusive) form of FIP presenting moderate abdominal distention due to peritoneal effusion. The abdominal distention is generally not evident in early stages, and may require imaging techniques to be confirmed.

Common signs of the dry or noneffusive form are mild and intermittent fever, decreased appetite, weight loss, stunted growth, depression, pale or yellow mucous membranes, and palpable abdominal organ enlargement.[73,131] Pyogranulomatous lesions develop in one or more abdominal organ, and the clinical signs will be associated with the affected organ, mimicking hepatic or kidney insufficiency, or intestinal tumors.[81] The pyogranulomatous lesions are detected on abdominal palpation as enlarged mesenteric lymph nodes and palpable nodular irregularities on the surface of kidneys and liver.[73,131] If granulomas form on the intestine, constipation, diarrhea, and/or vomiting may be the major clinical signs observed. Uveitis is the most common ocular abnormality documented in FIP cases, but other ocular lesions may be present, such as iritis, cuffing of the retinal vasculature, and keratic precipitates on the cornea (**Fig. 9**).[78,81,132] Neurologic signs can also be seen with FIP, the most common being abnormal mental status, ataxia, central vestibular signs, hyperesthesia, nystagmus, and seizures,[133–136] demonstrating that any part of the central nervous system can become affected in this disease.[137]

DIAGNOSIS

Almost half a century has passed since the first description of FIP in cats; nonetheless, the diagnosis of this syndrome remains one of the greatest challenges for veterinarians. Despite great advances in laboratory diagnostic techniques in the past decades, the diagnosis of FIP is still based on the combination of history of risk factors, signalment, clinical abnormalities, and laboratory findings.[81] With exception of histopathology and immunostaining, **no single laboratory test can definitely**

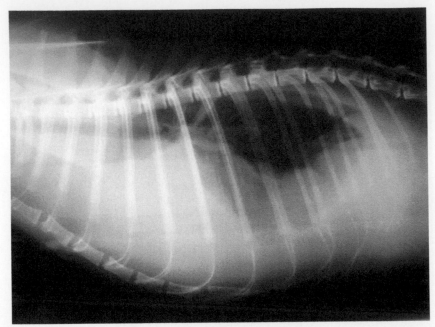

Fig. 8. Lateral thoracic radiograph image of a cat with pleural effusion due to FIP. (*Courtesy of* Daniel Gerardi, Universidade Federal do Rio Grande do Sul, Brazil.)

diagnose the FIP syndrome. Likewise, no diagnostic procedure can identify which FCoV-infected cats will go on to develop FIP. The diagnostic process starts with a good history and comprehensive physical examination.

Complete Blood Cell Count and Biochemical Profile

The complete blood cell count (CBC) and biochemical profile can be helpful in expanding the clinical picture of FIP. Often, as with most chronic illnesses in the feline patient, a nonregenerative anemia may be present. Other abnormalities may include but are not limited to lymphopenia, neutrophilia, thrombocytopenia, hyperbilirubinemia, and elevated aspartate aminotransferase (AST).[72,78,138–140]

Serum Proteins

Hyperproteinemia (>8.0 mg/dl) is a consistent finding, present in approximately 60% of the cats with FIP.[73] This is mainly because of elevated serum globulin levels, caused by a specific antibody response, presence of complement, and immune complexes in the bloodstream.[73,141,142] Hypoalbuminemia can be present associated with hepatic insufficiency or increased loss from endothelial leakage,[141] resulting in decrease in the albumin:globulin (A:G) ratio (**Table 2**). Low A:G ratios are strongly associated with FIP, but other causes of hyperglobulinemia should always be ruled out.[141,143]

Acute-Phase Proteins

Acute-phase proteins are a class of proteins whose plasma concentrations increase or decrease in response to inflammatory disorders. α_1-acid glycoprotein levels greater than 1.5 g/L in plasma or effusions are suggestive of FIP,[144] with diagnostic

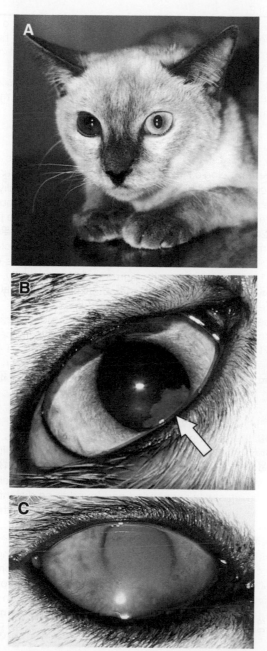

Fig. 9. (*A*) Anterior uveitis typically seen in noneffusive cases of FIP. Mild iridal neovascularization (rubeosis iridis) and hyphema are evident in the anterior chamber of the right eye (OD). (*B*) Fibrin formation, hypopyon, and evidence of mild diapedesis are suggestive of blood–ocular barrier breakdown associated with mild anterior uveitis. (*C*) Severe iritis, with rubeosis iridis, aqueous flare, hypopyon, and keratitic precipitates. These precipitates, known as "mutton-fat" precipitates, are suggestive of a chronic granulomatous disease process. (*A, courtesy of* Daniel Gerardi, Universidade Federal do Rio Grande do Sul, Brazil.)

Table 2
Accuracy of various diagnostic tests for FIP

Category	Test Type	Sensitivity (%)	Specificity (%)	PPV (%)	NPV (%)	Prevalence (%)	Ref.
Protein analysis	Total protein ≥8 g/dl	57	64	76	43	67	138,143,a
	Gamma-globulin ≥2.5 g/dl	70	86	90	61	65	143
	A:G ratio						
	≤0.8	80	82	92	61	72	143
	<0.45	25	98	64	90	13	139
	Protein electrophoresis	38	50	60	29	67	144
	α_1-Acid glycoprotein levels >1.5	85	100	100	75	70	192
Effusion analysis	Total protein >3.5 g/dl	87	60	77	71	72	142
	Gamma-globulin ≥1.0 g/dl	82	83	84	80	53	143
	A:G ratio						
	≤0.9	86	74	79	82	53	143
	≤0.5	62	89	86	68	53	143
	Rivalta test	98	80	84	97	51	143
	Presence of antibodies	86	85	86	85	51	143
	Cytology suggestive of FIP	90	71	89	73	72	142
	Antigen staining in macrophages	72	100	100	68	62	142,143,193,a
Serology	IFA (any titer)	85	57	44	90	28	143
	IFA (titer >1,600)	67	98	94	88	28	155,187,a
	ELISA	100	93	94	100	53	143
	Antigen–antibody complex	48	91	67	84	26	143
Viral nucleic acid detection	Nested RT-PCR						
	Serum	55	88	90	48	67	143,163,a
	Effusion	96	92	96	92	63	143,162,163,a
	mRNA RT-PCR						
	Blood	94	92	67	92	15	168–170,a

Abbreviations: A:G ratio, albumin to globulin ratio; ELISA, enzyme-linked immunosorbent assay; IFA, immunofluorescent antibody assay; mRNA, messenger RNA; NPV, negative predictive value; PPV, positive predictive value; RT-PCR, reverse transcriptase polymerase chain reaction.
a Calculated based on concatenated data from original studies.

accuracy provided in **Table 2**. However, risk factors and clinical signs should be taken into account for the appropriate interpretation, since other inflammatory conditions can also cause increase in this protein.[145] Therefore, in cats with clinical signs and supporting risk factors, a α_1-acid glycoprotein value above 1.5 g/L is consistent with FIP, whereas in asymptomatic cats, α_1-acid glycoprotein values equal to or above 3 g/L are needed to support the diagnosis of FIP.[145]

Effusion Fluid

In cats with the wet form of FIP, effusions from the abdomen or pleural space are typically clear, straw-colored, or viscous due to the high protein content (see Video 1 online [within this article at www.vetsmall.theclinics.com, November 2011 issue]). Sometimes the effusion can be red, pink, almost colorless, or even chylus.[82] It is characterized as nonseptic, modified transudate or pyogranulomateous exudate. Cytology generally documents low cell count (<5,000 nucleated cells/ml) consisting of neutrophils and macrophages, but with a high protein content (>3.5 g/dl).[82,131] A high A:G ratio in the effusion (>0.8) is unlikely to be seen in FIP syndrome, whereas a A:G ratio less than 0.45 is highly suggestive of effusive FIP.[131,146]

The Rivalta test, originally designed one century ago to differentiate transudates from exudates, provides good predictive values when compared to more expensive techniques (**Table 2**).[82,143] Detailed descriptions of how to perform this test are provided in written[78,81,131] and video resources elsewhere.[147] Due to its simplicity and low cost, the Rivalta test should be performed in any case of effusion in cats.[143] IFA can be used to detect macrophages infected with FCoV in effusions. Positive staining of macrophages is 100% predictive of FIP, but false-negative results can occur with low levels of infection.[142,143]

Serology

In the multicat environment, the quantification of FCoV antibodies is valuable for the following[70,82,98]:

- Identifying cats exposed to FCoV prior to their introduction into a FCoV-free cattery
- Screening a cattery for infection
- Testing a cat that has been in contact with a suspected FCoV shedder
- Establishing breeding programs based on FCoV status
- Classifying cats based on shedding level for the purpose of isolation in FCoV-eradication programs.

Although there are several assays currently available that detect antibodies to FCoV, **there is no serologic test capable of diagnosing the FIP syndrome, and serology cannot be used to differentiate between FECV and FIPV infections.** A positive titer only indicates that a given cat has been exposed to FCoV and cannot predict if the cat will ever develop FIP. Conversely, a negative titer is a good predictor of the absence of infection (90% negative predictive value).[143] Because the disease is caused by the FIPV, which arises from a mutant of the common FECV, control and prevention of the FIP syndrome must be directed first at control of its parent virus.[94] Therefore, knowledge of antibodies titers to FCoV can be helpful in controlling and eradicating the virus from multicat environments. Approximately one third of cats presenting with antibodies to FCoV shed FECV in the feces.[98] Cats with titers of 25 or less are often shedding low levels of FECV.[93] These cats frequently stop shedding when isolated from other cats.[94] Cats with titers of 400 or greater are frequently shedding high levels of FECV. When isolated, some of these cats will stop shedding, with concurrent decrease in titers. Cat with persistently high antibody titers generally are consistently shedding.[81,94] If isolation and stress reduction do not promote a decrease in shedding, removal of these consistently shedders from multicat environments should be taken into consideration.

It has been suggested that very high antibody titers (≥1,600) are good predictors of the development of FIP (94% positive predictive value, **Table 2**).[143] However, several studies have described cats with confirmed FIP in which no serologic response to FCoV was detected.[145,148,149] This is particularly true in cats with the wet form of FIP. It is suggested that large amounts of virus are present that can bind to antibodies, making them unavailable for the antibody test in these cases. An alternative explanation is that antibodies against FCoV are lost in the effusion when protein is translocated due to vasculitis.[82] The quantification of antibodies in effusions correlates with the presence of antibodies in blood,[150] suggesting effusions may be a more useful than testing sera.[141] However, other studies have shown no correlation between magnitudes of antibody titers with the occurrence of FIP.[82,143,151] Specific antibodies against FCoV may also be detected in CSF of cats with the neurologic form of FIP,[136] but the diagnostic value of their presence is limited because anti-FCoV antibodies were also detected in cats with brain tumors.[133] In addition, vaccination can also result in a positive titer and cannot be differentiated from natural exposure.[152]

The expression of the 7b gene was reported to be associated with FIPV infection.[153] Consequently, cats with clinical signs of FIP would have titers against 7b protein higher than cats infected only with FECV. Unfortunately, other studies suggest these findings may be artifactually related to the specific isolate tested. Furthermore, intact 7b genes were described in other field strains of FECV.[52,58] Testing for antibodies directed against the 7b protein was compared against the IFA in one study. The authors showed that the 7b protein assay had high sensitivity but poor specificity, with many false-positive results occurring in uninfected animals.[154] Therefore, **this test should not be used alone for the diagnosis of FIP**. Regardless of these findings, the 7b protein test has been advertised as "FIP Specific ELISA" by a commercial laboratory in the United States.

Several protocols, including enzyme-linked immunosorbent assay (ELISA),[155] kinetics-based ELISA,[156] virus neutralization assays,[157] and indirect IFA, have been developed to detect antibodies specific for FCoV.[67,92] The choice of the laboratory is important, since methodologies and antibody titer results can vary significantly among laboratories.[82] Clinicians should be encouraged to select a diagnostic service for which the methodology in use is supported by peer-reviewed publications. In addition, results should be provided as endpoint titers.[82,158] One should also understand that false-positive results can occur, for example due to antinuclear antibodies (ANA), which can be caused by concurrent infections (FIV, *Ehrlichia canis*), autoimmune disease, recent vaccination, or certain drugs, including thiamazole and methimazole.[158–160]

RT-PCR

The RT-PCR assay can detect FCoV in a variety of samples (feces, blood, effusion, cerebrospinal fluid, tissue, and saliva) with high sensitivity (**Table 2**).[93,161–163] In multicat environments, RT-PCR can be a valuable tool to identify continuous shedders as part of an FCoV management plan. However, repeated fecal RT-PCR tests are generally necessary to accurately document if a cat is shedding FCoV. In order to demonstrate that a cat has stopped shedding the virus, at least 5 consecutive monthly negative fecal tests should be obtained, or the cat should become seronegative by IFA.

Due to the inherit risk of false-negative and false-positive results, RT-PCR results are best interpreted in conjunction with serology results.[93]

RT-PCR cannot discriminate between FECV and FIPV due to the various single nucleotide polymorphisms (SNPs) and deletion mutations present in both biotypes, sometimes even identified from the same cat.[46,164,165] At the time of writing, no specific genetic determinants that trigger the evolution of FECV to FIPV or otherwise distinguish the 2 biotypes have been confirmed. Due to these particularities of FCoV, a specific RT-PCR for FIPV cannot, as yet, be designed.

Despite the FECV tropism for feline enterocytes, the enteric virus can be detected by RT-PCR in the bloodstream of healthy cats.[161] Therefore, **the detection of FCoV in blood does not indicate the presence of FIPV and cannot solely support the diagnosis of the FIP syndrome**. In addition, the presence of viremia does not appear to predispose the cats to the development of FIP.[161]

The presence of FCoV in effusions by as detected by RT-PCR is associated with the FIP syndrome, but reports of false-positive results indicate that the specificity is limited. The combined data from three initial studies indicated sensitivity of 96% and specificity of 92% for the diagnosis of FIP using RT-PCR to detect FCoV RNA in effusions from 23 FIP-confirmed cats and 13 cats with effusions due to other causes (**Table 2**). The detection of FCoV by RT-PCR in biopsy samples or fine needle aspirates of affected organs is considered suggestive of the systemic disease, if blood contamination of samples can be ruled out.[81] However, it is suggested that histopathologic examination and immunohistochemistry should be performed to confirm the diagnosis, since in one study, 51 of 84 (60.7%) cats without clinical signs of FIP were positive for FCoV in tissue samples by RT-PCR.[166]

mRNA RT-PCR

In 2005, a PCR procedure targeting the mRNA of the highly conserved M gene of FCoV was described with potential for detecting only replicating virus.[167] The concept was based on the assumption that during the pathogenesis of FIPV, the mutant virus replicates in peripheral blood monocytes and tissue macrophages. Therefore, detection of FCoV mRNA in blood samples would correlate with replication of FIPV and the development of FIP. Two studies in Europe and one in Malaysia have used this technique, with sensitivity ranging from 93% to 100%. However, the percentage of false negatives varied from 5% to 52%.[168-170] These variations may be associated with population selection, criteria used for diagnosis of FIP, and different RNA extraction procedures that may affect the quality of RNA template and downstream assays. The College of Veterinary Medicine at Auburn provides this PCR test for blood, effusion, and tissue, and results are provided in a semiquantitative scale. Unfortunately, at the time of writing, no epidemiologic data from the United States are available using the mRNA RT-PCR assay. Longitudinal studies are needed to determine if cats with replicating FCoV in the bloodstream have a higher risk for developing FIP in the future.

Histopathology

The gold standard and definitive diagnostic test available for FIP is provided by histopathologic examination. In the majority of cases, FIP can be diagnosed by gross and histopathologic lesions alone. The distinctive inflammatory infiltrates are characterized by varying degrees of severity and present with a combination of macrophages, lymphocytes, and plasma cells, mixed with lesser numbers of neutrophils.[82,83] The hallmark of the lesion is a perivascular granulomatous to pyogranulomatous inflammation and vasculitis. The vessels primarily affected are

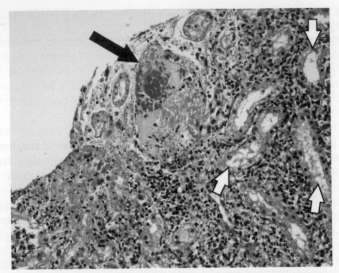

Fig. 10. Kidney. Superficial renal venules. Necrotic tubular epithelial cells (*white arrows*) with severe interstitial pyogranulomatous inflammation. The small venule (*black arrow*) contains an intravascular fibrin thrombus and with moderate mural vascular necrosis (hematoxylin-eosin, original magnification ×20).

small to medium-size veins (**Fig. 10**).[83] The perivascular macrophage-dominated infiltrate occasionally extends into the vessel wall, producing focal areas of necrosis and sporadic smooth muscle hyperplasia (**Fig. 11**). Vasculitis is one of the microscopic lesions that distinguishes the disease from other inflammatory infectious diseases.

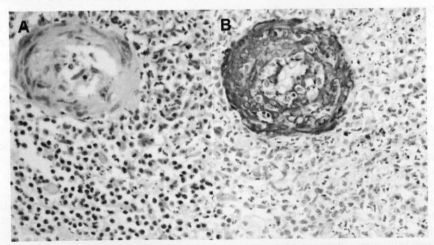

Fig. 11. Spinal cord. (*A*) There is severe pyogranulomatous inflammation that is most intense around the blood (hematoxylin-eosin, original magnification ×60). (*B*) The vessel wall is stained in brown and shows thickening of the wall by moderate to severe smooth muscle hyperplasia (smooth muscle actin with peroxidase stain, original magnification ×60).

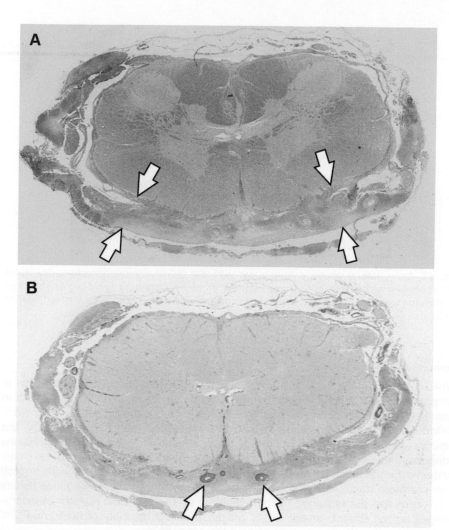

Fig. 12. Spinal cord. (*A*) Subgross cross-section with marked thickening of the meninges due to pyogranulomatous inflammation (between *white arrows*). (*B*) Immunohistochemistry for smooth muscle actin indicates marked medial thickening of the small or medium-size vessels due to smooth muscle hyperplasia (*white arrows*).

In cases of the noneffusive or dry form, brain, spinal cord, or eyes might be the only sites affected. Histopathologic lesions in the brain could include periventriculitis, ventriculitis, ependymitis, and/or leptomeningitis with vascular-oriented inflammatory reaction with or without vasculitis as the distinctive inflammatory lesion (**Fig. 12**). Lesions affecting the eyes have been reported as bilateral granulomatous anterior uveitis often accompanied by chorioretinitis.[171]

Recently, a nonpruritic intradermal cutaneous form of FIP has been described.[172,173] The skin lesions are described as slightly raised intradermal papules over the dorsal neck and on both lateral thoracic walls. In one of the cases reported, the patient was also infected with FIV.[172]

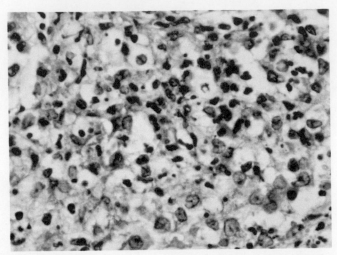

Fig. 13. Brain, lateral ventricle from a cat with FIP (FCoV immunohistochemistry stain). Macrophages within the lesion have intense cytoplasmic staining (*gold-brownish color*), confirming the presence of viral antigen (monoclonal antibody 1:400, original magnification ×60).

Immunostaining

When pathognomonic lesions are not present in histopathology, the detection of intracellular FCoV antigen in macrophages in effusions by immunofluorescence or in tissue by immunohistochemistry is the alternative diagnostic procedure (**Fig. 13**).[82] Unfortunately, these procedures cannot differentiate between FIPV and FECV, but positive antigen staining of macrophages in effusions or granulomatous lesions confirms the diagnosis for FIP.[81,143] In some instances, lesions can resemble systemic fungal infection, and it may be pertinent to rule this out with special histochemical stains. In the immunostaining of the effusion, false-negative results may occur and are explained by the possibility of an insufficient number of macrophages on the effusion smear or the presence of high quantity of host anti-FCoV antibodies in the effusion competing with the assay.[59,82]

PROGNOSIS

With the development of FIP, prognosis is poor to grave, with a reported survival time between 3 and 200 days.[174] All of these animals eventually die from the disease. Euthanasia is recommended when quality of life becomes poor.

TREATMENT OF FIP

Although treatment is focused on reducing the inflammatory and hyperimmune response, no studies have been published to prove any beneficial effects of corticosteroids. There have been several antivirals and immunosuppressants considered for use in FIP cases, and a review of the evidence-based data about therapy is provided elsewhere.[78] Of the antivirals, ribavirin and vidarabine, which are effective in inhibiting virus in cell culture, are toxic in cats. Human IFNα is contraindicated orally and is ineffective with subcutaneous administration.[78] Currently, feline interferon treatment is one of the options to treat FIPV-infected cats, although studies show differences in efficacy.[175] Of the immunosuppressants, prednisone/dexamethasone at immunosuppressive doses is the treatment of choice but such treatment is not curative and may only slow the progression of the disease.[78,176] Recently, a new immunostimulant named polyprenyl improved survival in 3 cats with the dry form of FIP, with 2 of them still alive 2 years after the diagnosis. Polyprenyl enhances cell-medicated immunity by upregulating biosynthesis of mRNA of Th-1 cytokines,[177] which is believed to be required to eliminate the FIP virus. Further studies with a larger number of cats are currently under way.

PREVENTION
Vaccination

A modified-live, nonadjuvanted, intranasal coronavirus vaccine is available that may provide some protection to cats that have not been previously exposed to FCoV. Preventable fractions between 0% and 75% have been reported.[178–181] Vaccination could be advantageous for cats with a negative FCoV titer, if they are entering a multicat environment known to be endemic for FCoV or to have been exposed to FCoV. However, its effectiveness is questionable in situations when cats have already been exposed, which frequently occurs in multicat environments. The vaccination is currently not recommended as a core vaccine in the feline patient.[182,183]

Co-infections

Since immunocompromised cats shed much more viruses[45] and perhaps have less ability to fight off mutant strains, screening and control of other infectious organisms, such as FeLV and FIV, in multicat environments are recommended for the management of FIP. It is a current practice in some shelters to keep FeLV- and FIV-infected individuals for "special needs adoptions." It is important for shelter managers and staff to understand the additional risks such a population poses to the rest of the feline residents and to ensure that measures are taken to minimize these risks. One might reconsider maintaining such populations in the shelter environment. A better option may be to house FeLV- and/or FIV-positive cats with an appropriate rescue organization, to separate them from the rest of the shelter population. Depopulation of FeLV- and/or FIV-positive cats is also an alternative.

Stress

Noise, overcrowding, and inefficient ventilation are a few of the many stress factors, especially in a shelter or cattery environments, that may contribute to the development of FIP in a given population. In the design and management of facilities that house cats, these issues should be addressed. To establish consistency and to introduce new approaches to infection control measures throughout a facility, having accessible "policies and procedures" may prove helpful in keeping compliance among the staff in instituting and maintaining appropriate protocols.[184]

Disinfection

FCoV can survive for 7 weeks in a dry environment and can be transmitted via feces and fomites, so proper cleaning and disinfection are essential in the management of the infection in feline populations. The majority of organic debris should be removed prior to use of disinfectants. A simple 1:32 dilution of sodium hypochlorite (equivalent to 1:10 dilution of the commercially available bleach) is an option but should be protected from light and should be prepared at the time of use. The majority of disinfectants effectively inactivates FCoV[81]; however, it has been suggested that some disinfects may be a more appropriate. Oxidizing agents (eg, Trifectant, Virkon-S, Oxy-Sept 333) are considered effective, whereas some of the quaternary ammonium compounds (eg, Roccal, Parvosol, DiQuat), biguanides (chlorhexidine), and phenolic compounds (eg, Lysol, TekTrol, Amphyl) have limited activity against enveloped viruses.[184] The virus is rarely found in saliva of healthy cats so contact with feeding bowls probably plays a minor role in transmission compared to the sharing of litter boxes among individuals.[93] Nonetheless, proper disinfection of all potentially contaminated surfaces is warranted.

MANAGEMENT
Cat Management After Exposure

If a single cat is diagnosed with FIP, it is recommended to wait at least 2 months before a new cat is introduced into the household so that FCoV infection is likely to be minimal or absent from the environment.[78] If FIP is diagnosed in a multicat household, there is no need to isolate the other cats as they have most likely already been exposed to FECV. If the other cats in the environment are genetically related, the risk of FIP to occur may be higher due to lineage predisposition.[75,78,79]

Multicat Environments

The key to control FCoV in a shelter/foster home is to minimize the viral load in the environment. Reducing the number of cats per room/cage; grouping high FCoV shedders, low shedders, and negative cats separately; decreasing stress; controlling concurrent illness; keeping surfaces and litter trays clean; and providing sufficient litter trays are the best methods to achieve this goal (**Table 3**).[70,78,81,176] Despite these precautions, the evaluation of the infection status of the population is still warranted for successful control of FCoV in a multicat environment.

In catteries, several methods have been attempted to minimize FIP outbreaks. Kittens are removed from the cattery (and from the mother if she has a positive titer for FCoV) and isolated at 3 to 4 weeks of age to prevent exposure to FCoV. This method may prove effective as kittens are protected from FCoV via maternal antibodies until about 4 to 6 weeks of age.[67,70] Although a genetic component for predisposition is not well established,[75] the removal of cats that has produced 2 or more litters affected by the disease from a breeding program is recommended.[82] Because the virus is very easily transmitted via fomites, isolation is not a particularly effective method of control.[78] Depopulation of shedders is generally not effective and requires specific diagnostic tests to identify shedders, which may not be cost effective for some catteries and shelters. Currently, complete elimination of FCoV in these multicat environments would seem to be virtually impossible.[176]

Outbreak Management

When an outbreak of FIP occurs in a shelter setting, several options should be considered, such as increased sanitation, isolation (segregation of infected and uninfected animals), depopulation, and adopters/community education. The characteristics of common methods for prevention and control of FIP outbreaks in multicat environments are presented at **Table 3**.

Even in shelters that follow strict sanitation or biosecurity guidelines, periodic reviewing and updating cleaning practices (especially in the event of an outbreak) are recommended. Good protocols that reduce stress and the amount of fomite transmission of FCoV are (1) to keep cats in the cage while cleaning, (2) daily "in-cage spot cleaning," and (3) deep cleaning of cages when the individual resident has changed.

Table 3
Common methods to prevent FCoV infection and control feline infectious peritonitis outbreaks in multicat environments

Method	Effectiveness	Advantages	Disadvantages	Comments
Individual cages	Effective	Decreases exposure to FCoV	Requires bigger infrastructure and personnel Decreases socialization of cats	If not an option consider monitoring potential shedders in group facilities.
In-cage spot cleaning	Effective	Decreases stress by preventing frequent rehousing of cats	Requires more frequent staff monitoring of litter trays	Not only may decrease the viral load in the environment but presents a more appealing environment for potential adopters.
Isolation or quarantine of cats exposed to FIP cases	Inefficient	None	True quarantine is hard to be performed Decreases socialization of cats	The majority of cats in the same environment are already infected with FCoV when FIP arises. It can take months for FIP to develop, and it occurs in a small percentage of the population
Staff workflow from new cats to longer term residents	Effective	Reduces exposure of more vulnerable population to shedders among longer term residents	Staff compliance with protocol may present a challenge	Fomites can easily transmit FCoV between different areas. This method will not eliminate but may reduce fomite transmission between populations.
Segregation by length of time	Partially effective	Limits exposure between populations Increases socialization	May be difficult to arrange distribution of populations within physical plant limitations	As younger cats are at an increase risk of infection, segregating the younger cats and kittens from adults helps limit their exposure to FCoV
Segregation by antibody status	Effective	Prevents exposure of naïve cats Increases socialization	Requires isolation of new cats until serology results are available	Expense of serology may be a limiting factor.
Grouping by shedding status	Effective	Prevents reinfection of cats Increases socialization	Requires frequent serology or fecal PCR testing to determine shedding status	Only 1/3 of the seropositive cats shed the virus. Repeated fecal PCR test are required to document shedding. Expenses of lab tests may be a limiting factor.

(continued on next page)

Table 3
(continued)

Method	Effectiveness	Advantages	Disadvantages	Comments
Isolation and removal of chronic shedders from facility	Partially effective	Decreases risk of FIP by reducing frequent re-exposure to FCoV	May require depopulation if chronic shedders are not adoptable. May increase risk of FIP in other cats at the adopters environment	Shedding decreases once the cat is isolated. Chronic shedders should be adopted only to single-cat households.
Visitor's flow from new cats to longer term residents	Partially effective	Reduces exposure of more vulnerable population to shedders among longer term residents	Keeping visitors consistent with protocol may present a challenge Predisposes new cats in the shelter to be adopted more frequently than long term residents	Visitors should be encouraged to adopt long term residents.
Vaccination	Partially effective	May decrease incidence of FIP in the long term	At the age of vaccination (16 weeks) the majority of cats in a shelter have already been exposed to FCoV	The vaccine is ineffective when cats have already had contact with FCoV. Not currently recommended for shelters.
Depopulation	Ineffective	Decreases amount of FCoV present in the environment Decreases the risk of exposure of new intakes to FCoV Prevents adoption of FCoV-infected cats	It must be followed by extensive disinfection of facility and introduction of strict biosecurity protocols. Poor shelter reputation regarding euthanasia of "healthy cats". Decrease moral of shelter staff attached to resident cats.	Depopulating only certain "sick" individuals is not effective as an apparently healthy cat may be chronic or intermittent shedder. Depopulating seropositive cats is not recommended due to the small number that may ever develop FIP. FCoV can easily become endemic again if other strict measures are not implemented.

A detailed approach for FIP outbreaks in shelters and foster homes has been published elsewhere.[81]

Isolation is inefficient when an outbreak occurs. As incoming kittens are at the greatest risk, the physical separation between exposed/at-risk cats and newly acquired ones is recommended. This separation should not only create a physical barrier but also involve client and staff flow within a facility (handling of new population first and then exposed cats last). These procedure may not eliminate infection with FCoV, but it will at least reduce exposure to the virus.[79]

Depopulation may be used to control FIP outbreaks, but it requires the removal of the exposed population, comprehensive disinfection of the facility and equipments, and adoption of strict biosecurity methods, which are unfeasible for most of the shelters. **Depopulation of cats seroreactive to FCoV is not recommended, since most cats will have antibodies against the virus, but very few will ever develop FIP.**[81] In addition, depopulation poses ethical, as well as public relation issues for any shelter.

Client Education

Although the incidence of FIP is fairly low, when outbreaks do occur, the impact on a facility can be profoundly damaging. When a cat adopted from a shelter develops FIP, it causes an emotionally and financially traumatic experience for the adopter, which can damage the reputation for the shelter. Ultimately, these cases can result in a lower adoption and higher euthanasia rates for the facility. Educating adopters about FCoV and FIP and the unfortunate consequences of infection in a multicat facility, prior to adopting a cat, is crucial in maintaining a good relationship with the public. Information regarding signs and symptoms is helpful in making a quicker diagnosis for the patient/client when such unfortunate scenarios arise.[79,81,82]

SUMMARY

An interdisciplinary approach is needed to better understand the relationship of FCoV and FIP. The epizoology and diagnostics assist in providing the stated management protocols aimed to decrease the risks of cats in shelters for developing FIP. Although FIP has been undeniably linked to FCoV infection, the mechanisms that permit the rather benign FECV to evolve into the FIPV are still unknown. As FIP is intimately connected to the immune responses of affected animals, the details of this interaction and the pathogenesis of FIPV will be valuable in designing therapeutic and prophy-lactic prevention, as will our understanding of prophylactic immunization. Currently, the best weapon for diminishing the occurrences of FIP in multicat environments is to use appropriate biosecurity protocols. Unfortunately, the highly infectious nature of the FECV and our lack of understanding of its evolution to FIPV causing either the dry or wet form of FIP make elimination of risk virtually impossible.

ACKNOWLEDGMENTS

The authors thank Drs Elizabeth Boynton and Linda Kidd for their review of this manuscript, Dr Christine Tindal Green for the description of the eye figures, and John Greenwood for his assistance.

REFERENCES

1. Rohrbach BW, Legendre AM, Baldwin CA, et al. Epidemiology of feline infectious peritonitis among cats examined at veterinary medical teaching hospitals. J Am Vet Med Assoc 2001;218(7):1111–5.

2. Cave TA, Thompson H, Reid SW, et al. Kitten mortality in the United Kingdom: a retrospective analysis of 274 histopathological examinations (1986 to 2000). Vet Rec 2002;151(17):497–501.

3. Decaro N, Buonavoglia C. An update on canine coronaviruses: viral evolution and pathobiology. Vet Microbiol 2008;132(3-4):221–34.

4. Garwes DJ. Transmissible gastroenteritis. Vet Rec 1988;122(19):462–3.

5. Perlman S, Dandekar AA. Immunopathogenesis of coronavirus infections: implications for SARS. Nat Rev Immunol 2005;5(12):917–27.

6. Sharpee RL, Mebus CA, Bass EP. Characterization of a calf diarrheal coronavirus. Am J Vet Res 1976;37(9):1031–41.

7. Ward JM. Morphogenesis of a virus in cats with experimental feline infectious peritonitis. Virology 1970;41(1):191–4.

8. Pedersen NC, Boyle JF, Floyd K. Infection studies in kittens, using feline infectious peritonitis virus propagated in cell culture. Am J Vet Res 1981;42(3):363–7.

9. Collisson EW, Pei J, Dzielawa J, et al. Cytotoxic T lymphocytes are critical in the control of infectious bronchitis virus in poultry. Dev Comp Immunol 2000;24(2-3): 187–200.

10. Masters PS. The molecular biology of coronaviruses. Adv Virus Res 2006;66:193–292.

11. Anderson LJ, Tong S. Update on SARS research and other possibly zoonotic coronaviruses. Int J Antimicrob Agents 2010;36 Suppl 1:S21–5.

12. Gorbalenya AE, Snijder EJ, Spaan WJ. Severe acute respiratory syndrome coronavirus phylogeny: toward consensus. J Virol 2004;78(15):7863–6.

13. Lai MMC, Perlman S, Anderson LJ. Coronaviridae. In: Knipe DM, Howley PM, editors. Fields virology, vol 1. Philadelphia: Lippincott William & Wilkins; 2007. p. 1305–35.

14. Pedersen NC, Ward J, Mengeling WL. Antigenic relationship of the feline infections peritonitis virus to coronaviruses of other species. Arch Virol 1978;58(1):45–53.

15. Wise AG, Kiupel M, Maes RK. Molecular characterization of a novel coronavirus associated with epizootic catarrhal enteritis (ECE) in ferrets. Virology 2006;349(1):164–74.

16. Gonzalez JM, Gomez-Puertas P, Cavanagh D, et al. A comparative sequence analysis to revise the current taxonomy of the family Coronaviridae. Arch Virol 2003;148(11):2207–35.

17. Gorbalenya AE, Enjuanes L, Ziebuhr J, et al. Nidovirales: evolving the largest RNA virus genome. Virus Res 2006;117(1):17–37.

18. Jacobs L, de Groot R, van der Zeijst BA, et al. The nucleotide sequence of the peplomer gene of porcine transmissible gastroenteritis virus (TGEV): comparison with the sequence of the peplomer protein of feline infectious peritonitis virus (FIPV). Virus Res 1987;8(4):363–71.

19. Herrewegh AA, Smeenk I, Horzinek MC, et al. Feline coronavirus type II strains 79-1683 and 79-1146 originate from a double recombination between feline coronavirus type I and canine coronavirus. J Virol 1998;72(5):4508–14.

20. Hohdatsu T, Nakamura M, Ishizuka Y, et al. A study on the mechanism of antibody-dependent enhancement of feline infectious peritonitis virus infection in feline macrophages by monoclonal antibodies. Arch Virol 1991;120(3-4):207–17.

21. Hohdatsu T, Okada S, Ishizuka Y, et al. The prevalence of types I and II feline coronavirus infections in cats. J Vet Med Sci 1992;54(3):557–62.

22. Pedersen NC, Evermann JF, McKeirnan AJ, et al. Pathogenicity studies of feline coronavirus isolates 79-1146 and 79-1683. Am J Vet Res 1984;45(12):2580–5.

23. Shiba N, Maeda K, Kato H, et al. Differentiation of feline coronavirus type I and II infections by virus neutralization test. Vet Microbiol 2007;124(3-4):348–52.

24. Rottier PJ. The molecular dynamics of feline coronaviruses. Vet Microbiol 1999;69(1-2):117-25.
25. Horsburgh BC, Brierley I, Brown TD. Analysis of a 9.6 kb sequence from the 3' end of canine coronavirus genomic RNA. J Gen Virol 1992;73(Pt 11):2849-62.
26. Motokawa K, Hohdatsu T, Hashimoto H, et al. Comparison of the amino acid sequence and phylogenetic analysis of the peplomer, integral membrane and nucleocapsid proteins of feline, canine and porcine coronaviruses. Microbiol Immunol 1996;40(6):425-33.
27. Wesley RD. The S gene of canine coronavirus, strain UCD-1, is more closely related to the S gene of transmissible gastroenteritis virus than to that of feline infectious peritonitis virus. Virus Res 1999;61(2):145-52.
28. Wang L, Junker D, Collisson EW. Evidence of natural recombination within the S1 gene of infectious bronchitis virus. Virology 1993;192(2):710-6.
29. Wang L, Junker D, Hock L, et al. Evolutionary implications of genetic variations in the S1 gene of infectious bronchitis virus. Virus Res 1994;34(3):327-38.
30. Wang L, Xu Y, Collisson EW. Experimental confirmation of recombination upstream of the S1 hypervariable region of infectious bronchitis virus. Virus Res 1997;49(2):139-45.
31. Zhang XW, Yap YL, Danchin A. Testing the hypothesis of a recombinant origin of the SARS-associated coronavirus. Arch Virol 2005;150(1):1-20.
32. De Groot RJ, Andeweg AC, Horzinek MC, et al. Sequence analysis of the 3'-end of the feline coronavirus FIPV 79-1146 genome: comparison with the genome of porcine coronavirus TGEV reveals large insertions. Virology 1988;167(2):370-6.
33. Banner LR, Lai MM. Random nature of coronavirus RNA recombination in the absence of selection pressure. Virology 1991;185(1):441-5.
34. Benetka V, Kubber-Heiss A, Kolodziejek J, et al. Prevalence of feline coronavirus types I and II in cats with histopathologically verified feline infectious peritonitis. Vet Microbiol 2004;99(1):31-42.
35. Duarte A, Veiga I, Tavares L. Genetic diversity and phylogenetic analysis of Feline Coronavirus sequences from Portugal. Vet Microbiol 2009;138(1-2):163-8.
36. Kummrow M, Meli ML, Haessig M, et al. Feline coronavirus serotypes 1 and 2: seroprevalence and association with disease in Switzerland. Clin Diagn Lab Immunol 2005;12(10):1209-15.
37. Pedersen NC, Allen CE, Lyons LA. Pathogenesis of feline enteric coronavirus infection. J Feline Med Surg 2008;10(6):529-41.
38. Pedersen NC, Black JW, Boyle JF, et al. Pathogenic differences between various feline coronavirus isolates. Adv Exp Med Biol 1984;173:365-80.
39. Tusell SM, Schittone SA, Holmes KV. Mutational analysis of aminopeptidase N, a receptor for several group 1 coronaviruses, identifies key determinants of viral host range. J Virol 2007;81(3):1201-73.
40. Tresnan DB, Holmes KV. Feline aminopeptidase N is a receptor for all group I coronaviruses. Adv Exp Med Biol 1998;440:69-75.
41. Benbacer L, Kut E, Besnardeau L, et al. Interspecies aminopeptidase-N chimeras reveal species-specific receptor recognition by canine coronavirus, feline infectious peritonitis virus, and transmissible gastroenteritis virus. J Virol 1997;71(1):734-7.
42. Kolb AF, Hegyi A, Maile J, et al. Molecular analysis of the coronavirus-receptor function of aminopeptidase N. Adv Exp Med Biol 1998;440:61-7.
43. Pedersen NC. Virologic and immunologic aspects of feline infectious peritonitis virus infection. Adv Exp Med Biol 1987;218:529-50.

44. Chang HW, de Groot RJ, Egberink HF, et al. Feline infectious peritonitis: insights into feline coronavirus pathobiogenesis and epidemiology based on genetic analysis of the viral 3c gene. J Gen Virol 2010;91(Pt 2):415–20.

45. Poland AM, Vennema H, Foley JE, et al. Two related strains of feline infectious peritonitis virus isolated from immunocompromised cats infected with a feline enteric coronavirus. J Clin Microbiol 1996;34(12):3180–4.

46. Vennema H, Poland A, Foley J, et al. Feline infectious peritonitis viruses arise by mutation from endemic feline enteric coronaviruses. Virology 1998;243(1):150–7.

47. Pedersen NC, Floyd K. Experimental studies with three new strains of feline infectious peritonitis virus FIPV-UCD2, FIPV-UCD3, and FIPV-UCD4. Compendium Continuing Education Practicing Veterinarians 1985;7:1001–11.

48. Rottier PJ, Nakamura K, Schellen P, et al. Acquisition of macrophage tropism during the pathogenesis of feline infectious peritonitis is determined by mutations in the feline coronavirus spike protein. J Virol 2005;79(22):14122–30.

49. Tekes G, Hofmann-Lehmann R, Bank-Wolf B, et al. Chimeric feline coronaviruses that encode type II spike protein on type I genetic background display accelerated viral growth and altered receptor usage. J Virol 2010;84(3):1326–33.

50. Dye C, Helps CR, Siddell SG. Evaluation of real-time RT-PCR for the quantification of FCoV shedding in the faeces of domestic cats. J Feline Med Surg 2008;10(2):167–74.

51. Tekes G, Hofmann-Lehmann R, Stallkamp I, et al. Genome organization and reverse genetic analysis of a type I feline coronavirus. J Virol 2008;82(4):1851–9.

52. Brown MA, Troyer JL, Pecon-Slattery J, et al. Genetics and pathogenesis of feline infectious peritonitis virus. Emerg Infect Dis 2009;15(9):1445–52.

53. Herrewegh AAPM, Vennema H, Horzinek MC, et al. The molecular genetics of feline coronaviruses: comparative sequence analysis of the ORF7a/7b transcription unit of different biotypes. Virology 1995;212(2):622–31.

54. Vennema H, Heijnen L, Rottier PJ, et al. A novel glycoprotein of feline infectious peritonitis coronavirus contains a KDEL-like endoplasmic reticulum retention signal. J Virol 1992;66(8):4951–6.

55. Dye C, Siddell SG. Genomic RNA sequence of Feline coronavirus strain FIPV WSU-79/1146. J Gen Virol 2005;86(Pt 8):2249–53.

56. Kennedy M, Boedeker N, Gibbs P, et al. Deletions in the 7a ORF of feline coronavirus associated with an epidemic of feline infectious peritonitis. Vet Microbiol 2001;81(3): 227–34.

57. Kennedy MA, Moore E, Wilkes RP, et al. Analysis of genetic mutations in the 7a7b open reading frame of coronavirus of cheetahs (Acinonyx jubatus). Am J Vet Res 2006;67(4):627–32.

58. Lin CN, Su BL, Huang HP, et al. Field strain feline coronaviruses with small deletions in ORF7b associated with both enteric infection and feline infectious peritonitis. J Feline Med Surg 2009;11(6):413–9.

59. Pedersen NC. A review of feline infectious peritonitis virus infection: 1963–2008. J Feline Med Surg 2009;11(4):225–58.

60. Pedersen NC. Serologic studies of naturally occurring feline infectious peritonitis. Am J Vet Res 1976;37(12):1449–53.

61. Cave TA, Golder MC, Simpson J, et al. Risk factors for feline coronavirus seropositivity in cats relinquished to a UK rescue charity. J Feline Med Surg 2004;6(2):53–8.

62. Addie DD, Dennis JM, Toth S, et al. Long-term impact on a closed household of pet cats of natural infection with feline coronavirus, feline leukaemia virus and feline immunodeficiency virus. Vet Rec 2000;146(15):419–24.

63. Pedersen NC, Sato R, Foley JE, et al. Common virus infections in cats, before and after being placed in shelters, with emphasis on feline enteric coronavirus. J Feline Med Surg 2004;6(2):83–8.

64. Luria BJ, Levy JK, Lappin MR, et al. Prevalence of infectious diseases in feral cats in Northern Florida. J Feline Med Surg 2004;6(5):287–96.

65. Addie DD, Toth S, Murray GD, et al. Risk of feline infectious peritonitis in cats naturally infected with feline coronavirus. Am J Vet Res 1995;56(4):429–34.

66. Foley JE, Poland A, Carlson J, et al. Risk factors for feline infectious peritonitis among cats in multiple-cat environments with endemic feline enteric coronavirus. J Am Vet Med Assoc 1997;210(9):1313–8.

67. Addie DD, Jarrett O. A study of naturally occurring feline coronavirus infections in kittens. Vet Rec 1992;130(7):133–7.

68. Herrewegh AA, Mahler M, Hedrich HJ, et al. Persistence and evolution of feline coronavirus in a closed cat-breeding colony. Virology 1997;234(2):349–63.

69. Spain CV, Scarlett JM, Houpt KA. Long-term risks and benefits of early-age gonadectomy in cats. J Am Vet Med Assoc 2004;224(3):372–9.

70. Hickman MA, Morris JG, Rogers QR. Elimination of feline coronavirus infection from a large experimental specific pathogen-free cat breeding colony by serologic testing and isolation. Feline practice 1995;23(3):96–102.

71. Pesteanu-Somogyi LD, Radzai C, Pressler BM. Prevalence of feline infectious peritonitis in specific cat breeds. J Feline Med Surg 2006;8(1):1–5.

72. Tsai HY, Chueh LL, Lin CN, et al. Clinicopathological findings and disease staging of feline infectious peritonitis: 51 cases from 2003 to 2009 in Taiwan. J Feline Med Surg 2011;13(2):74–80.

73. Norris JM, Bosward KL, White JD, et al. Clinicopathological findings associated with feline infectious peritonitis in Sydney, Australia: 42 cases (1990–2002). Aust Vet J 2005;83(11):666–73.

74. Bell ET, Malik R, Norris JM. The relationship between the feline coronavirus antibody titre and the age, breed, gender and health status of Australian cats. Aust Vet J 2006;84(1-2):2–7.

75. Foley JE, Pedersen NC. The inheritance of susceptibility to feline infectious peritonitis in purebreed catteries. Vet Pract 1996;24(1):14–22.

76. Hardy WD Jr. Immunopathology induced by the feline leukemia virus. Springer Semin Immunopathol 1982;5(1):75–106.

77. Cotter SM, Hardy WD Jr, Essex M. Association of feline leukemia virus with lymphosarcoma and other disorders in the cat. J Am Vet Med Assoc 1975;166(5): 449–54.

78. Addie D, Belak S, Boucraut-Baralon C, et al. Feline infectious peritonitis. ABCD guidelines on prevention and management. J Feline Med Surg 2009;11(7):594–604.

79. Hurley KF. Feline Infectious Peritonitis/Feline Enteric Coronavirus (FIP/FECV). 2011. Available at: http://www.sheltermedicine.com/shelter-health-portal/information-sheets/feline-infectious-peritonitisfeline-enteric-coronavirus-fip. Accessed May 8, 2001.

80. Potkay S, Bacher JD, Pitts TW. Feline infectious peritonitis in a closed breeding colony. Lab Anim Sci 1974;24(2):279–89.

81. Mullin CH. Feline Infectious Peritonitis. Infectious disease management in animal shelters 2009(20):319–30.

82. Hartmann K. Feline infectious peritonitis. Vet Clin North Am Small Anim Pract 2005;35(1):39–79, vi.

83. Kipar A, May H, Menger S, et al. Morphologic features and development of granulomatous vasculitis in feline infectious peritonitis. Vet Pathol 2005;42(3):321–30.

84. Andrew SE. Feline infectious peritonitis. Vet Clin North Am Small Anim Pract 2000;30(5):987–000.

85. Hagan WA, Bruner DW, Timoney JF. Hagan and Bruner's microbiology and infectious diseases of domestic animals. Ithaca (NY): Comstock Publishing Assoc; 1992.

86. Jacobse-Geels HE, Daha MR, Horzinek MC. Antibody, immune complexes, and complement activity fluctuations in kittens with experimentally induced feline infectious peritonitis. Am J Vet Res 1982;43(4):666–70.

87. Petersen NC, Boyle JF. Immunologic phenomena in the effusive form of feline infectious peritonitis. Am J Vet Res 1980;41(6):868–76.

88. Paltrinieri S, Cammarata Parodi M, Cammarata G, et al. Type IV hypersensitivity in the pathogenesis of FIPV-induced lesions. Zentralbl Veterinarmed B 1998;45(3): 151–9.

89. Wills-Karp M. Immunological mechanisms of allergic diseases. In: Paul WE, editor. Fundamental immunology. 6th edition. Philadelphia: Lippincott Williams & Wilkins; 2008. p. 1375–425.

90. Benacerraf B, Levine BB. Immunological specificity of delayed and immediate hypersensitivity reactions. J Exp Med 1962;115:1023–36.

91. Takano T, Ohyama T, Kokumoto A, et al. Vascular endothelial growth factor (VEGF), produced by feline infectious peritonitis (FIP) virus-infected monocytes and macrophages, induces vascular permeability and effusion in cats with FIP. Virus Res 2011;158(1-2):161–8.

92. Pedersen NC, Allen CE, Lyons LA. Pathogenesis of feline enteric coronavirus infection. J Feline Med Surg 2008;10(6):529–41.

93. Addie DD, Jarrett O. Use of a reverse-transcriptase polymerase chain reaction for monitoring the shedding of feline coronavirus by healthy cats. Vet Rec 2001;148(21): 649–53.

94. Addie DD, Paltrinieri S, Pedersen NC. Recommendations from workshops of the second international feline coronavirus/feline infectious peritonitis symposium. J Feline Med Surg 2004;6(2):125–30.

95. Harpold LM, Legendre AM, Kennedy MA, et al. Fecal shedding of feline coronavirus in adult cats and kittens in an Abyssinian cattery. J Am Vet Med Assoc 1999;215(7): 948–51.

96. Addie DD, Schaap IA, Nicolson L, et al. Persistence and transmission of natural type I feline coronavirus infection. J Gen Virol 2003;84(Pt 10):2735–44.

97. Kipar A, Meli ML, Baptiste KE, et al. Sites of feline coronavirus persistence in healthy cats. J Gen Virol 2010;91(Pt 7):1698–707.

98. Addie DD, Jarrett O. Feline coronavirus antibodies in cats. Vet Rec 1992;131(9): 202–3.

99. Gonon V, Duquesne V, Klonjkowski B, et al. Clearance of infection in cats naturally infected with feline coronaviruses is associated with an anti-S glycoprotein antibody response. J Gen Virol 1999;80(Pt 9):2315–7.

100. de Groot-Mijnes JD, van Dun JM, van der Most RG, et al. Natural history of a recurrent feline coronavirus infection and the role of cellular immunity in survival and disease. J Virol 2005;79(2):1036–44.

101. Hohdatsu T, Yamada H, Ishizuka Y, et al. Enhancement and neutralization of feline infectious peritonitis virus infection in feline macrophages by neutralizing monoclonal antibodies recognizing different epitopes. Microbiol Immunol 1993;37(6):499–504.

102. Dewerchin HL, Cornelissen E, Nauwynck HJ. Replication of feline coronaviruses in peripheral blood monocytes. Arch Virol 2005;150(12):2483–500.

103. Samuel CE. Antiviral actions of interferons. Clin Microbiol Rev 2001;14(4):778–809.

104. Kawai T, Akira S. Innate immune recognition of viral infection. Nat Immunol 2006; 7(2):131–7.
105. Pichlmair A, Reis e Sousa C. Innate recognition of viruses. Immunity 2007;27(3): 370–83.
106. Spiegel M, Pichlmair A, Martinez-Sobrido L, et al. Inhibition of Beta interferon induction by severe acute respiratory syndrome coronavirus suggests a two-step model for activation of interferon regulatory factor 3. J Virol 2005;79(4):2079–86.
107. Versteeg GA, Bredenbeek PJ, van den Worm SH, et al. Group 2 coronaviruses prevent immediate early interferon induction by protection of viral RNA from host cell recognition. Virology 2007;361(1):18–26.
108. Kiss I, Poland AM, Pedersen NC. Disease outcome and cytokine responses in cats immunized with an avirulent feline infectious peritonitis virus (FIPV)-UCD1 and challenge-exposed with virulent FIPV-UCD8. J Feline Med Surg 2004;6(2):89–97.
109. Takano T, Hohdatsu T, Hashida Y, et al. A "possible" involvement of TNF-alpha in apoptosis induction in peripheral blood lymphocytes of cats with feline infectious peritonitis. Vet Microbiol 2007;119(2-4):121–31.
110. Weiss RC, Scott FW. Antibody-mediated enhancement of disease in feline infectious peritonitis: comparisons with dengue hemorrhagic fever. Comp Immunol Microbiol Infect Dis 1981;4(2):175–89.
111. Olsen CW, Corapi WV, Ngichabe CK, et al. Monoclonal antibodies to the spike protein of feline infectious peritonitis virus mediate antibody-dependent enhancement of infection of feline macrophages. J Virol 1992;66(2):956–65.
112. Takano T, Azuma N, Hashida Y, et al. B-cell activation in cats with feline infectious peritonitis (FIP) by FIP-virus-induced B-cell differentiation/survival factors. Arch Virol 2009;154(1):27–35.
113. Huisman W, Martina BE, Rimmelzwaan GF, et al. Vaccine-induced enhancement of viral infections. Vaccine 2009;27(4):505–12.
114. Seo SH, Wang L, Smith R, et al. The carboxyl-terminal 120-residue polypeptide of infectious bronchitis virus nucleocapsid induces cytotoxic T lymphocytes and protects chickens from acute infection. J Virol 1997;71(10):7889–94.
115. Seo SH, Collisson EW. Specific cytotoxic T lymphocytes are involved in in vivo clearance of infectious bronchitis virus. J Virol 1997;71(7):5173–7.
116. Pedersen NC, Theilen G, Keane MA, et al. Studies of naturally transmitted feline leukemia virus infection. Am J Vet Res 1977;38(10):1523–31.
117. Cotter SM, Gilmore CE, Rollins C. Multiple cases of feline leukemia and feline infectious peritonitis in a household. J Am Vet Med Assoc 1973;162(12):1054–8.
118. Haagmans BL, Egberink HF, Horzinek MC. Apoptosis and T-cell depletion during feline infectious peritonitis. J Virol 1996;70(12):8977–83.
119. Kipar A, Kohler K, Leukert W, et al. A comparison of lymphatic tissues from cats with spontaneous feline infectious peritonitis (FIP), cats with FIP virus infection but no FIP, and cats with no infection. J Comp Pathol 2001;125(2-3):182–91.
120. Munder M, Mallo M, Eichmann K, et al. Murine macrophages secrete interferon gamma upon combined stimulation with interleukin (IL)-12 and IL-18: A novel pathway of autocrine macrophage activation. J Exp Med 1998;187(12):2103–8.
121. Frucht DM, Fukao T, Bogdan C, et al. IFN-gamma production by antigen-presenting cells: mechanisms emerge. Trends Immunol 2001;22(10):556–60.
122. Gessani S, Belardelli F. IFN-gamma expression in macrophages and its possible biological significance. Cytokine Growth Factor Rev 1998;9(2):117–23.
123. Sen E, Chattopadhyay S, Bandopadhyay S, et al. Macrophage heterogeneity, antigen presentation, and membrane fluidity: implications in visceral Leishmaniasis. Scand J Immunol 2001;53(2):111–20.

124. Salazar-Mather TP, Hamilton TA, Biron CA. A chemokine-to-cytokine-to-chemokine cascade critical in antiviral defense. J Clin Invest 2000;105(7):985–93.

125. Pien GC, Satoskar AR, Takeda K, et al. Cutting edge: selective IL-18 requirements for induction of compartmental IFN-gamma responses during viral infection. J Immunol 2000;165(9):4787–91.

126. Krukowski K, Eddy J, Kosik KL, et al. Glucocorticoid dysregulation of natural killer cell function through epigenetic modification. Brain Behav Immun 2011; 25(2):239–49.

127. Giordano A, Paltrinieri S. Interferon-gamma in the serum and effusions of cats with feline coronavirus infection. Vet J 2009;180(3):396–8.

128. Takano T, Hohdatsu T, Toda A, et al. TNF-alpha, produced by feline infectious peritonitis virus (FIPV)-infected macrophages, upregulates expression of type II FIPV receptor feline aminopeptidase N in feline macrophages. Virology 2007; 364(1):64–72.

129. Han S, Choi H, Ko MG, et al. Peripheral T cells become sensitive to glucocorticoid- and stress-induced apoptosis in transgenic mice overexpressing SRG3. J Immunol 2001;167(2):805–10.

130. Dhabhar FS. Enhancing versus suppressive effects of stress on immune function: implications for immunoprotection and immunopathology. Neuroimmunomodulation 2009;16(5):300–17.

131. Addie DD. Feline coronavirus infection. In: Greene CE, editor. Infectious diseases of the dog and cat, vol 3rd. St. Louis: Saunders Elsevier; 2006. p. 88–102.

132. Doherty MJ. Ocular manifestations of feline infectious peritonitis. J Am Vet Med Assoc 1971;159(4):417–24.

133. Boettcher IC, Steinberg T, Matiasek K, et al. Use of anti-coronavirus antibody testing of cerebrospinal fluid for diagnosis of feline infectious peritonitis involving the central nervous system in cats. J Am Vet Med Assoc 2007;230(2):199–205.

134. Marioni-Henry K, Vite CH, Newton AL, et al. Prevalence of diseases of the spinal cord of cats. J Vet Intern Med 2004;18(6):851–8.

135. Timmann D, Cizinauskas S, Tomek A, et al. Retrospective analysis of seizures associated with feline infectious peritonitis in cats. J Feline Med Surg 2008;10(1): 9–15.

136. Foley JE, Lapointe JM, Koblik P, et al. Diagnostic features of clinical neurologic feline infectious peritonitis. J Vet Intern Med 1998;12(6):415–23.

137. Diaz JV, Poma R. Diagnosis and clinical signs of feline infectious peritonitis in the central nervous system. Can Vet J 2009;50(10):1091–3.

138. Sparkes AH, Gruffydd-Jones T, Harbour DA. Feline infectious peritonitis: a review of clinico-pathological changes in 65 cases, and critical assessment of their diagnostic value. Vet Rec 1991;129:209–12.

139. Sparkes AH, Gruffydd-Jones TJ, Harbour DA. An appraisal of the value of laboratory tests in the diagnosis of feline infectious peritonitis. J Am Anim Hosp Assoc 1994;30:345–50.

140. Norsworthy GD. Feline infectious peritonitis. In: Norsworthy GD, Crystal MA, Grace SF, et al, editors. The feline patient, vol 3rd. Iowa: Wiley-Blackwell Publishing; 2006. p. 97–8.

141. Goodson T, Randell S, Moore L. Feline infectious peritonitis. Compend Contin Educ Vet 2009;31(10):E1–9.

142. Paltrinieri S, Parodi MC, Cammarata G. In vivo diagnosis of feline infectious peritonitis by comparison of protein content, cytology, and direct immunofluorescence test on peritoneal and pleural effusions. J Vet Diagn Invest 1999;11(4):358–61.

143. Hartmann K, Binder C, Hirschberger J, et al. Comparison of different tests to diagnose feline infectious peritonitis. J Vet Intern Med 2003;17(6):781–90.

144. Giori L, Giordano A, Giudice C, et al. Performances of different diagnostic tests for feline infectious peritonitis in challenging clinical cases. J Small Anim Pract 2011; 52(3):152–7.

145. Paltrinieri S, Giordano A, Tranquillo V, et al. Critical assessment of the diagnostic value of feline alpha1-acid glycoprotein for feline infectious peritonitis using the likelihood ratios approach. J Vet Diagn Invest 2007;19(3):266–72.

146. Shelly SM, Scarlett-Kranz J, Blue JT. Protein electrophoresis on effusions from cats as a diagnostic test for feline infectious peritonitis. Journal of the American Animal Hospital Association 1988;24:495–500.

147. Addie DD. The Rivalta Test in diagnosis of effusive Feline Infectious Peritonitis (FIP). [Online video]. 2010. Available at: http://www.youtube.com/user/DrDianeD Addie#p/u/4/XmOk2veunqA. Accessed May 12th, 2011.

148. Pedersen N. The history and interpretation of feline coronavirus serology. Feline Practice 1995;23:46–51.

149. Richards JR. Problems in the interpretation of feline coronavirus serology (specificity vs. sensitivity of test procedures). Feline Practice 1995;23:52–5.

150. Soma T, Ishii H. Detection of feline coronavirus antibody, feline immunodeficiency virus antibody, and feline leukemia virus antigen in ascites from cats with effusive feline infectious peritonitis. J Vet Med Sci 2004;66(1):89–90.

151. Kennedy MA, Brenneman K, Millsaps RK, et al. Correlation of genomic detection of feline coronavirus with various diagnostic assays for feline infectious peritonitis. J Vet Diagn Invest 1998;10(1):93–7.

152. Lappin MR, Turnwald GH. Microbiology and infectious diseases. In: Willard MD, Tvedten H, editors. Small animal clinical diagnosis by laboratory methods. 4th edition. St. Louis: Elsevier; 2004. p. 350–1.

153. Vennema H, Rossen JW, Wesseling J, et al. Genomic organization and expression of the 3' end of the canine and feline enteric coronaviruses. Virology 1992;191(1): 134–40.

154. Kennedy MA, Abd-Eldaim M, Zika SE, et al. Evaluation of antibodies against feline coronavirus 7b protein for diagnosis of feline infectious peritonitis in cats. Am J Vet Res 2008;69(9):1179–82.

155. Pratelli A. Comparison of serologic techniques for the detection of antibodies against feline coronaviruses. J Vet Diagn Invest 2008;20(1):45–50.

156. Barlough JE, Jacobson RH, Sorresso GP, et al. Coronavirus antibody detection in cats by computer-assisted kinetics-based enzyme-linked immunosorbent assay (KELA): field studies. Cornell Vet 1986;76(3):227–35.

157. Shiba N, Maeda K, Kato H, et al. Differentiation of feline coronavirus type I and II infections by virus neutralization test. Vet Microbiol 2007;124(3-4):348–52.

158. Addie D. Feline Coronavirus (Feline Infectious Peritonitis) Antibody tests. 2009. Available at: http://www.dr-addie.com/FCoVantibody.htm. Accessed 4/26/2011, 2011

159. Peterson ME, Kintzer PP, Hurvitz AI. Methimazole treatment of 262 cats with hyperthyroidism. J Vet Intern Med 1988;2(3):150–7.

160. Breitschwerdt EB, Abrams-Ogg AC, Lappin MR, et al. Molecular evidence supporting Ehrlichia canis-like infection in cats. J Vet Intern Med 2002;16(6):642–9.

161. Gunn-Moore DA, Gruffydd-Jones TJ, Harbour DA. Detection of feline coronaviruses by culture and reverse transcriptase-polymerase chain reaction of blood samples from healthy cats and cats with clinical feline infectious peritonitis. Vet Microbiol 1998;62(3):193–205.

162. Gamble DA, Lobbiani A, Gramegna M, et al. Development of a nested PCR assay for detection of feline infectious peritonitis virus in clinical specimens. J Clin Microbiol 1997;35(3):673–5.

163. Herrewegh AA, de Groot RJ, Cepica A, et al. Detection of feline coronavirus RNA in feces, tissues, and body fluids of naturally infected cats by reverse transcriptase PCR. J Clin Microbiol 1995;33(3):684–9.

164. Takano T, Tomiyama Y, Katoh Y, et al. Mutation of neutralizing/antibody-dependent enhancing epitope on spike protein and 7b gene of feline infectious peritonitis virus: influences of viral replication in monocytes/macrophages and virulence in cats. Virus Res 2011;156(1-2):72–80.

165. Pedersen N, Liu H, Dodd K, et al. Significance of Coronavirus Mutants in Feces and Diseased Tissues of Cats Suffering from Feline Infectious Peritonitis. Viruses 2009; 1(2):166–84.

166. Li X, Scott FW. Detection of feline coronaviruses in cell cultures and in fresh and fixed feline tissues using polymerase chain reaction. Vet Microbiol 1994;42(1):65–77.

167. Simons FA, Vennema H, Rofina JE, et al. A mRNA PCR for the diagnosis of feline infectious peritonitis. J Virol Methods 2005;124(1-2):111–6.

168. Can-Sahna K, Soydal Ataseven V, Pinar D, et al. The detection of feline coronaviruses in blood samples from cats by mRNA RT-PCR. J Feline Med Surg 2007;9(5): 369–72.

169. Sharif S, Arshad SS, Hair-Bejo M, et al. Evaluation of Feline Coronavirus Viraemia in Clinically Healthy and Ill Cats with Feline Infectious Peritonitis. Journal of Animal and Veterinary Advances 2011;10(1):18–22.

170. Simons FA, Vennema H, Rofina JE, et al. A mRNA PCR for the diagnosis of feline infectious peritonitis. J Virol Methods 2005;124(1-2):111–6.

171. Foley JE, Leutenegger C. A review of coronavirus infection in the central nervous system of cats and mice. J Vet Intern Med 2001;15(5):438–44.

172. Cannon MJ, Silkstone MA, Kipar AM. Cutaneous lesions associated with coronavirus-induced vasculitis in a cat with feline infectious peritonitis and concurrent feline immunodeficiency virus infection. J Feline Med Surg 2005;7(4):233–6.

173. Declercq J, De Bosschere H, Schwarzkopf I, et al. Papular cutaneous lesions in a cat associated with feline infectious peritonitis. Vet Dermatol 2008;19(5):255–8.

174. Ritz S, Egberink H, Hartmann K. Effect of feline interferon-omega on the survival time and quality of life of cats with feline infectious peritonitis. J Vet Intern Med 2007;21(6): 1193–7.

175. Ishida T, Shibanai A, Tanaka S, et al. Use of recombinant feline interferon and glucocorticoid in the treatment of feline infectious peritonitis. J Feline Med Surg 2004;6(2):107–9.

176. Hartmann K. Feline infectious peritonitis and feline coronavirus infection. In: Ettinger SJ, Feldman EC, editors. Textbook of veterinary internal medicine: diseases of the dog and the cat. vol 1. St. Louis: Saunders Elsevier; 2010. p. 940–5.

177. Legendre AM, Bartges JW. Effect of Polyprenyl Immunostimulant on the survival times of three cats with the dry form of feline infectious peritonitis. J Feline Med Surg 2009;11(8):624–6.

178. Hoskins J, Taylor H, Lomax T. Independent evaluation of a modified live feline infectious peritonitis virus vaccine under experimental conditions (Louisiana experience). Feline Practice 1995;23(3):72–3.

179. McArdle F, Bennett M, Gaskell RM, et al. Independent evaluation of a modified live FIPV vaccine under experimental conditions (University of Liverpool experience). Feline Practice 1995;23(3):67–71.

180. Scott F, Corapi W, Olsen C. Independent evaluation of a modified live FIPV vaccine under experimental conditions (Cornell experience). Feline Practice 1995;23(3): 74–6.
181. Gerber J. Overview of the development of a modified live temperature-sensitive FIP virus vaccine. Feline Practice 1995;23(3):62–6.
182. Richards JR, Elston TH, Ford RB, et al. The 2006 American Association of Feline Practitioners Feline Vaccine Advisory Panel report. J Am Vet Med Assoc 2006; 229(9):1405–41.
183. Day MJ, Horzinek MC, Schultz RD. WSAVA guidelines for the vaccination of dogs and cats. J Small Anim Pract 2010;51(6):1–32.
184. Peterson CA, Dvorak G, Spickler AR. Maddie's infection control manual for animal shelters for veterinary personnel. 1st edition. Ames (IA): Iowa State University, Center for Food Security and Public Health; 2008.
185. Bell ET, Toribio JA, White JD, et al. Seroprevalence study of feline coronavirus in owned and feral cats in Sydney, Australia. Aust Vet J 2006;84(3):74–81.
186. Holst BS, Englund L, Palacios S, et al. Prevalence of antibodies against feline coronavirus and Chlamydophila felis in Swedish cats. J Feline Med Surg 2006;8(3): 207–11.
187. Pratelli A, Yesilbag K, Siniscalchi M, et al. Prevalence of feline coronavirus antibodies in cats in Bursa province, Turkey, by an enzyme-linked immunosorbent assay. J Feline Med Surg 2009;11(10):881–4.
188. Sparkes AH, Gruffydd-Jones TJ, Harbour DA. Feline coronavirus antibodies in UK cats. Vet Rec 1992;131(10):223–4.
189. Muirden A. Prevalence of feline leukaemia virus and antibodies to feline immunodeficiency virus and feline coronavirus in stray cats sent to an RSPCA hospital. Vet Rec 2002;150(20):621–5.
190. Sharif S, Arshad SS, Hair-Bejo M, et al. Prevalence of feline coronavirus in two cat populations in Malaysia. J Feline Med Surg 2009;11(12):1031–4.
191. Kiss I, Kecskemeti S, Tanyi J, et al. Prevalence and genetic pattern of feline coronaviruses in urban cat populations. Vet J 2000;159(1):64–70.
192. Duthie S, Eckersall PD, Addie DD, et al. Value of alpha 1-acid glycoprotein in the diagnosis of feline infectious peritonitis. Vet Rec 1997;141(12):299–03.
193. Hirschberger J, Hartmann K, Wilhelm N, et al. [Clinical symptoms and diagnosis of feline infectious peritonitis]. Tierarztl Prax 1995;23(1):92–9.

Canine Noroviruses

Vito Martella, DVM*, Pierfrancesco Pinto, DVM, Canio Buonavoglia, DVM

KEYWORDS
• Norovirus • Calicivirus • Dogs • Enteritis

Noroviruses (NoVs) were first identified in humans in 1972 on immune electron microscopy observation of the stools of volunteers infected with filtrates of faecal samples collected from a nonbacterial gastroenteritis outbreak occurred in 1968 in Norwalk, Ohio, USA.[1] Nonenveloped, small, rounded viruses (SRVs), 27 nm in size, were observed in the fecal filtrates and specific antibodies were detected in both experimentally and naturally infected individuals, suggesting that the particles were the etiologic agent of Norwalk gastroenteritis.

On genetic characterization, NoVs have been classified as a distinct genus of the Caliciviridae family.[2] NoVs have been now recognized as the major etiologic agent of nonbacterial acute gastroenteritis worldwide and they are estimated to cause more than 1 million hospitalizations and up to 200,000 deaths in children younger than 5 years on an annual basis.[3] NoVs have been also identified in cows, pigs, mice, and carnivores, and the role of some animal species as potential source of novel human NoVs via interspecies transmission and eventually recombination has been hypothesized.[4]

ETIOLOGY

Caliciviruses are nonenveloped SRVs with a single-stranded, positive-sense, polyadenylated RNA genome of 7 to 8.5 kb.[5] Based on their genetic relationships and genome organization, caliciviruses have been classified into 4 genera: namely *Vesivirus, Lagovirus, Sapovirus,* and *Norovirus.*[5] More recently, other caliciviruses have been discovered and proposed as members of distinct genera: Nebraska-like viruses[6] (*Nebovirus*) in cows, rhesus caliciviruses,[7] Saint Valienè–like viruses in swine,[8] and avian caliciviruses.[9] Caliciviruses have been associated to a variety of clinical signs, ranging from gastroenteric disease to exanthematic lesions, to severe systemic diseases and hemorrhagic forms, and they are recognized as important pathogens in both humans and animals.

Disclosure: This work was financed by the grants "Calicivirus nei carnivori e nell'uomo: caratterizzazione molecolare, epidemiologia, implicazioni zoonosiche"—PRIN 2008 (20084F4P7X); "Analisi di stipiti norovirus del cane"—Fondi Ateneo 2009; and "Caratterizzazione molecolare di stipiti norovirus identificati nei carnivori e messa a punto di sistemi diagnostici"—Prin-Cofin 2007.
Dipartimento di Sanità Pubblica e Zootecnia, Università degli Studi Aldo Moro di Bari, S.p. per Casamassima km 3, 70010 Valenzano, Bari, Italy
* Corresponding author.
E-mail address: v.martella@veterinaria.uniba.it

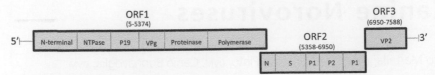

Fig. 1. Norovirus (strain Norwalk, accession M87661) genome organization. Proteolytic clivage map of the non-structural polyprotein encoded by ORF1. The NH2-terminal portion (N) of the highly conserved shell (S) domain and the protruding region (P) subdomains (P1 and P2) are also indicated.[15]

NoVs are important human enteric pathogens[3] and they have also been detected in the stools of livestock animals, although their role as pathogens in these animals remains controversial.[10,11] In mice, NoV is able to invade the central nervous system (CNS) in *STAT1*-deficient animals, causing fatal disease.[12] Mouse NoV has also been adapted to in vitro growth, thus providing an excellent model/surrogate for the study of human NoVs, which are noncultivatable.[13,14]

NoV genome is 7.5 to 7.7 kb in length and contains 3 distinct open reading frames (ORFs).[5] ORF1 encodes a large polyprotein that is post-translationally cleaved into 6 nonstructural proteins, including the RNA-dependent RNA polymerase (RdRp). ORF2 encodes the capsid protein VP1, while ORF3 encodes a small basic protein, VP2 **(Fig. 1)**.[5] The viral capsid contains 180 copies of VP1 protein and a few copies of VP2. The VP1 contains 2 main domains, S and P. The S (shell) domain is highly conserved and connected through the P1 subdomain to the highly variable P2 (protruding) subdomain.[15,16] The P2 region possesses several motifs that control binding to the host cell and virus antigenicity.[17,18]

NoVs are genetically and antigenically highly heterogeneous. Accumulation of punctate mutations and recombination drive their evolution, generating an impressive diversity. The highly conserved ORF1/ORF2 junction region is a preferential site for NoV recombination.[19] Recombination may create chimeric viruses with intermediate genetic features between the parental viruses, generating inconsistencies in the classification/nomenclature. A consistent and reliable classification of NoVs is based on the analysis of the complete capsid gene.[20] Strains within the same genotype (or cluster) share greater than 85% amino acid identity, while strains of different genotypes within the same genogroup share 55% to 85% amino acid identity.[20] Humans NoVs belong to genogroups (G) I, II, and IV.[4] In addition, NoVs classified as GII have been detected in pigs,[21,22] and GIII NoVs in large and small ruminants.[23,24] NoVs proposed as GV have been detected in mice.[12]

CALICIVIRUSES IN DOGS

Unlike calicivirus infections in cats,[25] canine caliciviruses are not regarded as important pathogens and they are not usually included in diagnostic algorithms for canine infectious diseases. Calicivirus-like particles have been occasionally identified by electron microscopy in specimens from dogs with fluid diarrhea and, in some instances, glossitis, balanitis, or vesicular vaginitis. Most isolates were feline caliciviruses (FCVs) and were likely acquired from cats.[26–30]

Thus far, there are only 2 documented reports on the identification of authentic canine caliciviruses in dogs. In 1985 a calicivirus was isolated from the feces of a 4-year-old dog with bloody diarrhea and central nervous system disturbance in Tennessee, USA. The virus was found to replicate in experimentally infected dogs and to elicit seroconversion, although disease was not reproduced. Also, the virus was antigenically unrelated to FCV and antibodies against the virus were identified in 76% of the canine sera collected.[31] However, it was not characterized molecularly and its taxonomic status remains uncertain. In 1990, another calicivirus was identified in Japan in a 2-month-old pup with intermittent watery diarrhea.[32] The virus, strain 48, was found to be antigenically and genetically unrelated to FCV and was tentatively proposed as a "true" canine calicivirus (CaCV) and included in the *Vesivirus* genus.[33,34] Antibodies to CaCV 48 have been detected in 57% of dogs in Japan[35] and in 36.5% of dogs in Korea.[36]

NOROVIRUSES IN DOGS

The first evidence of NoV in carnivores was documented in 2006 in a captive lion cub that died of severe hemorrhagic enteritis at 4 weeks of age in Pistoia, Italy.[37] The animal tested negative to all potential lion viral pathogens, and on bacteriologic investigations it was found to be infected by toxigenic *Clostridia*. Unexpectedly, NoV RNA was detected in the intestinal tract and, on genomic characterization, the virus was found to resemble human GIV NoVs (Alphatron-like), with 69.3% to 70.1% amino acid identity in the full-length capsid protein, and it was proposed as a distinct NoV genotype, GIV.2, while human Alphatron-like NoVs are GIV.1. Human GIV.1 NoVs are usually identified only sporadically in the human population, although they may be commonly detected in sewage samples from treatment plants,[38,39] indicating that there are open gaps in the understanding of their ecology and in the diagnosis.

As lions are susceptible to the majority of canine and feline pathogens, the detection of NoV in lions raised the question of whether domestic carnivores represented the source of infection for the captive lion cub. By expressing in baculovirus the capsid protein of the lion NoV, virus-like particles (VLPs) were produced and used to set up an ELISA, revealing specific antibodies in 16.1% of feline and 4.8% of canine sera.[40] Also, by screening a collection of stools from dogs with gastroenteritis in Italy in 2007, NoV was detected in 2.2% (4 of 183) of the pups.[41,42] The age of the pups ranged between 60 and 70 days and 3 of 4 pups were also co-infected by canine parvovirus. These direct and indirect pieces of evidence confirmed that domestic carnivores might harbor NoVs.

Shortly after the first identification, additional evidence about the circulation of NoVs in dogs has been documented. During an epidemiologic study in 2008 in Greece, a cluster of NoV infection was identified in a kennel in Thessaloniki in 6 pups, 2.5 to 3 months old, that were housed together,[43] suggesting the highly infectious nature of canine NoVs for young pups. All the NoV-infected animals were also co-infected by canine coronavirus.

In a 1-year survey in Portugal in 2008 of dogs from municipal shelters, veterinary clinics, and pet shops, NoV was detected in the stools of 25 of 63 (40%) of dogs with diarrhea and 4 (0%) of 42 asymptomatic animals. In most cases, the NoV-infected dogs displayed mixed infections by either canine parvovirus or coronavirus or both.[44]

Also, NoV RNA was detected in 3 of 106 stools collected from pups with parvovirus gastroenteritis in 2007 in the United Kingdom (Martella and colleagues, unpublished information, 2011). These findings indicate the canine NoVs circulate in several European countries.

GENETIC HETEROGENEITY IN CANINE NoVs

Thus far, 6 canine NoV strains have been analyzed molecularly. Sequence information has been gathered on the RdRp region, at the 3′ end of ORF1, the full-length capsid protein (ORF2), and the minor basic protein (ORF3). The prototype canine NoV strain, Bari/170/07/ITA,[41] resembles the virus lion NoV Pistoia/387/06/ITA, as the 2 viruses share 96.7% amino acid identity in the RdRp and 90.1% amino acid identity in the capsid protein. Likewise, the Greek strain Thessaloniki/30/2008/GRC resembles the canine virus Bari/170/07/ITA, both in the RdRp (100% amino acid identity) and the capsid gene (99.4% amino acid identity).[43]

A large insertion of 20 residues can be observed in the P2 hypervariable domain of GIV.2 animal NoVs with respect to GIV.1 human viruses. By homology modeling and 3-dimensional alignment, the P insertion appears to form a loop protruding from the compact barrel-like structure of the P2 subdomain and exposed on the outer surface of the capsid.

Interestingly, another canine NoV strain, Bari/91/07/ITA, although sharing the same pol (RdRp) type as strains Dog/Bari/170/07/ITA and Lion/Pistoia/387/06/ITA, possesses a novel ORF2 gene, with the highest identity (57.8% amino acid) to the unclassified human strain Chiba/040502/04/JAP. This canine virus is distantly related (36.0%–54.5% amino acid identity) to all other NoVs,[42] suggesting the existence in dogs of NoVs with a novel capsid genotype. The UK strain FD210/07/GBR resembles both in the RdRp (98.5% amino acid identity) and the capsid (95.0% amino acid identity) canine virus Bari/91/07/ITA.

The Portuguese NoV strain Viseu/C33/08/PRT and the UK strain FD53/07/GBR display a third capsid genotype. These viruses are related to each other (99.5% amino acid identity in the RdRp and 98.6% amino acid in the VP1), while they have only 63.1% to 63.9% amino acid identity in the full-length VP1 to the strain Bari/91/07/ITA and FD210/07/GBR (**Fig. 2**, **Table 1**).

PATHOGENIC POTENTIAL OF CANINE NoVs

The pathogenicity of canine NoVs in experimental infections in gnotobiotic or specific-pathogen-free (SPF) animals has not been assessed. Viral shedding could be monitored in a naturally infected pup with mixed infection by NoV and canine parvovirus type-2. The pup recovered from the disease 4 days after hospitalization but NoV was shed at detectable levels for 3 weeks.[41] Prolonged NoV shedding after infection/disease has been documented for weeks or even months in human patients.[45,46] Likewise, murine NoV shedding can last for several weeks in immune-competent mice,[12,47] and this has been interpreted as a mechanism of virus persistence in the host population.

In most cases, NoV-infected dogs were also co-infected by other pathogens. That mixed infections can elicit mechanisms of synergism, as observed between coronaviruses and parvoviruses,[48,49] cannot be ruled out. Interestingly, the frequency of detection of NoV has been found to differ significantly between symptomatic and asymptomatic dogs in a 1-year survey in Portugal.[44] Interpretation of these findings is not clear, as several factors can influence the course of NoV infection. As canine NoVs appear to display a number of capsid genotypes, there could be differences in the biological properties (eg, virulence, ability to bind to canine cellular receptors, and so on) among the various NoV strains. In addition, mechanisms of genetic resistance could alter the outcome of NoV infection in some canine breeds, thus confounding the picture. Experimental human infection studies with the prototype Norwalk virus (GI.1) showed that the study participants were repeatedly susceptible or resistant to symptomatic infection following repeated virus challenge.[50] Subsequent studies have revealed that human NoVs recognize histoblood group antigens (HBGAs) as receptors or co-receptors. HGBAs are complex carbohydrates present on the surface of red blood cells and mucosal epithelia, or free in biological fluids such as milk and

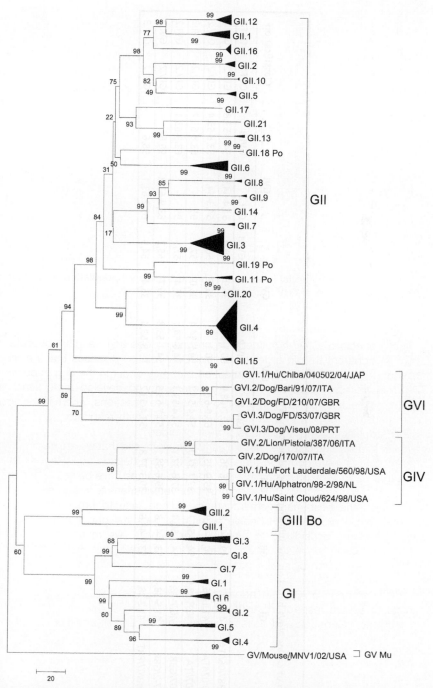

Fig. 2. Phylogenetic tree constructed on the full-length amino acid sequence of the capsid protein. The tree was constructed using a selection of NoV strains representative of the genogroups I to V. bo, bovine; po, porcine; mu, murine; hu, human.

Table 1
Classification of canine NoVs based on the full-length capsid protein VP1

| Genogroup | GI | GII | GIII | GIV | | GV | GVI | | | Classification | |
Genotype				GIV.1	GIV.2		GVI.1	GVI.2	GVI.3	ORF1	ORF2
Lion/Pistoia/387/06/ITA	41,6-37,8	49,7-45,8	36,6-36,5	69,2-68,9	90,1	36,9	50,0	54,4-54,5	54,1-53,8	GIV.2	GIV.2
Dog/Bari/170/07/ITA	41,1-36,9	50,2-45,9	35,9-35,1	68,0-67,7	90,1	36,6	50,0	54,3-54,0	53,8-53,4	GIV.2	GIV.2
Dog/Bari/91/07/ITA	40,8-38,0	54,4-50,2	37,7-37,0	54,4-54,2	54,5-54,4	36,0	57,8	95	63,8-63,2	GIV.2	GVI.2
Dog/FD/210/07/GBR	40,7-38,1	54,7-50,4	37,6-37,1	53,4-53,3	54,6-54,1	36,4	57,5	95	63,9-63,1	GIV.2	GVI.2
Dog/FD/53/07-2/GBR	41,5-38,4	53,4-48,8	39,6-38,1	53,7-53,5	54,1-53,8	36,7	55,2	63,9-63,8	98,6	GIV.2	GVI.3
Dog/C33-Viseu/07/PRT	41,2-38,1	53,9-48,6	39,3-37,8	53,4-53,2	53,8-53,4	36,4	54,9	63,2-63,1	98,6	GIV.2	GVI.3

saliva. HGBAs are synthesized under the control of highly polymorphic ABO, Lewis, and secretor gene families. Different NoV genotypes variously recognize these antigens, and the recognition patterns have been found to correlate with susceptibility to infection and illness.[51–54] The global spread and predominance of pandemic GII.4 NoV variants have been related to the broad range of recognized HBGA types.[51] Similar mechanisms appear to influence genetic resistance of pigs to NoV infection under experimental conditions.[55]

DIAGNOSIS

Several sets of primers have been designed for molecular diagnosis of human NoVs in different diagnostic regions (A–C) spanning the ORF1 and ORF2.[56] Diagnostic tools can be greatly affected by NoV genetic diversity.[57] In most cases, diagnosis of canine NoV was accomplished using broadly reactive primers sets targeting diagnostic region A within the RdRp, such as p289-p290 or JV12Y/YV13I.[58,59] However, it has been shown that designing more specific primers can allow increasing significantly the detection rates of canine NoVs (from 1.9% to 27.6%).[60]

Several unsuccessful attempts have been made to adapt to in vitro cultivation the prototype canine NoV strain Bari/170/07/ITA, using both canine and feline cell lines and primary cells. With the exception of murine NoVs,[13] NoVs appear to be noncultivatable in vitro.[14,61] Replication of human NoVs in vitro has been demonstrated in a 3-dimensional organoid model of human small intestinal epithelium, displaying a high level of cellular differentiation.[62] However, these results have not been reproduced in other laboratories.

An ELISA has been set up using the baculovirus-expressed capsid protein of the GIV.2 lion NoV.[40] This assay was successfully used to assess exposure of domestic carnivores to NoVs. However, considering the extent of the genetic heterogeneity of canine NoVs, generating synthetic antigens based on other capsid genotypes (GVI.2 and GVI.3) would be necessary to portray a more precise picture.

ZOONOTIC POTENTIAL OF CANINE NoVs

Dogs are regarded as vectors of viral, bacterial, or parasitic zoonosis,[63] but the risks linked to transmission of enteric viruses are almost ignored. However, several pieces of evidences indicate that enteric viruses may have a zoonotic potential: (1) infection of young children by rotavirus strains of canine and feline origin has been documented repeatedly[64]; (2) having dogs in or near a home has been recognized as a risk factor for acquisition of IgA antibodies specific for NoV in infants in a seroepidemiologic study conducted in rural Mexico[65]; and (3) a calicivirus gastroenteritis outbreak occurred in a nursing home in Exeter, UK, in 1983 and was found to be epidemiologically linked to the household dog. Acute gastroenteric disease in the dog occurred 24 hours before the human index case and antibodies specific for the human caliciviruses were identified in the dog, thus suggesting a possible association.[66] (4) Also, under experimental conditions, NoVs have been found to be able to cross the host species barriers. A GII.4 human NoV was able to infect and induce diarrhea in gnotobiotic piglets and calves,[11,10] thus indicating that heterologous infections can occur. (5) In addition, NoV strains genetically similar to the canine virus Bari/91/07/ITA (88.9% nucleotides and 98.9% amino acid identities in a short fragment spanning the 5′ end of ORF2) have been detected in oysters destined for raw consumption in Japan (strains Yamaguchi/C34/03/JAP, Yamaguchi/24B/02/JAP, and Yamaguchi/24C/02/JAP[67]). This could indicate that canine-like GVI NoVs are common in some geographic settings and that they can contaminate the coastal areas and accumulate at detectable levels in bivalve molluscs destined for raw consumption. Contamination of shellfish by animal (porcine and bovine) enteric caliciviruses, alone or in conjunction with human viruses, has been demonstrated in 22% of oysters in United States.[68] However, while the impact of sewage pollution on the water environment by livestock may be relevant, especially in the areas of high livestock production, it is difficult to explain the presence of canine-like NoVs in oysters. A possible explanation for this is that similar viruses are harbored in other animal species or in settled human populations. (6) Finally, human GIV (Alphatron-like) NoVs are genetically much more related to animal GIV NoVs (GIV.2) than to GI and GII human NoVs, suggesting points of intersection during their evolution. The modalities of this intersection are uncertain but likely they were favored by the strict social interactions between humans and pets.

SUMMARY

NoV are regarded as emerging pathogens in humans, and the creation of worldwide surveillance networks has allowed the researchers to gather important epidemiologic information and to gain unforeseen insights into the mechanisms of NoV evolution. The discovery of NoVs in carnivores and the genetic relationship between them and some human viruses raise interesting questions inherent in the ecology of these viruses and the possibilities of interspecies transmission. Also, it will be interesting to assess whether and to which extent NoVs impact on pet health.

REFERENCES

1. Kapikian AZ, Wyatt RG, Dolin R, et al. Visualization by immune electron microscopy of a 27-nm particle associated with acute infectious nonbacterial gastroenteritis. J Virol 1972;10(5):1075–81.
2. Xi JN, Graham DY, Wang KN, et al. Norwalk virus genome cloning and characterization. Science 1990;250(4987):1580–3.
3. Patel MM, Hall AJ, Vinjé J, et al. Noroviruses: a comprehensive review. J Clin Virol 2009;44(1):1–8.
4. Koopmans M. Progress in understanding norovirus epidemiology. Curr Opin Infect Dis 2008;21(5):544–52.
5. Green KY. Caliciviridae: the noroviruses. In: Knipe DM, Howley PM, editors. Fields virology. 5th edition. Philadelphia: Wolters Kluwer Health/Lippincott Williams and Wilkins; 2006. p. 949–79.
6. Smiley JR, Chang KO, Hayes J, et al. Characterization of an enteropathogenic bovine calicivirus representing a potentially new calicivirus genus. J Virol 2002; 76(20):10089–98.
7. Farkas T, Sestak K, Wei C, et al. Characterization of a rhesus monkey calicivirus representing a new genus of Caliciviridae. J Virol 2008;82(11):5408–16.
8. L'Homme Y, Sansregret R, Plante-Fortier E, et al. Genomic characterization of swine caliciviruses representing a new genus of Caliciviridae. Virus Genes 2009; 39(1):66–75.
9. Wolf S, Reetz J, Otto P. Genetic characterization of a novel calicivirus from a chicken. Arch Virol 2011. Available at: http://www.ncbi.nlm.nih.gov/pubmed/21404111. Accessed March 21, 2011.
10. Souza M, Azevedo MSP, Jung K, et al. Pathogenesis and immune responses in gnotobiotic calves after infection with the genogroup II.4-HS66 strain of human norovirus. J Virol 2008;82(4):1777–86.
11. Cheetham S, Souza M, Meulia T, et al. Pathogenesis of a genogroup II human norovirus in gnotobiotic pigs. J Virol 2006;80(21):10372–81.

12. Karst SM, Wobus CE, Lay M, et al. STAT1-dependent innate immunity to a Norwalk-like virus. Science 2003;299(5612):1575–8.
13. Wobus CE, Karst SM, Thackray LB, et al. Replication of Norovirus in cell culture reveals a tropism for dendritic cells and macrophages. PLoS Biol 2004;2(12):e432.
14. Duizer E, Schwab KJ, Neill FH, et al. Laboratory efforts to cultivate noroviruses. J Gen Virol 2004;85(Pt 1):79–87.
15. Prasad BV, Hardy ME, Dokland T, et al. X-ray crystallographic structure of the Norwalk virus capsid. Science 1999;286(5438):287–90.
16. Chen R, Neill JD, Estes MK, et al. X-ray structure of a native calicivirus: structural insights into antigenic diversity and host specificity. Proc Natl Acad Sci U S A 2006;103(21):8048–53.
17. Siebenga JJ, Vennema H, Renckens B, et al. Epochal evolution of GGII.4 norovirus capsid proteins from 1995 to 2006. J Virol 2007;81(18):9932–41.
18. Tan M, Jiang X. Norovirus and its histo-blood group antigen receptors: an answer to a historical puzzle. Trends Microbiol 2005;13(6):285–93.
19. Bull RA, White PA. Mechanisms of GII.4 norovirus evolution. Trends Microbiol 2011. Available at: http://www.ncbi.nlm.nih.gov/pubmed/21310617. Accessed March 23, 2011.
20. Zheng D-P, Ando T, Fankhauser RL, et al. Norovirus classification and proposed strain nomenclature. Virology 2006;346(2):312–23.
21. van Der Poel WH, Vinjé J, van Der Heide R, et al. Norwalk-like calicivirus genes in farm animals. Emerging Infect Dis 2000;6(1):36–41.
22. Wang Q-H, Han MG, Cheetham S, et al. Porcine noroviruses related to human noroviruses. Emerging Infect Dis 2005;11(12):1874–81.
23. Oliver SL, Dastjerdi AM, Wong S, et al. Molecular characterization of bovine enteric caliciviruses: a distinct third genogroup of noroviruses (Norwalk-like viruses) unlikely to be of risk to humans. J Virol 2003;77(4):2789–98.
24. Wolf S, Williamson W, Hewitt J, et al. Molecular detection of norovirus in sheep and pigs in New Zealand farms. Vet Microbiol 2009;133(1-2):184–9.
25. Radford AD, Coyne KP, Dawson S, et al. Feline calicivirus. Vet Res 2007;38(2):319–35.
26. Crandell RA. Isolation and characterization of caliciviruses from dogs with vesicular genital disease. Arch Virol 1988;98(1-2):65–71.
27. Evermann JF, McKeirnan AJ, Smith AW, et al. Isolation and identification of caliciviruses from dogs with enteric infections. Am J Vet Res 1985;46(1):218–20.
28. Martella V, Pratelli A, Gentile M, et al. Analysis of the capsid protein gene of a feline-like calicivirus isolated from a dog. Vet Microbiol 2002;85(4):315–22.
29. San Gabriel MC, Tohya Y, Sugimura T, et al. Identification of canine calicivirus capsid protein and its immunoreactivity in western blotting. J Vet Med Sci 1997;59(2):97–101.
30. Evermann JF, Bryan GM, McKiernan AJ. Isolation of a calicivirus from a case of canine glossitis. Canine Pract 1981;8:36–9.
31. Schaffer FL, Soergel ME, Black JW, et al. Characterization of a new calicivirus isolated from feces of a dog. Arch Virol 1985;84(3-4):181–95.
32. Mochizuki M, Kawanishi A, Sakamoto H, et al. A calicivirus isolated from a dog with fatal diarrhoea. Vet Rec 1993;132(9):221–2.
33. Matsuura Y, Tohya Y, Nakamura K, et al. Complete nucleotide sequence, genome organization and phylogenic analysis of the canine calicivirus. Virus Genes 2002;25(1):67–73.
34. Roerink F, Hashimoto M, Tohya Y, et al. Organization of the canine calicivirus genome from the RNA polymerase gene to the poly(A) tail. J Gen Virol 1999;80(Pt 4):929–35.

35. Mochizuki M, Hashimoto M, Roerink F, et al. Molecular and seroepidemiological evidence of canine calicivirus infections in Japan. J Clin Microbiol 2002;40(7): 2629–31.

36. Jang HK, Tohya Y, Han KY, et al. Seroprevalence of canine calicivirus and canine minute virus in the Republic of Korea. Vet Rec 2003;153(5):150–2.

37. Martella V, Campolo M, Lorusso E, et al. Norovirus in captive lion cub (Panthera leo). Emerging Infect Dis 2007;13(7):1071–3.

38. La Rosa G, Iaconelli M, Pourshaban M, et al. Molecular detection and genetic diversity of norovirus genogroup IV: a yearlong monitoring of sewage throughout Italy. Arch Virol 2010;155(4):589–93.

39. La Rosa G, Pourshaban M, Iaconelli M, et al. Detection of genogroup IV noroviruses in environmental and clinical samples and partial sequencing through rapid amplification of cDNA ends. Arch Virol 2008;153(11):2077–83.

40. Di Martino B, Marsilio F, Di Profio F, et al. Detection of antibodies against norovirus genogroup GIV in carnivores. Clin Vaccine Immunol 2010;17(1):180–2.

41. Martella V, Lorusso E, Decaro N, et al. Detection and molecular characterization of a canine norovirus. Emerging Infect Dis 2008;14(8):1306–8.

42. Martella V, Decaro N, Lorusso E, et al. Genetic heterogeneity and recombination in canine noroviruses. J Virol 2009;83(21):11391–6.

43. Ntafis V, Xylouri E, Radogna A, et al. Outbreak of canine norovirus infection in young dogs. J Clin Microbiol 2010;48(7):2605–8.

44. Mesquita JR, Barclay L, Nascimento MSJ, et al. Novel norovirus in dogs with diarrhea. Emerging Infect Dis 2010;16(6):980–2.

45. Atmar RL, Opekun AR, Gilger MA, et al. Norwalk virus shedding after experimental human infection. Emerging Infect Dis 2008;14(10):1553–7.

46. Siebenga JJ, Beersma MFC, Vennema H, et al. High prevalence of prolonged norovirus shedding and illness among hospitalized patients: a model for in vivo molecular evolution. J Infect Dis 2008;198(7):994–1001.

47. Hsu CC, Riley LK, Wills HM, et al. Persistent infection with and serologic cross-reactivity of three novel murine noroviruses. Comp Med 2006;56(4):247–51.

48. Appel MJ. Does canine coronavirus augment the effects of susbequent parvovirus? Vet Med 1988;83:360–6.

49. Pratelli A, Tempesta M, Roperto FP, et al. Fatal coronavirus infection in puppies following canine parvovirus 2b infection. J Vet Diagn Invest 1999;11(6):550–3.

50. Parrino TA, Schreiber DS, Trier JS, et al. Clinical immunity in acute gastroenteritis caused by Norwalk agent. N Engl J Med 1977;297(2):86–9.

51. Tan M, Xia M, Chen Y, et al. Conservation of carbohydrate binding interfaces: evidence of human HBGA selection in norovirus evolution. PLoS ONE 2009;4(4): e5058.

52. Hutson AM, Atmar RL, Graham DY, et al. Norwalk virus infection and disease is associated with ABO histo-blood group type. J Infect Dis 2002;185(9):1335–7.

53. Hutson AM, Atmar RL, Marcus DM, et al. Norwalk virus-like particle hemagglutination by binding to histo-blood group antigens. J Virol 2003;77(1):405–15.

54. Chakravarty S, Hutson AM, Estes MK, et al. Evolutionary trace residues in noroviruses: importance in receptor binding, antigenicity, virion assembly, and strain diversity. J Virol 2005;79(1):554–68.

55. Cheetham S, Souza M, McGregor R, et al. Binding patterns of human norovirus-like particles to buccal and intestinal tissues of gnotobiotic pigs in relation to A/H histo-blood group antigen expression. J Virol 2007;81(7):3535–44.

56. Vinjé J, Hamidjaja RA, Sobsey MD. Development and application of a capsid VP1 (region D) based reverse transcription PCR assay for genotyping of genogroup I and II noroviruses. J Virol Methods 2004;116(2):109–17.

57. Mattison K, Grudeski E, Auk B, et al. Multicenter comparison of two norovirus ORF2-based genotyping protocols. J Clin Microbiol 2009;47(12):3927–32.

58. Jiang X, Huang PW, Zhong WM, et al. Design and evaluation of a primer pair that detects both Norwalk- and Sapporo-like caliciviruses by RT-PCR. J Virol Methods 1999;83(1-2):145–54.

59. Vennema H, de Bruin E, Koopmans M. Rational optimization of generic primers used for Norwalk-like virus detection by reverse transcriptase polymerase chain reaction. J Clin Virol 2002;25(2):233–5.

60. Mesquita JR, Barclay L, Nascimento MSJ, et al. Novel norovirus in dogs with diarrhea. Emerging Infect Dis 2010;16(6):980–2.

61. Lay MK, Atmar RL, Guix S, et al. Norwalk virus does not replicate in human macrophages or dendritic cells derived from the peripheral blood of susceptible humans. Virology 2010;406(1):1–11.

62. Straub TM, Höner zu Bentrup K, Orosz-Coghlan P, et al. In vitro cell culture infectivity assay for human noroviruses. Emerging Infect Dis 2007;13(3):396–403.

63. Heyworth JS, Cutt H, Glonek G. Does dog or cat ownership lead to increased gastroenteritis in young children in South Australia? Epidemiol Infect 2006;134(5):926–34.

64. Martella V, Bányai K, Matthijnssens J, et al. Zoonotic aspects of rotaviruses. Vet Microbiol 2010;140(3-4):246–55.

65. Peasey AE, Ruiz-Palacios GM, Quigley M, et al. Seroepidemiology and risk factors for sporadic norovirus/Mexico strain. J Infect Dis 2004;189(11):2027–36.

66. Humphrey TJ, Cruickshank JG, Cubitt WD. An outbreak of calicivirus associated gastroenteritis in an elderly persons home. A possible zoonosis? J Hyg (Lond) 1984;93(2):293–9.

67. Nishlda T, Nishio O, Kato M, et al. Genotyping and quantitation of noroviruses in oysters from two distinct sea areas in Japan. Microbiol Immunol 2007;51(2):177–84.

68. Costantini V, Loisy F, Joens L, et al. Human and animal enteric caliciviruses in oysters from different coastal regions of the United States. Appl Environ Microbiol 2006;72(3):1800–9.

Canine Papillomaviruses

Christian E. Lange, PhD, DVM[a,b,]*, Claude Favrot, DVM, MS[a]

KEYWORDS
- Canine • Papilloma • Virus • Infection • Wart • Tumor

Papillomaviruses (PVs) can infect epithelia and induce proliferative disorders. Different types of canine PVs have been found to be associated with distinct pathologies including exophytic warts as in canine oral papillomatosis, endophytic warts, and pigmented plaques and, in some cases, squamous cell carcinomas.

ETIOLOGY

PVs are double-stranded DNA viruses with a circular genome of about 8000 base pairs that is contained in a nonenveloped 50- to 55-nm icasahedral capsid. The capsid consists of the 2 structural proteins, L1 and L2, at a ratio of 30:1 and exposes primarily pentamers of L1 to the outside.[1–3] All genetic information in the PV genome is encoded on the same DNA strand, and usually 6 to 8 open reading frames (ORFs) can be identified.[4] Those ORFs are the late ones, L1 and L2, and the early ones, E1, E2, E4, E6, and E7. While L1, L2, E1, and E2 are present in all PVs, E4 is not always easily identified, as it is contained within the E2 ORF. E6 and E7 are present in most but not all known PVs. Some, like the members of the genus *Alpha-Papillomaviruses*, also contain an E5 ORF.[5]

Originally, PVs had been allocated to the family Papovaviridae together with the polyomaviruses because of similarities in genome and capsid structure.[3] As genome size and organization were found to differ and no significant sequence homologies could be identified, this categorization was abandoned and the taxonomic families Polyomaviridae and Papillomaviridae were established. The current classification of PVs within the Papillomaviridae family is based on nucleotide sequence identities of the L1 ORF. The categories genus (<60% identities), species (more than 60% identities), type (more than 70% identities), subtype (more than 90% identities), and variant (more than 98% identities) were introduced for further description of PV isolates.[5] To date 29 PV genera have been recognized containing almost 200 distinct

The authors have nothing to disclose.
[a] Dermatology Department, Clinic for Small Animal Internal Medicine, Vetsuisse Faculty, University of Zurich, Winterthurerstrasse 260, CH-8057 Zurich, Switzerland
[b] Institute of Virology, Vetsuisse Faculty, University of Zurich, Winterthurerstrasse 266a, CH-8057 Zurich, Switzerland
* Corresponding author.
E-mail address: clange@vetclinics.uzh.ch

Vet Clin Small Anim 41 (2011) 1183–1195
doi:10.1016/j.cvsm.2011.08.003
0195-5616/11/$ – see front matter © 2011 Elsevier Inc. All rights reserved.

Table 1
Canine papillomaviruses and clinical symptoms

Virus	PV Genus	Described Clinical Symptoms
CPV1	Lambda	Asymptomatic infections, exophytic papillomas, endophytic papillomas, invasive SCCs
CPV2	Tau	Exophytic papillomas, endophytic papillomas, invasive SCCs
CPV3	Chi	Pigmented plaques, in situ SCC, invasive SCC
CPV4	Chi	Pigmented plaques
CPV5	Chi	Pigmented plaques
CPV6	Lambda	Endophytic papillomas
CPV7	Tau	Exophytic papillomas, in situ SCC

PV types.[6] The number of known PVs is growing constantly, but so far more than half of the published sequences derive from PVs infecting the human host.

PVs are species-specific pathogens, and the target tissues of most of them are keratinizing and mucous membranes. However, there are exceptions. The bovine PVs BPV1 and BPV2 naturally infect the cow as well as the horse and can experimentally also infect rodents.[7,8] It also appears that the PV involved in feline sarcoids is of bovine origin.[9–11] PVs induce a broad spectrum of benign epithelial neoplasias but are also known to be involved in the development of malignant neoplasias or are suspected to be.[12–14]

PV infections in dogs have repeatedly been described since the late 19th century, and thus far the entire sequences of 7 canine PVs (CPVs) have been published as well as several short stretches of other putative CPVs.[14–22] The 7 genomes of CPVs have been allocated to 3 different PV genera: *Lambda, Tau,* and *Chi* (**Table 1**). While *Lambda* contains also PVs of other carnivore species, *Tau* and *Chi* contain only CPVs so far.[6]

EPIDEMIOLOGY

The primary target cells of infectious PV particles are epithelial cells. Not all epithelial cells are, however, capable of cell division, which is mandatory for PVs to establish persisting infections. In case of the squamous epithelium, such cells are only found in the basal cell layer, protected by several layers of differentiated and differentiating keratinocytes. It was concluded that PVs require sites of injuries to be able to make contact with those basal cells.[23–25] The virus seems to enter the cell mainly by clathrin-dependent receptor–mediated endocytosis after binding to α6 integrin.[26–28] During the following first phase of a PV infection, there is an initial amplification of the viral DNA in the nucleus, whereas thereafter it is copied about once per cell cycle in synchrony with the host genome.[29] This phase is also characterized by a lack of clinical symptoms. It has been demonstrated, that in case of experimental infections, this phase lasts at least 4 weeks before the onset of apparent symptoms.[15,30] Not all natural infections seem to involve the development of overt symptoms, though, and viral DNA can be detected on the clinically health skin of humans and several animal species.[31,32] Dogs have as well been shown to harbor the DNA of PVs in the absence of clinical symptoms to a high proportion (more than 50%) on their skin.[33] It is, however, not clear whether those are cases of subclinical infections or if dogs just carry PVs or their DNA on their skin. A study on the prevalence of antibodies against CPV1 and CPV3 indicates that, depending on the population and the cut-off value chosen, up to about 50% may have had contact with at least 1 of these 2 PVs.[34]

The immune system of the host plays an important role in the outcome of PV infections, where the cellular immunity is mainly responsible for virus eradication while the humoral immunity protects the organism against reinfections. This is probably true for PV infections in all species.[35-37] Thus, PV infections pose a greater threat for immunocompromised than for immunocompetent animals. This was supported by several reports, especially by the observation of a severe outbreak of CPV2-associated papillomatosis in a population of dogs with severe combined immunodeficiency (SCID).[13] Also, reports of corticosteroid- or cyclosporine A–induced cases of papillomatosis support the role of the immune response in the dog.[38-41] There are also indications that breed predispositions putatively associated with an inherited immune defect may exist, although the available data are very limited. The pug, as perhaps the best-documented example, seems to be prone to develop pigmented plaques.[19,42,43]

PATHOGENESIS

The whole PV life cycle is closely linked to its host cells and thus to the differentiation program of the squamous epthelium.[44,45] Most of the early genes are expressed primarily in the basal and suprabasal levels of the epidermis, while the 2 late genes are exclusively expressed in the spinous and granular cell layers.[46] Consequently, the assembly of virions occurs in the upper stratum granulosum and stratum corneum. The infective viruses are probably released due to normal death of cells in these layers, as PVs are not lytic viruses.[47] In case of canine oral papillomatosis, hyperplasia develops in the stratum spinosum after the initial phase of subclinical infection, and wart formation with acanthosis and hyperkeratosis occurs.[30] Most cytopathic effects such as intracytoplasmic pseudoinclusions, koilocytosis, and clumped keratohyalin granules can primarily be observed in the mid and upper epidermis, while intranuclear inclusions are only present in the upper epidermis.[48] Spontaneous wart regression at 4 to 8 weeks after the onset of symptoms is part of the common course of PV infections inducing exophytic warts like oral paplillomatosis.[30] However, age and immune status of the dog determine the outcome of such infections. While in young dogs transient infections seem to be the rule, older and/or immunosuppressed dogs not only have a higher risk of developing clinical disease but also suffer from persistent infection and neoplastic transformation.[13]

The outcome of PV infections probably depends on factors in addition to host immunity and genetic background. Among those influential factors may be the intrinsic pathogenicity of the involved PV type, subtype, or variant, as well as putative external factors.[49] While the connection between PVs and benign neoplasias, primarily the canine oral papillomatosis, is well established, making a direct causal link between CPV infection and the development of malignant neoplastic transformation is rather difficult. Although there is some epidemiologic evidence for such a correlation, definite proof from in vitro experiments is missing.[13,14,20,22,50,51] The individual differences in the outcome of PV infections can be illustrated based on an described outbreak of papillomatosis in a group of X-linked SCID dogs. Although all individuals were of the same breed, similarly immunocompromised and infected by the same pathogen (CPV2), the range of diagnosed lesions included exophytic and endophytic papillomas as well as, in some cases, in situ and even invasive squamous cell carcinomas (SCCs).[13] In case of CPV3, which was isolated from a Rhodesian ridgeback, pigmented plaques, in situ and invasive SCC were found alongside in the same dog putatively marking different stages of PV infection.[14] Although a serologic study indicated the prevalence of the virus, no further cases associated with this virus have been described yet.[34] Even the mechanisms involved in the

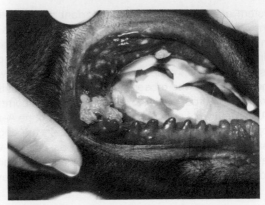

Fig. 1. Young flat-coated retriever with fringed oral papillomas.

relatively well-studied CPV1 infections that are responsible for canine oral papillomatosis seem to be understood only partially.

CLINICAL FINDINGS

Dogs may display a variety of CPV-associated skin disorders including classic warts with exophytic or endophytic growth, pigmented plaques, hyperkeratotic to horny lesions, and, in some cases, in situ or invasive SCCs (**Table 1**).[13,14,16,19,20,22,39,43,50,52–65]

Canine Oral Papillomatosis

Mainly young dogs are affected by canine oral papillomatosis, which appears in a broad spectrum of forms in the oral cavity but is not restricted to it.[15,30] It is typically characterized by cauliflower like exophytic warts, but the benign tumors may as well be fringed or nodular (**Fig. 1**). The mainly affected tissue is the oral mucosa including the lips and mucocutaneous junctions. Tongue and esophagus are only occasionally afflicted. In some cases, the eyelids are also affected and papillomas infrequently occur on the haired skin in this context. Often these papillomas come in small numbers, but occasionally severe manifestations of oral papillomatoses are seen (**Fig. 2**). In larger dog colonies, outbreaks affect a varying proportion of animals.[66] The virus involved in this oral papillomatosis complex was originally named canine oral papillomavirus (COPV), but other names were also sometimes used. In order to avoid confusion and for more uniformity in PV nomenclature, it was recently suggested to use the term *canine papillomavirus 1* (CPV1).[6] Although CPV1 is primarily involved in the transient oral papillomatosis, it has also been reported to be possibly involved in nonregressing lesions and the development of SCCs and endophytic papillomas.[21,50,67] Oral papillomatosis has also been observed in the coyote (*Canis latrans*) and the wolf (*Canis lupus*). As they are closely related to the domestic dog, it can be expected that the same virus is involved in the development of the lesions.[68–72]

Inverted Papillomas

Inverted papillomas or endophytic warts are characterized by a growth downward into the skin. This development results in raised and smooth nodules with a central pore filled with keratin. In histology endophytic, papillary projections of the epidermis

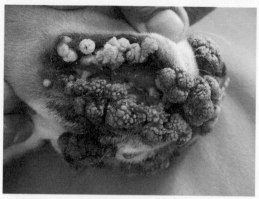

Fig. 2. Young beagle with severe oral papillomatosis.

extending into the dermis are typical. Cytopathic effects are usually present in the form of clumped keratohyaline granules, koilocytes, and, less frequently, basophilic or eosinophilic inclusions. Four different subtypes have been described in dogs. Classic inverted papillomas, which were initially described by Campbell et al,[58] have a diameter of 1- to 2-cm and are rather large, cup-shaped, grayish nodules with a large central pore (**Fig. 3**). They are typically found at the abdomen in small numbers or as solitary lesions. Shimada et al[61] described a second type of inverted papilloma where the lesions have a diameter of about 4 mm. They present as dome-shaped flesh-colored papillomas, which may be disseminated over the whole body. A third type described by Le Net et al[39] is characterized by even smaller (2 mm) disseminated black papules that display intracytoplasmatic eosinopylic inclusions on histopathologic assessment. A fourth type described by Goldschmidt et al,[13] that mainly resembles classic inverted papillomas, seems to be prone to induce interdigital lesions. Distinct PV types have been isolated from each of these lesions, but except for perhaps CPV2-associated papillomas, data are limited.[13,18,21]

Pigmented Plaques

Canine pigmented plaques consist of small (1 mm) to medium-sized (1 cm), dark, plaquelike hyperkeratotic lesions that predominantly show up at the limbs, axillae, or

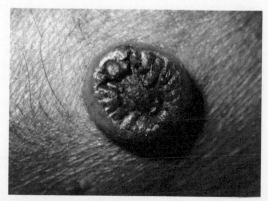

Fig. 3. Classic inverted papilloma at the abdomen of a flat-coated retriever.

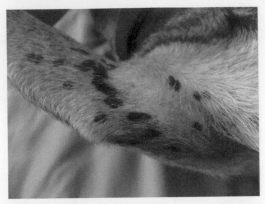

Fig. 4. Pigmented plaques in a pug.

abdomen (**Fig. 4**). They are usually very flat but may be slightly raised and usually appear in clusters. Pigmented plaques were initially referred to as lentiginosis profuse.[42] However, as the association between CPV and this condition was demonstrated, it was hypothesized that it could be the canine counterpart of human epidermodysplasia verruciformis.[73] Some major differences exist, though, between these conditions, and any premature comparison should consequently be avoided.[48] In contrast to typical exophytic or endophytic papillomas, canine pigmented plaques show little tendency for spontaneous regression. In pugs, this condition has repeatedly been reported, and the DNA of CPV4 was connected to it in all tested cases. Progression into malignant lesions was not reported in the pug.[19,73–75] In the case of CPV3 infection and in the case of at least one other uncharacterized PV, a causal relation between virus, pigmented plaques, and in situ and invasive SCC seems to be evident (**Fig. 5**).[14,22,51] CPV5 was also discovered in a dog with pigmented plaques but no signs of cancerous transformation were noticed. All viruses thus far connected with pigmented lesions are or seem to belong to the PV genus *Chi*.[14,19,20,22]

DIAGNOSIS

The diagnosis of CPV-associated disorders depends on the type of disorder but may in general be based on gross appearance of the lesions and the epidemiologic

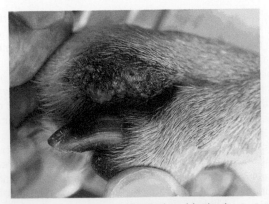

Fig. 5. *In situ* squamous cell carcinoma in a Rhodesian ridgeback.

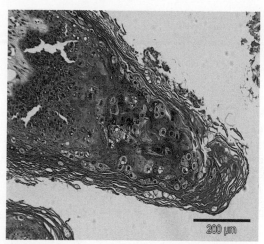

Fig. 6. Histopathology of oral papillomatosis (hematoxylin-eosin stain).

background. The methods most frequently used are classic histopathology and polymerase chain reaction (PCR).

Canine oral papillomatosis has a very obvious clinical presentation and may therefore be diagnosed without any laboratory testing, when observed in young dogs. Because other cases of suspected PV-induced papillomatosis are not as distinct in terms of morphology and epidemiology, full-thickness excision biopsy samples of entire lesions including some adjacent normal tissue should be obtained to perform histologic examination.

Classic warts usually reveal hyperplasia of the epidermis with extensive orthokeratotic hyperkeratosis. Typical features are clumped keratohyalin granules in the stratum spinosum, koilocytes (keratinocytes with swollen, clear cytoplasm and a pyknotic nucleus), clear cells (keratinocytes with swollen, blue-gray cytoplasm and enlarged nuclei), and intranuclear inclusion bodies (**Fig. 6**).[48] In endophytic papillomas, centripetal papillary projections of hyperplastic squamous epithelium with a central core of keratin layers and parakeratotic cells are typically observed.[21] The stratum spinosum is usually found to show irregular hyperplasia and contains moderate numbers of mitotic figures and dysplastic cells. The subcorneal epithelium displays a variable number of koilocytes, which may have basophilic intranuclear inclusions and a few large keratohyalin granules.[58] In the case of the subtype described by Le Net et al, however, large eosinophilic intranuclear inclusions are apparent.[39]

In pigmented plaques, moderate acanthosis with scalloped configuration, hyperpigmentation, and clumped keratohyalin granules in the stratum spinosum are typically found, while koilocytes as well as viral inclusions are usually not observed (**Fig. 7**).[48]

PCR assays have been established for the detection of CPV DNA and can be applied to test material from biopsy or cytobrush samples.[33] The assays are very sensitive, and short stretches of the viral genome may be determined using direct sequencing. However, as PV DNA may be found independent of clinical symptoms, PCR results have to be interpreted with caution and should be correlated with histopathology, clinical lesions, and epidemiologic data if available.

Additional methods that can be very helpful in verifying a diagnosis of CPV-associated papillomatosis are immunohistochemistry, in situ hybridization, electron

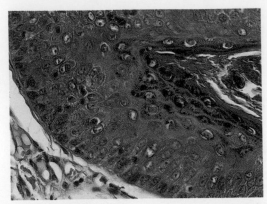

Fig. 7. Histopathology of a pigmented plaque (hematoxylin-eosin stain).

microscopy, and rolling circle amplification. Immunohistochemistry is a very informative method. It requires a decent amount of viral protein to provide a signal, but when positive, it clearly proves viral activity. However, no CPV-specific antibodies are commercially available. Antibodies against conserved regions of PV proteins have been used in the past. In situ hybridization can be used to locate nucleic acids of the virus in fixed tissues, thus determining the infected tissues and cells, and to show viral transcription when targeting RNA. Electron microscopy can be used to actually visualize characteristic viral structures to prove productive infection. Finally, rolling circle amplification is a method to amplify whole viral genomes independent of the sequence, which can be applied to fresh, but not fixed, samples. It enables the detection and characterization of already known as well as of unknown PVs as long as the circular form of PV DNA is not dissolved.

TREATMENT AND PREVENTION

The transient character of canine oral papillomatosis was already demonstrated more than 100 years ago.[15] As transience is probably a feature of most PV-induced lesions, putative therapeutic approaches for papillomas should be reviewed with caution. Spontaneous regression and therapeutic effect are, under these circumstances, hard to discriminate, and the statement that "the credit claimed for some methods of treatment may be undeserved" remains relevant.[15] Most papillomas will spontaneously regress within 1 to 2 months. The treatment of choice for papillomas that do not regress and cause severe problems due to their size or location is surgery. It should nevertheless be kept in mind that surgical excision has been reported to be associated with latent infection and increased recurrence.[76,77] Medical treatments with interferons as well as with the immune modulator imiquimod have been suggested, but so far no studies on their effectiveness in canine papillomatoses have been published.

It was shown in 1898 and repeatedly confirmed that dogs that had suffered from oral papillomatosis are apparently protected from reinfections.[15,35,78–80] The use of inactivated crude wart extract as a prophylactic vaccine had been demonstrated to be effective in preventing oral papillomatosis, and such techniques have repeatedly been used to protect larger dog populations from clinical papillomatosis.[35,81] More recent approaches to develop effective and save vaccines in the lab are very promising. Viruslike particles consisting exclusively of CPV1 L1 capsid protein could be produced.[82] It was also possible to induce cellular and humoral immunity by the administration of plasmids coding for a few genes or a single gene of CPV1.[83–86] While preventative vaccines against some human PVs involved in the development of cervix carcinomas are now on the market, commercial vaccines against CPVs are not available.

SUMMARY

PVs can infect epithelia and induce proliferative disorders. Different types of CPVs have been found to be associated with distinct pathologies including exophytic warts as in canine oral papillomatosis, endophytic warts, and pigmented plaques and, in some cases, squamous cell carcinomas. Virus infection is followed by a phase of subclinical infection before the onset of symptoms. A diagnosis can in some cases be made clinically but should be verified if there are any doubts. Most papillomas do regress spontaneously within a few months. Preventative vaccination is possible but not on the market.

REFERENCES

1. Crawford LV, Crawford EM. A comparative study of polyoma and papilloma viruses. Virology 1963;21:258–63.
2. Baker TS, Newcomb WW, Olsen NH, et al. Structures of bovine and human papillomaviruses. Analysis by cryoelectron microscopy and three-dimensional image reconstruction. J Biophys 1991;60:1445–56.
3. Belnap DM, Olson NH, Cladel NM, et al. Conserved features in papillomavirus and polyomavirus capsids. J Mol Biol 1996;259:249–63.
4. Chen EY, Howley PM, Levinson AD, et al. The primary structure and genetic organisation of the bovine papillomavirus 1 genome. Nature 1982;299:529–34.
5. de Villiers E, Fauquet C, Broker T, et al. Classification of papillomaviruses. Virology 2004;324:17–27.
6. Bernard H, Burk R, Chen Z, et al. Classification of papillomaviruses (PVs) based on 189 PV types and proposal of taxonomic amendments. Virology 2010;401:70–9.
7. Black PH, Hartley JW, Rowe WP. Transformation of bovine tissue culture cells by bovine papillomavirus. Nature 1963;199:1016–18.
8. Dvoresky I, Shober R, Chattopadhyay SK, et al. A quantitative in vitro focus assay for bovine papilloma virus. Virology 1980;103:369–75.
9. Munday JS, Knight CG, Howe L. The same papillomavirus is present in feline sarcoids from North America and New Zealand but not in any non-sarcoid feline samples. J Vet Diagn Invest 2010;22:97–100.
10. Munday JS, Knight CG. Amplification of feline sarcoid-associated papillomavirus DNA sequences from bovine skin. Vet Dermatol 2010;21:341–4.
11. Orbell GM, Young S, Munday JS. Cutaneous sarcoids in captive African lions associated with feline sarcoid-associated papillomavirus infection. Vet Pathol. [Epub ahead of print].
12. zur Hausen H. Papillomaviruses in human cancers. Proc Assoc Am Physicians 1999;111:581–7.
13. Goldschmidt MH, Kennedy JS, Kennedy DR, et al. Severe papillomavirus infection progressing to metastatic squamous cell carcinoma in bone marrow-transplanted X-linked SCID dogs. J Virol 2006;80:6621–8.
14. Tobler K, Favrot C, Nespeca G, et al. Detection of the prototype of a potential novel genus in the family Papillomaviridae in association with canine epidermodysplasia verruciformis. J Gen Virol 2006;87:3551–7.

15. M'Fadeyan J, Hobday F. Not on the experimental transmission of warts in the dog. J Comp Pathol Ther 1898;11:341–4.
16. Delius H, Van Ranst MA, Jenson AB, et al. Canine oral papillomavirus genomic sequence: a unique 1.5-kb intervening sequence between the E2 and L2 open reading frames. Virology 1994;204:447–52.
17. Zaugg N, Nespeca G, Hauser B, et al. Detection of novel papillomaviruses in canine mucosal, cutaneous and in situ squamous cell carcinomas. Vet Dermatol 2005;16: 290–8.
18. Yuan H, Ghim S, Newsome J, et al. An epidermotropic canine papillomavirus with malignant potential contains an E5 gene and establishes a unique genus. Virology 2007;359:28–36.
19. Tobler K, Lange C, Carlotti DN, et al. Detection of a novel papillomavirus in pigmented plaques of four pugs. Vet Dermatol 2008;19:21–5.
20. Lange C, Tobler K, Ackermann M, et al. Three novel canine papillomaviruses support taxonomic clade formation. J Gen Virol 2009;90:2615–21.
21. Lange CE, Tobler K, Brandes K, et al. Canine inverted papillomas associated with DNA of four different papillomaviruses. Vet Dermatol 2010;21:287–91.
22. Munday JS, O'Connor KI, Smits B. Development of multiple pigmented viral plaques and squamous cell carcinoma in a dog infected by a novel papillomavirus. Vet Dermatol 2011;22:104–10.
23. Oriel JD. Natural history of genital warts. Br J Vener Dis 1971;47:1–13.
24. Dürst M, Bosch FX, Glitz D, et al. Inverse relationship between human papillomavirus (HPV) type 16 early gene expression and cell differentiation in nude mouse epithelial cysts and tumors induced by HPV-positive human cell lines. J Virol 1991;65:796–804.
25. zur Hausen H. Papillomavirus infections: a major cause of human cancers. Biochim Biophys Acta 1996;1288:F55–78.
26. Evander M, Frazer IH, Payne E, et al. Identification of the alpha6 integrin as a candidate receptor for papillomaviruses. J Virol 1991;71:2449–56.
27. Sibbet G, Romero-Graillet C, Menguzzi G, et al. $\alpha6$ integrin is not the obligatory cell receptor for bovine papillomavirus type 4. J Gen Virol 2000;81:327–34.
28. Day PM, Lowy DR, Schiller JT. Papillomaviruses infect cells via a clathrin-dependent pathway. Virology 2004;307:1–11.
29. Gilbert DM, Cohen SN. Bovine papilloma virus plasmids replicate randomly in mouse fibroblsts throughout S phase of the cell cycle. Cell 1987;50:59–68.
30. Chambers VC, Evans CA. Canine oral papillomatosis. I. Virus assay and observations on the various stages of the experimental infection. Cancer Res 1959;19:1188–95.
31. Antonsson A, Forslund O, Ekberg H, et al. The ubiquity and impressive genomic diversity of human skin papillomaviruses suggest a commensalic nature of these viruses. J Virol 2000;74:11636–41.
32. Antonsson A, Hansson B. Healthy skin of many animal species harbors papillomaviruses which are closely related to their human counterparts. J Virol 2002;76: 12537–42.
33. Lange CE, Zollinger S, Tobler K, et al. The clinically healthy skin of dogs is a potential reservoir for canine papillomaviruses. J Clin Microbiol 2011;49:707–9.
34. Lange CE, Tobler K, Favrot C, et al. Detection of antibodies against epidermoplasia verruciformis-associated canine papillomavirus 3 in sera of dogs from Europe and Africa by enzyme-liked immunosorbent assay. Clin Vaccine Immunol 2009;16:66–72.
35. Chambers VC, Evans CA, Weiser RS. Canine oral papillomatosis. II. Immunologic aspects of the disease. Cancer Res 1960;20:1083–93.

36. Suzich JA, Ghim SJ, Palmer-Hill FJ, et al. Systemic immunization with papillomavirus L1 protein completely prevents the development of viral mucosal papillomas. Proc Natl Acad Sci USA 1995;92:11553–7.

37. Frazer IH. Immunology of papillomavirus infection. Curr Opin Immunol 1996;8: 484–91.

38. Sundberg JP, Smith EK, Herron AJ, et al. Involvement of canine oral papillomavirus in generalized oral and cutaneous verrucosis in a Chinese shar pei dog. Vet Pathol 1994;31:183–7.

39. Le Net J-L, Orth G, Sunberg JP, et al. Multiple pigmented cutaneous papules associated with a novel canine papillomavirus in an immunosuppressed dog. Vet Pathol 1997;34:8–14.

40. Callan MB, Preziosi D, Mauldin E. Multiple papillomavirus-associated epidermal hamartomas and squamous cell carcinomas in situ in a dog following chronic treatment with prednisolone and cyclosporine. Vet Dermatol 2005;16:338–45.

41. Favrot C, Olivry T, Werner AH, et al. Evaluation of papillomaviruses associated with cyclosporine-induced hyperplastic verrucous lesions in dogs. Am J Vet Res 2005;66: 1764–9.

42. Briggs OM. Lentiginosis profusa in the pug: three case reports. J Small Anim Pract 1985;26:675–80.

43. Nagata M, Nanko H, Moriyana A, et al. Pigmented plaques associated with papillo-mavirus infection in dogs. Is this epidermodysplasia verruciformis? Vet Dermatol 1995;6:179–81.

44. Bedell MA, Hudson JB, Golub TR, et al. Amplification of human papillomavirus genomes in vitro is dependent on epithelial differentiation. J Virol 1991;65:2254–60.

45. Ozbun MA, Meyers C. Human paapillomavirus type 31b E1 and W2 transcript expression correlates with vegetative viral genome amplification. Virology 1998;248: 218–30.

46. Doorbar J. The papillomavirus life cycle. J Clin Virol 2005;32:7.

47. Lehr E, Brown DR. Infection with the oncogenic human papillomavirus type 59 alter protein components of the cornified cell envelope. Virology 2003;309:53–60.

48. Gross TL, Ihrke PJ, Walder EJ, et al. Hyperplastic diseases of the epidermis. In: Gross TL, Ihrke PJ, Walder EJ, et al, editors. Skin diseases of the dog and cat. Oxford: Blackwell Publishing; 2005. P. 136–60.

49. Howley PM, Lowy DR. Papillomaviruses. In: Knipe DM, Howley PM, editors. Fields virology, 5th edition. Philadelphia: Lippincott Williams & Wilkins; 2007. p. 2299–354.

50. Teifke JP, Löhr CV, Shirasawa H. Detection of canine oral papillomavirus-DNA in canine oral squamous cell carcinomas and p53 overexpressing skin papillomas of the dog using the polymerase chain reaction and non-radioactive in situ hybridization. Vet Microbiol 1998;60:119–30.

51. Stokking LB, Ehrhart EJ, Lichtensteiger CA, et al. Pigmented epidermal plaques in three dogs. J Am Anim Hosp Assoc 2004;40:411–7.

52. Watrach AM. The ultrastructure of canine cutaneous papilloma. Cancer Res 1969; 29:2079–84.

53. Tokita H, Konishi S. Studies on canine oral papillomatosis. II. Oncogenicity of canine oral papillomavirus to various tissues of dog with special reference to eye tumour. Nippon Juigaku Zasshi 1975;37:109–20.

54. Hare CL, Howard EB. Canine conjunctivocorneal papillomatosis: a case report. J Am Anim Hosp Assoc 1977;13:688–90.

55. Belkin PV. Ocular lesions in canine oral papillomatosis (a case report). Vet Med Small Anim Clin 1979;74:1520–7.

56. Bonney CH, Koch SA, Confer AW, et al. A case report: a conjunctival papilloma with evidence of a viral etiology. J Small Anim Pract 1980;21:183–8.

57. Sundberg JP, Junge RE, Lancester WD. Immunoperoxidase localisation of papillomaviruses in hyperplastic and neoplastic epithelial lesions of animals. Am J Vet Res 1984;45:1441–6.

58. Campbell KL, Sundberg JP, Goldschmidt MH, et al. Cutaneous inverted papillomas in dogs. Vet Pathol 1988;25:67–71.

59. Kubo M. A case report of canine cutaneous papilloma. J Jpn Vet Med Assoc 1992;45:109–12.

60. Narama I, Ozaki K, Maeda H, et al. Cutaneous papilloma with viral replication in an old dog. J Vet Med Sci 1992;54:387–9.

61. Shimada A, Shinya K, Awakura T, et al. Cutaneous papillomatosis associated with papillomavirus infection in a dog. J Comp Pathol 1993;108:103–7.

62. Sansom J, Barnett KC, Blunden AS, et al. Canine conjunctival papilloma: a review of five cases. J Small Anim Pract 1996;37:84–6.

63. DeBey BM, Balgladi-Swanson M, Kapil S, et al. Digital papillomatosis in a confined Beagle. J Vet Diagn Invest 2001;13:346–8.

64. Platter BL, Hostetter JM. Cutaneous viral papilloma with local extension and sublingual cyst formation in a dog. J Vet Diagn Invest 2009;21:551–4.

65. Munday JS, French AF, MacNamara AR. The development of multiple cutaneous inverted papilloma following ovariohisterectomy in a dog. N Z Vet J 2010;58:168–71.

66. Penberthy J. Contagious warty tumours in dogs. J Comp Pathol Ther 1898;11:363–5.

67. Nicholls PK, Klaunberg BA, Moore RA, et al. Naturally occurring, nonregressing canine oral papillomavirus infection: host immunity, virus characterisation, and experimental infection. Virology 1999;265:365–74.

68. Trainer DO, Knowlton FF, Karstadt L. Oral papillomatosis in the coyote. Bull Wildl Dis Assoc 1968;4:52–4.

69. Broughton E, Graesser FE, Carbyn LN, et al. Oral papillomatosis in the coyote in western Canada. J Wildl Dis 1970;6:180–1.

70. Greig AS, Charkton KM. Electron microscopy of the virus of oral papillomatosis in the coyote. J Wildl Dis 1973;9:359–61.

71. Nellis CH. Prevalence of oral papilloma-like lesions in coyotes in Alberta. Can J Zool 1973;51:900.

72. Samuel WM, Chalmers GA, Gunson JR. Oral papillomatosis in coyotes (Canis latrans) and wolves (Canis lupus) of Alberta. J Wildl Dis 1978;14:165–9.

73. Nagata M. Canine papillomatosis. In: Bonagura JD, editor. Kirk's current veterinary therapy XIII. Philadelphia: WB Saunders; 2000. p. 569–71.

74. Tanabe C, Kano R, Nagata M, et al. Molecular characteristics of cutaneous papillomavirus from the canine pigmented epidermal nevus. J Vet Med Sci 2000;62,1189–92.

75. Narama I, Kobayashi Y, Yamagami T, et al. Pigmented cutaneous papillomatosis (pigmented epidermal nevus) in three pug dogs; histopathology, electron microscopy and analysis of viral DNA by the polymerase chain reaction. J Comp Pathol 2005;132: 132–8.

76. Collier LL, Collins BK. Excision and cryosurgical ablation of severe periocular papillomatosis in a dog. J Am Vet Med Assoc 1994;2004:881–5.

77. Bredal WP, Thoresen SI, Rimstad E, et al. Diagnosis and clinical course of canine oral papillomavirus infection. J Small Anim Pract 1996;37:138–42.

78. DeMonbreun WA, Goodpasteur EW. Infectious oral papillomatosis in dogs. Am J Clin Pathol 1932;8,43–5.

79. Konishi S, Tokita H, Ogata H. Studies on canine oral papillomatosis. I. Transmission and characterisation of the virus. Nippon Juigaku Zasshi 1972;34:263–8.
80. Ghim S, Newsome J, Bell J, et al. Spontaneous regression in oral papillomas induces systemic antibodies that neutralize canine oral papillomavirus. Exp Mol Pathol 2000; 68:147–51.
81. Bell JA, Sunberg JP, Ghim S, et al. A formalin-inactivated vaccine protects against mucosal papillomavirus infection: a canine model. Pathobiology 1994;62:194–8.
82. Chen Y, Ghim S, jenson AB, et al. Mutant canine oral papillomavirus L1 capsid proteina which form virus.like particles but lack native conformational epitopes. J Gen Virol 1998;79:2137–46.
83. Moore RA, Nicholls PK, Santos EB, et al. Absence of canine oral papillomavirus DNA following prophylactic L1 particle-mediated immunotherapeutic delivery vaccination. J Gen Virol 2002;83:2299–301.
84. Moore RA, Santos EB, Nicholls PK, et al. Intraepithelial DNA immunisation with a plasmid encoding a codon optimized COPY E1 gene sequence but not the wild-type gene sequence completely protects against mucosal challenge with infectious COPV in beagles. Virology 2002;304:451–9.
85. Moore RA, Walcott S, White KL, et al. Therapeutic immunization with COPV early genes by epithelial DNA delivery. Virology 2003;314:630–35.
86. Stanley MA, Moore RA, Nicholls PK, et al. Intra-epithelial vaccination with COPV L1 DNA by particle-mediated DNA delivery protects against mucosal challenge with infectious COPV in beagle dogs. Vaccine 2001;19:2783–92.

Feline Immunodeficiency Virus: Disease Association Versus Causation in Domestic and Nondomestic Felids

Joanna White, BVSc, MACVSc[a],*, Alison Stickney, BVSc, MVs, MACVSc[a], Jacqueline M. Norris, BVSc, PhD[b]

KEYWORDS

- Immunodeficiency virus, feline • Animals, domestic
- Animals, nondomestic • HIV

Since its discovery,[1] feline immunodeficiency virus (FIV) has been the focus of substantial and sustained research efforts, partially in recognition of its potential role as an animal model for human immunodeficiency virus (HIV).[2] Whereas there have been considerable insights into the pathophysiology and immunologic responses to FIV infection, important questions remain regarding the impact of FIV infection on an individual cat and its likely association with specific disease syndromes.

PATHOPHYSIOLOGY

FIV-induced immune dysfunction is characterized by a paradoxical state involving immune hyperactivation and immune suppression. As the disease progresses, FIV-infected cats eventually lose the ability to mount an effective cell-mediated immune response against opportunistic pathogens. Early reports of immune dysfunction demonstrated reduced blastogenesis of peripheral blood mononuclear cells following mitogen stimulation in FIV-infected cats compared with uninfected cats.[3–6] Many studies have since attempted to further characterize the immune dysfunction, concluding that it is multifactorial. Loss of CD4+ T cells and associated reductions in cytokines, chronic antigenic stimulation and anergy, activation of immune regulatory Treg cells, and dendritic cell dysfunction are the major mechanisms by which immune dysfunction can occur in FIV-infected cats.[5,7]

---

[a] Institute of Veterinary, Animal, and Biomedical Sciences, Massey University, Tennent Drive, Palmerston North 4412, New Zealand
[b] Faculty of Veterinary Science, University of Sydney, NSW 2006, Australia
* Corresponding author.
E-mail address: J.White@massey.ac.nz

Vet Clin Small Anim 41 (2011) 1197–1208
doi:10.1016/j.cvsm.2011.07.003
0195-5616/11/$ – see front matter © 2011 Published by Elsevier Inc.

DIAGNOSIS

Commercially available in-house test kits have been the main method of diagnosing FIV status in domestic cats by identifying feline antibodies to FIV gag (p24 or p15) or transmembrane protein (gp40). The sensitivity (82%–100%) and specificity (98%–100%) of these tests is generally considered to be high,[8] but their predictive value is affected by the prevalence of FIV in the population, and cats testing positive with an in-house test should have their diagnosis confirmed.[9] Western blot studies to identify a range of specific antibodies to FIV have generally been considered to be the gold standard for the detection of FIV antibodies but are technically demanding, and indeterminate results are occasionally seen, at least in people tested for HIV.[10,11]

The introduction of a vaccine to protect against FIV in domestic cats has complicated the diagnosis of FIV. Vaccine administration results in the production of antibodies that are detected by commercially available in-house tests and Western blots.[12] An enzyme-linked immunosorbent assay (ELISA) has been developed to detect antibodies specifically against formaldehyde-inactivated virus, and this has been suggested as a method of discriminating between vaccinated cats and FIV-infected cats.[13] However, this assay requires further validation, and to the authors' knowledge is not yet commercially available.

Nucleic acid amplification has been used with increasing frequency to detect viral nucleic acid in blood. Commercial assays qualitatively and more recently quantitatively detect proviral DNA incorporated into the host genome, but experimentally, viral load can also be quantified using real-time polymerase chain reaction (PCR). Following the release of the FIV vaccine, nucleic acid amplification was suggested as an effective way to distinguish between vaccinated and infected cats. However, there have been concerns regarding the sensitivity and specificity of some commercially available PCR assays.[14] False-negative results may occur as a result of sequence variation between isolates, and it is important that primers are designed to detect maximally conserved regions of the genome. The assays are generally extremely sensitive and can detect as few as 1 to 10 copies of viral DNA per sample.[14] Consequently, it is imperative that these assays are performed with technical precision, because contamination of samples can easily lead to false-positive results. Sensitivity and specificity of PCR varies between laboratories and is dependent on factors such as primer design, reagents, and the technical proficiency of the laboratory staff. As the expertise and technology in nucleic acid amplification methods grows, the commercial assays will likely improve and become more reliable for practical use in the diagnosis of FIV. Continued surveillance of the sensitivity and specificity of commercial diagnostic tests is required by independent researchers, especially when the methodology remains confidential and therefore not subject to peer scrutiny.

In non-domestic cats nested PCR, western blots, and antibody tests specific to the FIV gag (p24 or p15) have been evaluated for use in the African lion and found to be highly sensitive, however studies evaluating antibody tests centered on transmembrane protein (gp40) are currently lacking.[15] Given the significant genetic differences within and between clades infecting each feline species, extrapolations from findings in domestic cats needs to be done with caution.

The difficulty of evaluating test performance (sensitivity and specificity) in the absence of an obvious gold standard can be addressed statistically. Bayesian analysis combines prior knowledge regarding test performance including uncertainties (prior distribution), and new test results to estimate a distribution of possible values for test performance in the absence of a gold standard.[16] Bayesian analysis has been applied to FIV diagnostic tests including immunomigration, ELISA, and real-time PCR.[17] Sensitivity and specificity range from 94% to 99.7% and 91% to 98%, respectively, for immunomigration and ELISAs and from 85% to 97% (sensitivity) and 98.8% to 99.9% (specificity) for real-time PCR. The authors have observed, as was demonstrated in this study, equivocal results with the in-house tests and that equivocal results were excluded from the analysis.[17]

DISEASE ASSOCIATIONS IN DOMESTIC CATS

Domestic cats experimentally infected with FIV can develop marked immune dysfunction with severe and progressive respiratory and intestinal disease.[5,18] However, the relationship between seropositivity and disease, especially among naturally infected cats, is less clear. Whereas some surveys have found FIV-positive cats at increased risk of illness,[19] others have demonstrated a similar prevalence of FIV infection among "healthy" and "sick" cats.[20–23]

Severe clinical signs did not develop in experimentally infected animals even with prolonged follow up (6.5 years), although some clinicopathologic differences were noted between FIV negative and positive cats.[24] Fewer secondary infections could be expected when specific pathogen-free cats are experimentally infected with FIV, but observations of naturally infected cats showed that progression to symptomatic FIV infection, feline AIDS, or even persistent clinical disease was not invariable.[25–27]

A case-control study that compared disease associations and outcomes in sick cats found an increased likelihood of death in FIV-positive cats compared with FIV-negative cats.[28] Since then, two cohort studies have compared the survival times of naturally infected FIV-positive with FIV-negative cats and found no statistical difference in survival in either a closed household[25] or among pet cats at Canadian teaching hospitals.[29] In the latter study, control cats were age and sex matched, removing these as potential confounders from the survival analysis.

It is difficult to determine the effect FIV infection will have on an individual cats' survival based on the previous studies. Studies of naturally occurring disease may underestimate the role of FIV because of the potentially prolonged asymptomatic period.[30] Surveys and case control studies are also limited by the inability to determine the temporal relationship between infection and disease. Prospective cohort studies following naturally infected FIV-positive and FIV-negative cats for a period of time would be the ideal way to determine true disease associations, and these studies have been performed,[25] but the asymptomatic period makes this type of study potentially difficult. The proportion of cats that will ultimately develop AIDS or symptomatic FIV infection or with infectious and neoplastic complications of FIV is unknown.[31] For rare diseases, cohort studies are inefficient and potentially expensive.

Hematologic abnormalities are frequently reported in FIV-infected cats, both in the asymptomatic and symptomatic stages of infection.[26,32–38] Nonregenerative anemia, leucocytosis, leucopenia, and thrombocytopenia have all been described, but cytopenias affecting multiple cell lineages seems to be most common. In particular, neutropenia is frequently reported in FIV-infected cats, and this may occur as early as 21 days postinfection.[32]

The mechanism of FIV-induced cytopenias is likely to be multifactorial and result from direct or indirect suppression of hematopoiesis or secondary factors such as opportunistic infection and neoplasia.[39] Direct infection of the bone marrow stromal cells with FIV and subsequent changes in cytokine expression can result in suppression of hematopoiesis.[38] Recently, direct infection of bone marrow progenitor cells (as demonstrated by PCR and immunocytochemistry) has also been implicated in the pathogenesis of peripheral blood cytopenia.[30] Myelodysplasia of various cell lines has been reported in association with the hematologic abnormalities in asymptomatic and symptomatic FIV-infected cats. Unlike feline leukemia virus–associated myelodysplastic syndrome, FIV-associated myelodysplasia does not typically progress to leukemia. One investigator has suggested that the bone marrow changes may be more accurately termed FIV myelopathy rather than myelodysplastic syndrome.[30]

Oral cavity disease has been identified as an important limitation on quality of life for FIV-positive cats. In a large cohort of cats, diseases identified in FIV-positive cats included pyrexia, gingivitis or stomatitis, and respiratory tract signs.[40] A case-control study investigating the prevalence and severity of oral cavity disease in cats from a veterinary teaching hospital and private shelter found that FIV-positive cats were more likely to have oral disease and to have more severe disease than FIV-negative cats. The relationship between FIV infection and disease severity was only significant in cats from the shelter, and there were notable differences in the severity of oral disease between all cats, complicating interpretation of the data.[41] Similarly, oral disease of all forms was more common among FIV-positive than age-matched FIV-negative cats.[29] In contrast, a comparison of cats with and without gingivostomatitis found no increased risk of FIV infection among affected cats.[42] Some of these differences may be due to differences in case definitions: oral disease encompasses a spectrum of disease severity from mild periodontal disease to severe, diffuse gingivostomatitis resulting in anorexia and weight loss. For potentially multifactorial diseases such as those in the oral cavity, determining the contribution of infectious agents such as FIV requires consideration of other potential causes of disease (eg, age, diet, and breed).

The relationship between FIV infection and toxoplasmosis has been investigated repeatedly. Several surveys have identified coinfection of Toxoplasma gondii and FIV in naturally exposed cats but without necessarily confirming a relationship between the two infections or identifying clinicopathologic differences between cats seropositive for T gondii with and without FIV infection.[43,44] When regression methods have been used to account for the variability in seropositivity due to age, FIV-positive cats were more likely to be seropositive for T gondii than FIV-negative cats.[20,45] Because risk factors for both infections include being male and exposure to outdoors, these surveys cannot determine whether the increased likelihood of both infections is simply due to increased exposure.

Immunologic mechanisms to explain a potential disease association between FIV infection and toxoplasmosis have also been studied. Among naturally infected cats, FIV-positive cats with positive toxoplasmosis serology were more likely to have immunoglobulin M antibodies, lower immunoglobulin G antibodies, and reduced lymphocyte responsiveness to T gondii antigens.[46] Variation in experimental methods may be the cause of differences in clinical outcome. For example, differences may be predictable when cats are exposed to T gondii soon after FIV infection[7] compared with 12 months after FIV infection,[47] when kittens are infected or when animals are infected intravenously with either agent.[48] More work is required to clarify if a disease association exists between FIV and toxoplasmosis in naturally exposed cats.

Several descriptive studies identified kidney disease among FIV-positive cats.[21,49–52] Because kidney disease is a common disease of all cats, this result was perhaps not surprising and, in the absence of a control population, unremarkable. Renal disease in FIV-positive animals is biologically plausible based on the microscopic renal abnormalities in a small number of FIV-positive cats[49,53]; the presence of FIV antigen (p24) within tubular, glomerular or interstitial cells[50]; and the presence of nephropathies in people with HIV.[54] In people infected with HIV, patient cofactors play a notable role in disease development, with race being a predictor of the type of renal disease associated with HIV.[55]

Two case-control studies of naturally infected cats have identified an association between FIV infection and indicators of renal disease including azotemia, proteinuria,[53] and small kidneys,[51] but no associations were identified in a third study.[56] Specific pathogen-free cats experimentally infected with FIV were more likely to have evidence of renal disease than FIV-negative control cats.[24,53]

Observations from case-control studies confirm a complicated relationship between FIV and kidney disease that appears to be age dependent. FIV does not influence initial disease severity but does adversely affect survival times. Among cats with chronic kidney disease, younger cats were more likely to be FIV-positive than cats without chronic kidney disese,[57] and the presence FIV infection increased the hazard of death 2-fold (J. White thesis, unpublished observations, 2011).

Among all the studies attempting to associate FIV infection with disease, the most convincing are those reports describing neurologic disease and lymphoma. The first reported cases of FIV in cats described neurologic abnormalities. These cats displayed behavioral changes with compulsive roaming and abnormal facial movements. Since then, similar reports of neurologic signs have been described in both naturally and experimentally infected cats, independent of secondary infections affecting the nervous system. The majority of reported clinical signs can be attributed to cortical and subcortical neuronal dysfunction,[58] with behavioral changes predominating. Affected cats may show signs of dementia, loss of social behavior, aggression, loss of toilet training, altered sleep patterns, and compulsive roaming behavior.[1,31,59,60] Facial twitching, ataxia, reduced peripheral sensory and motor conduction, seizures, and gait abnormalities have also been described.[1,61–64] Cats may lose the ability to learn new tasks, and this has been attributed to impaired cognition.[63]

FIV enters the central nervous system when infected macrophages or monocytes cross the blood-brain or blood-cerebrospinal fluid (CSF) barrier. The neurotropism of FIV has been confirmed following isolation of virus in brain tissue and CSF, the finding of anti-FIV antibodies within the CSF, and CSF pleocytosis in affected cats.[60,65,66] Neurotropism is strain dependent, and brain-derived isolates are primarily monocytotropic.[65] The pathogenesis of neurologic disease is likely to be multifactorial, but affected cats have progressive neuronal loss and higher levels of excitatory neurotoxic compounds.[66] It is thought that FIV sensitizes neurons to the effects of glutamate and inhibits glutamate uptake by astrocytes, leading to increased intracellular calcium, neuronal swelling, and death.[67] Neuronal glutamate toxicity can be induced in vitro with purified envelope glycoprotein, suggesting that the mechanism is indirect and does not require whole, infectious virions.[68] FIV-induced neurologic disease seems to parallel overall disease progression and decline in CD4/CD8 ratio, but pathologic changes have also been described in asymptomatic FIV-positive cats.[61]

FIV infected cats with immunodeficiency may develop neoplasia due to reduced immune suppression of the cell-mediated immune response. Recently however, a direct role for FIV in oncogenesis has also been demonstrated.[69] An oncogenic role has been best described in cases of lymphoma, and an association between lymphoma and FIV is now well-recognized.[70–75] The majority of reports describe predominately B cell lymphoma in FIV-infected cats, with a large proportion of the tumors being extranodal.[70,73,75] FIV is thought to induce lymphoma via both direct and indirect mechanisms. Indirectly, chronic antigenic stimulation with FIV leads to activation of B cells, which may undergo malignant transformation if replication errors occur.[76] A direct mechanism has also been proposed whereby the insertion of provirus into the host genome leads to loss of a tumor suppressor gene[69] or activation of an oncogene. One study demonstrated the presence of provirus within a clone of malignant lymphocytes, which is supportive of a direct role of FIV in oncogenesis.[76]

Some of the differences in disease expression in the published literature may reflect host, virus, or experimental method variation. As a generalization, it is unusual for an infectious agent to be a "sufficient cause," in other words one that, acting alone, always produces disease.[77] The role of concurrent disease and age has been clearly demonstrated experimentally. Specific pathogen-free cats experimentally infected with FIV developed B cell lymphoma, neurologic disease, and wasting syndromes, whereas cats with a more typical history of exposure to other infectious agents developed chronic stomatitis and upper respiratory disease.[78] The role of age has also been demonstrated experimentally, with young animals showing greatest susceptibility to disease compared with young adult and older cats.[79] Variation in virulence due to FIV strain or subtype is possible, and warrants further study, but at least one reported difference in FIV strain virulence[80] became markedly less apparent when cats of comparable age were infected.[81] The severity of clinical signs that develops after experimental FIV infection is dependent on the dose of FIV administered.[82]

Overall, the disease-causing potential of FIV would seem to be less than that of HIV. The diseases that are described in FIV-positive cats also occur in FIV-negative cats, and the existence of any association, let alone the presence of any causative pathway, remains to be confirmed for many diseases, with lymphoma and neurologic disease being the most obvious exceptions.

DISEASE IN NONDOMESTIC FELIDS

FIV strains have been present in the nondomestic cat population longer than in domestic cats,[83] however, the relationship between FIV infection and disease causation or association is less clear. Whereas FIV infects many feline species, selective pressures within each host species have resulted in development of predominantly species-specific strains named in accordance with the infecting felid species such as FIV-Ple (African lion), FIV-Aju (cheetah), FIV-Ppa (leopard), FIV-Pco (puma), FIV-Pon (jaguar), and so on.[84] Although interspecies transmission among the nondomestic felids is not impossible, it is rare.[85,86] Therefore, the role of FIV in disease causation needs to be made on an individual felid species level using an evidence-based approach.

There are numerous potential obstacles in accurately assessing the role of FIV in the cause of disease in non domestic felids, making comparisons between infected and noninfected populations in the same environmental settings difficult. For example, prevalence of FIV in African lions in many African countries ranges from 68% to 100%, whereas 22% to 40% of African cheetahs mainly in the Serengeti population and 26% to 46% of the leopards are infected with their respective FIV.[84,87-89] Second, in the wild it is difficult to monitor infected populations longitudinally, and as a consequence there are limited studies in nondomestic felids.[90] Finally, the same issues arise as with domestic cats in differentiating the role of FIV as a direct agent of disease, a secondary agent resulting from immune suppression, or simply an incidental finding.

Host-virus symbiosis, or adaptation resulting from the natural selection of resistant felids and the attenuation of FIV over the extended time frame of their relationship, has been suggested as a possible explanation for the absence of obvious clinical manifestations in many FIV-infected nondomestic felids.[89,91] However, it is unwise to assume this explanation to be true of all FIV subtypes in all felid species, and so the possibility of FIV-associated disease in nondomestic felids has remained a possibility, and researchers in the last decade have actively sought the answer to this question. Indeed, when comparing FIV-Ple subtypes B and E of African lions in Africa for their usage of the important primary attachment receptors (CD134) and coreceptors (CXCR4) on activated $CD4^+$ T lymphocytes, McEwan and colleagues[92] found that only FIV-Ple subtype E was able to use these receptors, as is the case in domestic cats, indicating differences in their likely in vivo pathogenicity and cell trophism.

Immunologic dysfunction similar to that seen in domestic cats, such as decrease in $CD4^+$ lymphocytes or a reduction in the overall $CD4^+/CD8^+$ ratio, has been seen in African lions and pumas infected with FIV-Ple and FIV-Pco, respectively. However, increases in $CD5^-$ and $CD4^-/CD8^-$ cells as well as the $CD8^+$ B^{low} subset indicated evidence of host adaption to the virus and was suggested as a reason for the asymptomatic infection.[90]

Analogous to the lentiviral encephalopathy in domestic cats and humans, an association between FIV-Ple and neurologic disease was reported in three African lions displaying lymphocytes subset alterations and progressive behavioral, locomotor, and neuroanatomic abnormalities in the absence of other known neuropathogens. Proviral tissue loads were low in brain tissue, suggestive of a non specific encephalopathy rather than the direct effects of viral replication.[93]

Recently, Roelke and colleagues[94] found further evidence to challenge the belief that FIV does not cause apparent pathology in nondomestic felids. In a longitudinal study over 6 years of various clinical, biochemical, histologic, and serologic parameters of FIV-Ple–positive and –negative African lions in Botswana, several important abnormalities similar to those caused by lentivirus infection in HIV were found in the FIV-Ple–positive lions. These abnormalities included lymphadenopathy, gingivitis, and tongue papillomas, whereas clinicopathologic findings included abnormal red blood cell parameters, elevated gamma globulin, depleted lymphoid cells within spleen and lymph node biopsies, and mild elevations of liver indices. These researchers concluded that prolonged FIV-Ple infections in free-range lions could result in adverse clinical, immunologic, and pathologic outcomes. These types of studies would be easy to mirror in the many captive lion and other felids populations in which monitoring for disease is in many places diligent and fastidious, lending themselves to longitudinal comparisons between FIV-positive and -negative populations.

Similarly, Brown and colleagues[95] monitored a group of 28 free-ranging Pallas' cats in a long-term ecology study in Mongolia from 2000 to 2007, collecting serial blood samples and ultimately necropsy tissues. They found the seroprevalence of FIV-Oma was 25%, and sequence analysis showed a monophyletic virus with little genetic diversity between cats. FIV-positive cats were found to have severe lymphoid depletion in the spleen and moderate lymphoid depletion in the lymph nodes. Continued monitoring of clinical correlates is recommended in this threatened species.

SUMMARY

There are common issues and constraints on our ability to clearly establish the association between FIV infection and the pathogenesis of disease in both domestic and nondomestic felids. Because of the importance of secondary or concurrent infections in the pathogenesis of disease associated with FIV, use of experimental models may not yield answers in domestic cats and is certainly not feasible in non domestic felids, many of which are endangered species. Therefore, researchers might consider early surveillance programs across varied populations and detailed, cohort studies of naturally infected animals to provide further insights. The power of these studies would be enhanced, especially in more unusual presumed disease associations, if a multicenter approach was taken.

REFERENCES

1. Pedersen NC, Ho EW, Brown ML, et al. Isolation of a T-lymphotropic virus from domestic cats with an immunodeficiency-like syndrome. Science 1987;235(4790):790–3.

2. Bendinelli M, Pistello M, Lombardi S, et al. Feline immunodeficiency virus: an interesting model for AIDS studies and an important cat pathogen. Clini Microbiol Rev 1995;8(1):87–112.

3. Taniguchi A, Ishida T, Konno A, et al. Altered mitogen response of peripheral blood lymphocytes in different stages of feline immunodeficiency virus infection. Nihon Juiquaku Zasshi 1990;52(3):513–8.

4. Lin DS, Bowman DD, Jacobson RH, et al. Suppression of lymphocyte blastogenesis to mitogens in cats experimentally infected with feline immunodeficiency virus. Vet Immunol Immunopathol 1990;26(2):183–9.

5. Torten M, Franchini M, Barlough JE, et al. Progressive immune dysfunction in cats experimentally infected with feline immunodeficiency virus. J Virol 1991;65(5):2225–30.

6. Bishop SA, Williams NA, Gruffydd-Jones TJ, et al. Impaired T-cell priming and proliferation in cats infected with feline immunodeficiency virus. AIDS 1992;6(3):287–93.

7. Lin DS, Bowman DD, Jacobson RH. Immunological changes in cats with concurrent Toxoplasma gondii and feline immunodeficiency virus infections. J Clin Microbiol 1992;30(1):17–24.

8. Hartmann K, Griessmayr P, Schulz B, et al. Quality of different in-clinic test systems for feline immunodeficiency virus and feline leukaemia virus infection. J Feline Med Surg 2007;9:439–45.

9. Levy J, Crawford C, Hartmann K, et al. 2008 American Association of Feline Practitioners' feline retrovirus management guidelines. J Feline Med Surg 2008;10(3):300–16.

10. Mylonakis E, Paliou M, Lally M, et al. Laboratory testing for infection with the human immunodeficiency virus: established and novel approaches. Am J Med 2000;109(7):568–76.

11. Yilmaz G. Diagnosis of HIV infection and laboratory monitoring of its therapy. J Clin Virol 2001;21(3):187–96.

12. Levy JK, Crawford PC, Slater MR. Effect of vaccination against feline immunodeficiency virus on results of serologic testing in cats. J Am Vet Med Assoc 2004;225(10):1558–61.

13. Levy JK, Crawford PC, Kusuhara H, et al. Differentiation of feline immunodeficiency virus vaccination, infection, or vaccination and infection in cats. J Vet Intern Med 2008;22(2):330–4.

14. Crawford PC, Slater MR, Levy JK. Accuracy of polymerase chain reaction assays for diagnosis of feline immunodeficiency virus infection in cats. J Am Vet Med Assoc 2005;226(9):1503–7.

15. Adams HM, Vuuren S, Kania AM, et al. Sensitivity and specificity of a nested polymerase chain reaction for detection of lentivirus infection in lions (Panthera leo). J Zoo Wildl Med 2010;41:608–15.

16. Browne W, Stryhn H. Introduction to bayesian analysis. In: Dahoo I, Martin W, H Stryhn H, editors. Veterinary epidemiologic research. Charlottetown (Canada): VER Inc; 2010. p. 637–61.

17. Pinches MDG, Diesel G, Helps CR, et al. An update on FIV and FeLV test performance using a bayesian statistical approach. Vet Clin Pathol 2007;36(2):141–7.

18. Matsumura S, Ishida T, Washizu T, et al. Pathologic features of acquired immunodeficiency-like syndrome in cats experimentally infected with feline immunodeficiency virus. J Vet Med Sci 1993;55(3):387–94.

19. Muirden A. Prevalence of feline leukaemia virus and antibodies to feline immunodeficiency virus and feline coronavirus in stray cats sent to an RSPCA hospital. Vet Rec 2002;150(20):621–5.

20. Akhtardanesh B, Ziaali N, Sharifi H, et al. Feline immunodeficiency virus, feline leukemia virus and Toxoplasma gondii in stray and household cats in Kerman-Iran: Seroprevalence and correlation with clinical and laboratory findings. Res Vet Sci 2010;89(2):306–10.

21. Norris JM, Bell ET, Hales L, et al. Prevalence of feline immunodeficiency virus infection in domesticated and feral cats in eastern Australia. J Feline Med Surg 2007;9(4):300–8.
22. Hitt ME, Spangler L, McCarville C. Prevalence of feline immunodeficiency virus in submissions of feline serum to a diagnostic laboratory in Atlantic Canada. Can Vet J 1992;33(11):723–76.
23. Robertson ID, Robinson WF, Alexander R, et al. Feline immunodeficiency virus and feline leukaemia virus in cats. Australian Veterinary Practitioner 1990;20(2):66–9.
24. Hofmann-Lehmann R, Holznagel E, Ossent P, et al. Parameters of disease progression in long-term experimental feline retrovirus (feline immunodeficiency virus and feline leukemia virus) infections: hematology, clinical chemistry, and lymphocyte subsets. Clin Diagn Lab Immunol 1997;4(1):33–42.
25. Addie D, Dennis JM, Toth S, et al. Long-term impact on a closed household of pet cats of natural infection with feline coronavirus, feline leukaemia virus and feline immunodeficiency virus. Vet Rec 2000;146(15):419–24.
26. Shelton GH, Linenberger ML, Persik MT, et al. Prospective hematologic and clinico-pathologic study of asymptomatic cats with naturally acquired feline immunodeficiency virus infection. J Vet Intern Med 1995;9(3):133–40.
27. Ishida T, Taniguchi A, Matsumura S, et al. Long-term clinical observations on feline immunodeficiency virus infected asymptomatic carriers. Vet Immunol Immunopathol 1992;35(1–2):15–22.
28. Shaw SE, Robertson ID, Robinson WF, et al. Feline immunodeficiency virus: disease associations. Australian Veterinary Practitioner 1990;20(4):194–8.
29. Ravi M, Wobeser GA, Taylor SM, et al. Naturally acquired feline immunodeficiency virus (FIV) infection in cats from western Canada: Prevalence, disease associations, and survival analysis. Can Vet J 2010;51(3):271–6.
30. Fujino Y, Horiuchi H, Mizukoshi F, et al. Prevalence of hematological abnormalities and detection of infected bone marrow cells in asymptomatic cats with feline immunodeficiency virus Infection. Vet Microbiol 2009;136(3–4):217–25.
31. Pedersen NC, Yamamoto JK, Ishida T, et al. Feline immunodeficiency virus infection. Vet Immunol Immunopathol 1989;21(1):111–29.
32. Sprague WS, TerWee JA, VandeWoude S. Temporal association of large granular lymphocytosis, neutropenia, proviral load, and FasL mRNA in cats with acute feline immunodeficiency virus infection. Vet Immunol Immunopathol 2010;134(1–2): 115–21.
33. Sparkes AH, Hopper CD, Millard WG, et al. Feline immunodeficiency virus infection. Clinicopathologic findings in 90 naturally occurring cases. J Vet Intern Med 1993;7(2): 85–90.
34. Hopper CD, Sparkes AH, Gruffyd-Jones TJ, et al. Clinical and laboratory findings in cats infected with feline immunodeficiency virus. Vet Rec 1989;125(13):341–6.
35. Fleming EJ, McCaw DL, Smith JA, et al. Clinical, hematologic, and survival data from cats infected with feline immunodeficiency virus: 42 cases (1983–1988). J Am Vet Med Assoc 1991;199(7):913–6.
36. Kohmoto M, Uetsuka K, Ikeda Y, et al. Eight-year observation and comparative study of specific pathogen-free cats experimentally infected with feline immunodeficiency virus (FIV) subtypes A and B: terminal acquired immunodeficiency syndrome in a cat infected with FIV petaluma strain. J Vet Med Sci 1998;60(3):315–21.
37. Deniz A. Evaluation of clinical findings, some hematological and biochemical findings, and age and sex status in feline immunodeficiency virus (FIV) seropositive cats with clinical symptoms and without clinical symptoms. Turkish Journal of Veterinary & Animal Sciences 2001;25(4):409–19.

38. Gleich S, Hartmann K. Hematology and serum biochemistry of feline immunodeficiency virus-infected and feline leukemia virus-infected cats. J Vet Intern Med 2009; 23(3):552–8.

39. Shelton GH, Linenberger ML. Hematologic abnormalities associated with retroviral infections in the cat. Semin Vet Med Surg (Small Anim) 1995;10(4):220–33.

40. Hosie MJ, Robertson C, Jarrett O. Prevalence of feline leukaemia virus and antibodies to feline immunodeficiency virus in cats in the United-Kingdom. Vet Rec 1989; 125(11):293–7.

41. Tenorio AP, Franti AP, Madewell BR, et al. Chronic oral infections of cats and their relationship to persistent oral carriage of feline calici-, immunodeficiency, or leukemia viruses. Vet Immunol Immunopathol 1991;29(1–2):1–14.

42. Quimby JM, et al. Evaluation of the association of Bartonella species, feline herpesvirus 1, feline calicivirus, feline leukemia virus and feline immunodeficiency virus with chronic feline gingivostomatitis. J Feline Med Surg 2008;10(1):66–72.

43. Dubey JP, Lappin MR, Kwok OCH, et al. Seroprevalence of Toxoplasma gondii and concurrent Bartonella spp. feline immunodeficiency virus, and feline leukemia virus infections in cats from Grenada, West Indies. J Parasitol 2009;95(5):1129–33.

44. O'Neil SA, Lappin MR, Reif JS, et al. Clinical and epidemiological aspects of feline immunodeficiency virus and Toxoplasma gondii coinfections in cats. J Am Anim Hosp Assoc 1991;27(2):211–20.

45. Dorny P, Speybroeck N, Verstraete S, et al. Serological survey of Toxoplasma gondii, feline immunodeficiency virus and feline leukaemia virus in urban stray cats in Belgium. Vet Rec 2002;151(21):626–9.

46. Lappin MR, Marks A, Greene CE, et al. Effect of feline immunodeficiency virus infection on Toxoplasmosis gondii-specific humoral and cell-mediated immune responses of cats with serological evidence of Toxoplasmosis. J Vet Intern Med 1993;7(2):95–100.

47. Lappin MR, George JW, Pedersen NC, et al. Primary and secondary Toxoplasma gondii infection in normal and feline immunodeficiency virus-infected cats. J Parasitol 1996;82(5):733–42.

48. Davidson MG, Rottman JB, English RV, et al. Feline immunodeficiency virus predisposes cats to acute generalized toxoplasmosis. Am J Pathol 1993;143(5):1486–97.

49. Poli A, Abramo F, Taccini E, et al. Renal involvement in feline immunodeficiency virus infection: a clinicopathological study. Nephron 1993;64(2):282–8.

50. Poli A, Abramo F, Matteucci D, et al. Renal involvement in feline immunodeficiency virus infection: p24 antigen detection, virus isolation and PCR analysis. Vet Immunol Immunopathol. 1995;46(1–2):13–20.

51. Thomas JB, Robinson WF, Chadwick BJ, et al. Association of renal disease indicators with feline immunodeficiency virus infection. J Am Anim Hosp Assoc 1993;29(4): 320–6.

52. Tozon N. Proteinuria in clinical diagnostic of renal disease in cats infected with feline immunodeficiency virus. Slov Vet Res 2000;37(1/2):53–66.

53. Levy JK. CVT update: Feline immunodeficiency virus. In: Bonagura JD, editor. Kirk's current veterinary therapy XIII: small animal practice. Saunders: Philadelphia; 2000. p. 284–91.

54. Weiner NJ, Goodman JW, Kimmel PL. The HIV-associated renal diseases: current insight into pathogenesis and treatment. Kidney Int 2003;63(5):1618–31.

55. Kimmel PL. The nephropathies of HIV infection: pathogenesis and treatment. Curr Opin Nephrol Hypertens 2000;9(2):117–22.

56. Arjona A, Escolar E, Soto I, et al. Seroepidemiological survey of infection by feline leukemia virus and immunodeficiency virus in Madrid and correlation with some clinical aspects. J Clin Microbiol 2000;38(9):3448–9.

57. White JD, Malik R, Norris JM, et al. Association between naturally occurring chronic kidney disease and feline immunodeficiency virus infection status in cats. J Am Vet Med Assoc 2010;236(4):424–9.

58. Podell M, March PA, Buck WR, et al. The feline model of neuroAIDS: understanding the progression towards AIDS dementia. J Psychopharmacol 2000;14(3):205–13.

59. Prosperogarcia O, Herold N, Phillips TR, et al. Sleep patterns are disturbed in cats infected with feline immunodeficiency virus. Proc Natl Acad Sci U S A 1994;91(26): 12947–51.

60. Phillips TR, Prospero-Garcia O, Puaoi DL, et al. Neurological abnormalities associated with feline immunodeficiency virus-infection. J Gen Virol 1994;75:979–87.

61. Power C, Moench T, Peeling J, et al. Feline immunodeficiency virus causes increased glutamate levels and neuronal loss in brain. Neuroscience 1997;77(4):1175–85.

62. Power C, Buist R, Johnston JB, et al. Neurovirulence in feline immunodeficiency virus-infected neonatal cats is viral strain specific and dependent on systemic immune suppression. J Virol 1998;72(11):9109–15.

63. Steigerwald ES, Sarter M, March P, et al. Effects of feline immunodeficiency virus on cognition and behavioral function in cats. J Acquir Immune Defic Syndr 1999;20(5): 411–9.

64. Phillips TR, Prospero-Garcia O, Wheeler DW, et al. Neurologic dysfunctions caused by a molecular clone of feline immunodeficiency virus, FIV-PPR. J Neurovirol 1996; 2(6):388–96.

65. Dow SW, Poss ML, Hoover EA. Feline immunodeficiency virus—a neurotropic lentivirus. J Acquir Immune Defic Syndr Hum Retrovirol 1990;3(7):658–68.

66. Podell M, Hayes K, Oglesbee M, et al. Progressive encephalopathy associated with CD4/CD8 inversion in adult FIV-infected cats. J Acquir Immune Defic Syndr Hum Retrovirol 1997;15(5):332–40.

67. Gruol D, Yu N, Parsons KL, et al. Neurotoxic effects of feline immunodeficiency virus, FIV-PPR. J Neurovirol 1998;4(4):415–25.

68. Bragg DC, Meeker RB, Duff BA, et al. Neurotoxicity of FIV and FIV envelope protein in feline cortical cultures. Brain Res 1999;816(2):431–7.

69. Beatty J, Terry A, MacDonald J, et al. Feline immunodeficiency virus integration in B-cell lymphoma identifies a candidate tumor suppressor gene on human chromosome 15q15. Cancer Res 2002;62(24):7175–80.

70. Hutson CA, Rideout BA, Pedersen NC. Neoplasia associated with feline immunodeficiency virus-infection in cats of southern California. J Am Vet Med Assoc 1991; 199(10):1357–62.

71. Callanan JJ, Mccandish IA, O'Noil B, et al. Lymphosarcoma in experimentally induced feline immunodeficiency virus infection [corrected]. Vet Rec 1992;130(14):293–5.

72. Barr MC, Butt MT, Anderson KL, et al. Spinal lymphosarcoma and disseminated mastocytoma associated with feline immunodeficiency virus infection in a cat. J Am Vet Med Assoc 1993;202(12):1978–80.

73. Poli A, Abramo F, Baldinotti F, et al. Malignant lymphoma associated with experimentally induced feline immunodeficiency virus infection. J Comp Pathol 1994;110(4): 319–28.

74. Shelton GH, Grant CK, Cotter SM, et al. Feline immunodeficiency virus and feline leukemia virus infections and their relationships to lymphoid malignancies in cats: a retrospective study (1968–1988). J Acquir Immune Defic Syndr 1990;3(6):623–30.

75. Gabor LJ, Love DN, Malik R, et al. Feline immunodeficiency virus status of Australian cats with lymphosarcoma. Aust Vet J 2001;79(8):540–5.

76. Beatty JA, Callanan JJ, Terry A, et al. Molecular and immunophenotypical characterization of a feline immunodeficiency virus (FIV)-associated lymphoma: a direct role for FIV in B-lymphocyte transformation? J Virol 1998;72(1):767–71.

77. Dahoo I, Martin W, Stryhn H. Introduction and causal concepts. In: Veterinary epidemiologic research. Dahoo I, Martin W, Stryhn H, editors. Charlottetown (Canada): VER Inc; 2010. p. 1–23.

78. English RV, Nelson P, Johnson CM, et al. Development of clinical disease in cats experimentally infected with feline immunodeficiency virus. J Infect Dis 1994;170(3):543–52.

79. George JW, Pedersen NC, Higgins J. The effect of age on the course of experimental feline immunodeficiency virus infection in cats. AIDS Res Hum Retroviruses 1993;9(9): 897–905.

80. Diehl LJ, Mathiason-Dubard CK, O'Neil LL, et al. Induction of accelerated feline immunodeficiency virus disease by acute-phase virus passage. J Virol 1995;69(10):6149–57.

81. Pedersen NC, Leutenegger CM, Woo J, et al. Virulence differences between two field isolates of feline immunodeficiency virus (FIV-APetaluma and FIV-CPGammar) in young adult specific pathogen free cats. Vet Immunol Immunopathol 2001;79(1/2):53–67.

82. Hokanson RM, TerWee J, Choi InSoo, et al. Dose response studies of acute feline immunodeficiency virus PPR strain infection in cats. Vet Microbiol 2000;76(4):311–27.

83. Pecon-Slattery J, Troyer JL, Johnson WE, et al. Evolution of feline immunodeficiency virus in Felidae: implications for human health and wildlife ecology. Vet Immunol Immunopathol 2008;123(1–2):32–44.

84. Troyer JL, Pecon-Slattery J, Roelke ME, et al. Seroprevalence and genomic divergence of circulating strains of feline immunodeficiency virus among Felidae and Hyaenidae species. J Virol 2005;79(13):8282–94.

85. Troyer JL, VandeWoude S, Pecon-Slattery J, et al. FIV cross-species transmission: an evolutionary prospective. Vet Immunol Immunopathol 2008;123(1–2):159–66.

86. Franklin SP, Troyer JL, Terwee JA, et al. Frequent transmission of immunodeficiency viruses among bobcats and pumas. J Virol 2007;81(20):10961–9.

87. Driciru M, Siefert L, Prager KC, et al. A serosurvey of viral infections in lions (Panthera leo), from Queen Elizabeth National Park, Uganda. J Wildl Dis 2006;42(3):667–71.

88. Olmsted RA, Langley R, Roelke ME, et al. Worldwide prevalence of lentivirus infection in wild feline species: epidemiologic and phylogenetic aspects. J Virol 1992;66(10): 6008–18.

89. Brown EW, Miththapala S, O'Brien SJ. Prevalence of exposure to feline immunodeficiency virus in exotic felid species. J Zoo Wildlife Med 1993;24(3):357–64.

90. Roelke ME, Pecon-Slattery J, Taylor S, et al. T-lymphocyte profiles in FIV-infected wild lions and pumas reveal CD4 depletion. Journal Wildl Dise 2006;42(2):234–48.

91. Brown EW, Yuhki N, Packer C, et al. A lion lentivirus related to feline immunodeficiency virus— epidemiologic and phylogenetic aspects. J Virol 1994;68(9):5953–68.

92. McEwan WA, McMonagle EL, Logan N, et al. Genetically divergent strains of feline immunodeficiency virus from the domestic cat (Felis catus) and the African lion (Panthera leo) share usage of CD134 and CXCR4 as entry receptors. J Virol 2008; 82(21):10953–8.

93. Brennan G, Podell MD, Wack R, et al. Neurologic disease in captive lions (Panthera leo) with low-titer lion lentivirus infection. J Clin Microbiol 2006;44(12):4345–52.

94. Roelke ME, Brown MA, Troyer JL, et al. Pathological manifestations of feline immunodeficiency virus (FIV) infection in wild African lions. Virology 2009;390(1):1–12.

95. Brown MA, Munkhtsog JL, Troyer S, et al. Feline immunodeficiency virus (FIV) in wild Pallas' cats. Vet Immunol Immunop 2010;134:90–5.

Canine Brucellosis Management

Chelsea L. Makloski, DVM, MS

KEYWORDS

• Brucellosis • *Brucella canis* • Infertility • Abortion

Infertility in dogs is a growing concern in breeding kennels. There are a number of bacteria, viruses, and husbandry practices that must be considered to determine the cause of decreased litter sizes, abortions, weak puppies, and lack of pregnancy, but brucellosis should be at the top of the differential list.

Brucella canis, the causative agent of canine brucellosis, is the leading cause of infertility in domestic canids, more specifically, breeding kennels worldwide.[1] This small, rough, gram-negative coccobacillus intracellular bacterium[2] was first isolated by Leland Carmichael in 1966.[1–3] It has had a huge impact on the canine breeding industry economically, costing some clients tens of thousands of dollars in loss of litters and breeding stock, veterinary and diagnostic costs, and reputation, in this author's experience.

B canis is an intracellular bacterium that has a predilection for steroid-producing tissues such as the testicles, epididymi, and prostate of male dogs and the uterus of female dogs. In addition to these tissues, this bacterium will also be found in the eyes, spinal column, liver, spleen, and lymph nodes on a regular basis. Due to this, canine brucellosis may be manifested as infertility as well as chronic, poorly responding uveitis,[4,5] discospondylitis within the thoracic and lumbar vertebrae,[6–9] and meningitis.[10] These other clinical signs may be seen in spayed and neutered pets that may never present for infertility issues.

EPIDEMIOLOGY

In recent years, this disease appears to becoming more prevalent in breeding kennels across the country. Oklahoma alone has seen an increase in the domestic dog population from 2% in 1994 through 1995 to 13% in 2002 through 2003, with numbers continuing to rise today.[11] This may be due to the growing number of breeding kennels; the buying, selling, and trading of infected dogs; and the increased incidence of semen shipped around the country and world. Some reports indicate that stray and feral dogs are predominant reservoirs of the bacteria,[1,12] which may be the case in many Third World countries, but recent research from northern Oklahoma In which stray dogs from a local shelter were tested indicates that less than 2% of the stray population are serologically positive with none of the dogs having been culture positive (Makloski and colleagues, unpublished data).

The author has nothing to disclose.

JEH Equine Reproduction Specialists, 1030 Roland Road, PO Box 650, Whitesboro, TX 76273, USA
E-mail address: cmakloski.jehers@yahoo.com

TRANSMISSION

This bacterium primarily enters the body through contact of the genital, oronasal, and conjunctival mucosa but may also enter though skin lesions. The most common mode of transmission is venereal, although dogs can become infected when they are exposed to or ingest infected fetal membranes, aborted fetuses, vulvar discharge, or urine from infected dogs.[13–15] Artificial insemination will protect male dogs from contracting the disease from infected females, but this reproductive technique will not protect the female if inseminated with infected semen. Many of the commonly used commercial semen extenders do not inhibit the growth of B canis even after cooling to 37°F for 5 days in some cases (Makloski and colleagues, unpublished research). Some puppies, if not infected in utero, which will most likely occur, can become infected by ingesting milk from lactating females as the somatic cell count is normally very high in canine milk[13] and this is an intracellular bacterium. Although it is rare, transmission can occur via saliva and tears.[16]

Infection can also occur via fomites such as water and food bowls, equipment, and clothing. This bacterium may survive in the environment for several months in conditions of high humidity, low temperatures, and no sunlight, especially if organic material is present. B canis can also withstand drying and can survive in dust and soil.[17]

CLINICAL SIGNS

The most common clinical sign associated with B canis is infertility. It is important to collect a thorough history from the owner and determine if there are actually fertility issues or if poor management is the culprit. In many cases, poor management may lead to a canine brucellosis outbreak in breeding kennels.

In the female, outward signs of B canis infection are limited. The classic symptom of canine brucellosis in the bitch is a late-term abortion (45–55 days' gestation), resulting in the birth of stillborn puppies that are often autolysed, having subcutaneous edema, congestion and hemorrhage of the subcutaneous abdominal region, serosanguinous peritoneal fluid loss with focal infiltration of lymphoid cells, and degenerative lesions in the liver, spleen, kidneys, and intestines[16] (**Fig. 1**). The bitch will continue to excrete vulvar discharge with high numbers of bacteria for several weeks after the abortion or parturition.[3] If the puppies survive, they may be weak and

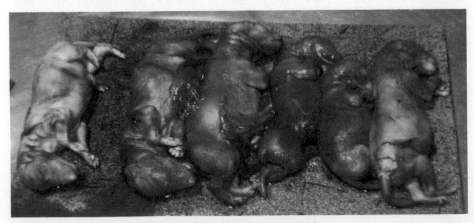

Fig. 1. Puppies from a late-term abortion (56 days' gestation).

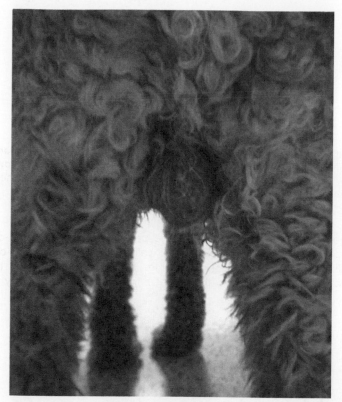

Fig. 2. Scrotal asymmetry. Note the stud dog's left testicle is smaller than the right testicle. Further diagnostics revealed a small atrophied left testicle and epididymis and the right testicle was small with an enlarged epididymis (epididymitis).

die within a few hours or weeks of birth. Some apparently normal puppies will survive but show clinical signs or test positive for the disease as they age, sometimes waiting until puberty.[18] Females may also exhibit embryo resorption or conception failure.[16]

Males may have more obvious signs of *B canis*. During the acute stages of the disease, many male dogs may have epididymitis, which results in swelling of the epididymis and leads to pain and discomfort in the scrotum. This may lead to licking of the scrotum, then scrotal edema, dermatitis, and scrotal asymmetry in unilateral cases **(Fig. 2)**. Chronically, the epididymis will decrease in size, as will the testes. Orchitis is an infrequent clinical sign but will result in testicular necrosis[19] **(Figs. 3** and **4)**. Testicular damage initiates the development of antisperm antibodies that may be found in the blood and prostatic fluid at about 11 to 14 weeks postinfection. Autoagglutination of the sperm can then be visualized starting at approximately 18 weeks postinfection.[20,21] *B canis* also localizes in the prostate of the male, which may lead to classic clinical signs of prostatitis **(Fig. 5)**, including enlarged and painful prostate and difficulty urinating and defecating.

In addition to these clinical signs, clinicians and owners may observe chronic, unresponsive uveitis, discospondylitis, and low-grade meningitis as previously discussed.

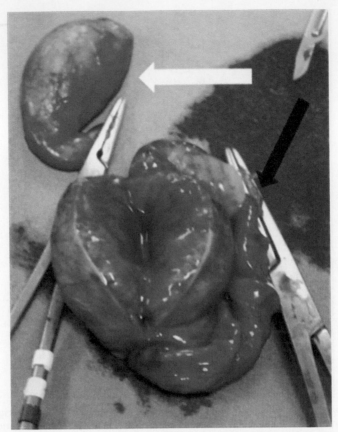

Fig. 3. Testicles that where removed due to illness, pain, and scrotal asymmetry. The patient had tested positive on RSAT prior to surgery. The confirmatory AGIDcpa was also positive and culture of the testicular tissues indicated that the testicle was infected with *B canis*. Note the normal-sized testicle indicated by the white arrow and the necrotic tissue of the affected testicle indicated by the black arrow. The spermatic cord is also engorged, as well as the epididymis.

DIAGNOSIS

Diagnosis of canine brucellosis can be difficult, and as diagnosticians, veterinarians cannot rely solely on one testing modality. The most common historical finding is infertility, but veterinarians must remember that many patients are adopted from shelters or purchased from breeding kennels as a family pet and may be spayed or neutered, so there is no known history of infertility in these cases. A thorough physical exam is necessary to gain basic information on vision, weight, locomotion, discharge, or any palpable swellings. Routine blood work and urinalysis may be collected but are often unremarkable in this disease.

Positive blood culture is a definitive diagnosis for *B canis*. Dogs are generally bacteremic starting 4 to 6 weeks after oronasal exposure and may remain bacteremic for 1 to 5 years.[22] The number of organisms in the circulating leukocytes may be low, making multiple samples necessary. Previous antibiotic therapy may make culturing difficult. Tissues from canine abortions, vaginal discharge, semen, lymph node, and bone marrow aspirates and urine are also great areas to collect culture samples. Due

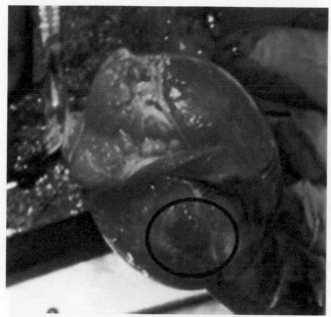

Fig. 4. Testicular abscess infected with *B canis*.

to the slow growth rate, bacterial overgrowth, and the intracellular component of this bacterium, a negative culture does not rule out the disease (**Fig. 6**).

The use of real-time polymerase chain reaction (PCR) will detect the DNA of the *B canis* organism, whether it is alive or dead.[23,24] This is an area where bacterial cultures are limited. Only live organisms may grow and replicate on culture media. If there are not enough live organisms, then the bacterial culture may be considered negative, but the patient may be harboring the organism. PCR diagnostic testing is a new tool that may be used to diagnose *B canis*. Semen, vaginal swabs, uterine swabs, and urine are appropriate samples to submit for PCR. Whole blood can also be submitted, but due to the limited time of bacteremia, this may not be an adequate sample.[25]

Serologic testing in the dog can be very challenging but can be helpful in screening for the disease. *B canis* has a rough, not smooth, plasma membrane as *B abortus, B melitensis,* and *B suis* possess.[2] The surface antigens of this bacterium make serologic tests highly sensitive, but the specificity is low, making the occurrence of false-positive results very high. Given this information, it has come as a surprise that a significant amount of false-negative results have also been encountered.[1] This may be due to the limitations of the serologic and microbiologic tests, but it may also be due to recent or chronic infection.

The serology tests include the rapid slide agglutination test (RSAT; developed in 1974), which is a rapid commercially available countertop diagnostic test that can be used in-house for a quick diagnosis or screening (**Fig. 7**). Results can be available within 2 minutes. The RSAT may cross-react with antibodies from *Bordetella, Pseudomonas, Moraxella*-type organisms, and other gram-negative bacteria. To decrease some of this cross reaction, 2-mercaptoethanol (2-ME) drops are added to increase the specificity of the RSAT; this is often referred to as

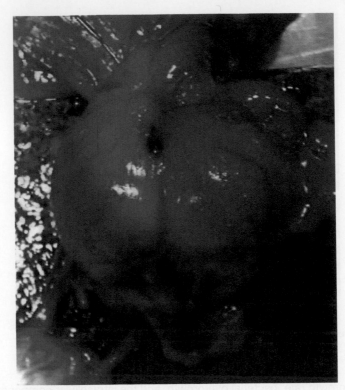

Fig. 5. Canine prostate from an infected stud dog.

the 2-ME RSAT. The tube agglutination test (TAT) detects antibodies in the serum and can be quantitative; samples with titers less than 1:200 should be retested in 2 weeks. The agar gel immunodiffusion test is used to confirm positive results from the RSAT, 2-ME RSAT, and TAT. There are 2 types of agar gel immunodiffusion tests—the first is the cell wall antigen test and the second is the more specific cytoplasmic protein antigen test. Both of these tests are more specific than the RSAT, 2-ME RSAT, and TAT and should be used to confirm any positive results before taking action.

There are 2 other types of serology tests that have been used: the indirect fluorescent antibody (IFA) test and enzyme-linked immunosorbent assay (ELISA). The IFA sensitivity is uncertain so some infected dogs may go undetected with this test. In research, the ELISA is more specific than the IFA and can detect positive dogs within 30 days of infection.[1] Unfortunately, there are no labs conducting this test commercially in the United States at this time.

B suis[26] and B abortus have infected dogs when the animals ingest contaminated fetal membranes or fluid or an aborted fetus.[1] These Brucella spp are smooth bacteria and do not cross-react with the traditional serologic tests generally used to diagnose B canis.

In addition to the discrepancies in the types of diagnostic tests, there is also a substantial lag time between the initial exposure and infection to seroconversion and/or a positive blood culture: 8 to 12 weeks and 4 to 6 weeks, respectively. Bacteremia may last for 1 to 5 years, while chronically infected dogs may remain

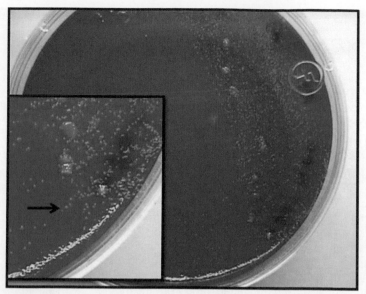

Fig. 6. Slow-growing culture and small colonies.

serologically positive for 5 years or more before dropping below detectable levels.[27] Although the chronically infected dog may be serologically negative, the organism may still be harbored within lymph nodes, liver, spleen, prostate, or other reproductive tissues and may recrudesce at anytime.

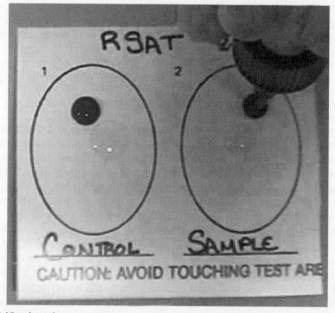

Fig. 7. RSAT (Card test).

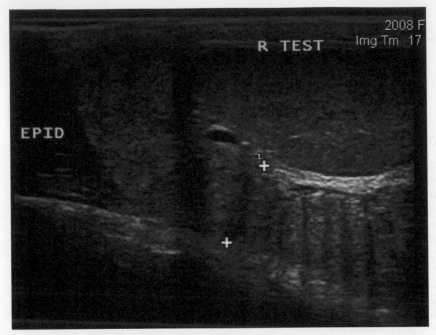

Fig. 8. Testicular ultrasound revealing epididymitis.

Diagnostic imaging such as radiography and ultrasound are modalities that can be used frequently in veterinary clinics today and may reveal lesions that may be suspicious for *B canis*. Such lesions may include unifocal or multifocal areas of inflammation of the intervertebral spaces that do not appear to affect vertebrae.[9] Occasionally, some soft tissue abnormalities in the female, such as stump pyometra,[27] may be seen on radiography or ultrasound. Real-time ultrasound of the male reproductive tract may reveal inflammation or lesions within the testicles, epididymi, or prostate (**Figs. 8** and **9**). These lesions do not provide a definitive diagnosis but should prompt the examiner to pursue further serologic or culture diagnostics.[1]

TREATMENT

Quarantine of the facility will be necessary during an outbreak and treatment. In some states, this may be state mandated, but in many, this is a voluntary quarantine. This quarantine would include that there are no new canine additions, that no dogs should be sold or relocated from the premises, and that all breeding should be suspended until the quarantine is lifted. It may be necessary to quarantine positive dogs from suspect and negative dogs on the same premises. In this event, it would be necessary to follow strict guidelines to not carry the disease from one dog to the next. This would include separate feeding and watering dishes, caring for the negative dogs first then the suspect and then the positive dogs last. It is important that the dogs do not share turnout areas as this bacteria can survive in the environment for many days and weeks.

Several antibiotic therapies have been attempted, but there are no known cures for this disease. This bacteria is sequestered inside cells and it is difficult for antibiotics to penetrate and eradicate this organism from a body. The disease may recrudesce at times of stress and the animal can be a source of infection for other dogs and

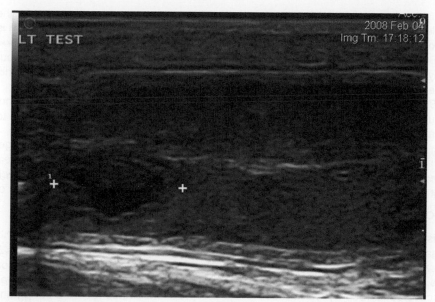

Fig. 9. Testicular abscess in a *B canis*–positive dog.

humans. This is why antibiotic therapy is not encouraged and euthanasia is the treatment of choice among veterinarians and kennel owners.

When treatment is attempted, the patients should be spayed or neutered, and studies have shown that single-antibiotic regimens are unsuccessful.[13,28,29] Combination therapy has had better results such as doxycycline (10 mg/kg po q 12 hours), gentamicin (5 mg/kg SC q 24 hours for 7 days and repeated every 3 weeks), and rifampin (5 mg/kg po q 24 hours) for 3 months.[30] Some success has been reported using enrofloxacin (5 mg/kg po q 24 hours) alone with similar efficacy to that of combination therapy.[31] After this antibiotic trial, retest and repeat until the patient has a negative test. After reaching a negative serology test, continue to test every 4 to 6 months and repeat treatment as necessary. It is also important to isolate these treated dogs from other dogs and breeding animals. The cost of antibiotic therapy and diligence of the testing protocol may deter many owners from trying to treat. It is also important to counsel owners and kennel workers that the therapy is not curative and the dog may be a risk to other dogs and humans, especially young children, older persons, and immunocompromised individuals.

PREVENTION

As with many diseases, prevention is the best treatment. It is important to quarantine and test all new additions to kennels. Due to the lag time with many of the diagnostic tests available, it is recommended that the new additions remain isolated from the general population for 8 to 12 weeks and that they be tested and found to be negative upon arrival and before coming out of quarantine.

For outside breedings, artificial insemination will decrease the male dog's exposure to the disease and should be used when possible. Artificial insemination will not protect females from the disease, so testing the male dog prior to breeding is recommended. Periodic testing of all of the dogs twice a year in kennels is recommended. This could be during a heat cycle in the female and then on an every-6-month-period for the males. This kennel screening can help decrease exposure in the event a positive dog is introduced to the kennel and may decrease losses.

Buying dogs from and breeding to dogs in reputable kennels are encouraged, but may not decrease exposure. Routine diagnostic testing is the only way to monitor this disease in a population.

B canis is susceptible to 1% sodium hypochlorite, 70% ethanol, iodine/alcohol solutions, glutaraldehyde, and formaldehyde, and these solutions may be used to clean facilities and equipment to decrease the spread of the disease.

REPORTING

B canis is a reportable disease in many states. It is important to be aware of your state's regulations and report the disease appropriately.

ZOONOSIS

This organism is also of zoonotic concern. The symptoms manifested by this organism are not as severe as those seen with other *Brucella* organisms, such as *B abortus*, *B melintensis,* and *B suis*. The Centers for Disease Control and Prevention has had 30 human cases of canine brucellosis reported since this bacterium was discovered in 1966 by Carmichael.[13] The seroprevalence rates reported in humans include 13% in Mexico, 0.3% in Germany, 0.4% in US military populations, 0.6% in Florida residents, and 67.9% in Oklahoma residents according to the Center for Food Security and Public Health at Iowa State University. The high seroprevalence rate in Oklahoma was determined by testing several hospitalized and nonhospitalized individuals at the Oklahoma Health Sciences Center in the 1970s.[29] While these data may be very outdated, many believe this organism is underreported in human medicine due to the varying symptoms humans may display, ranging from flulike symptoms to endocarditis and septicemia. Unlike dogs, humans do respond well to antibiotic therapy and often clear this bacterium after long-term treatment.

REFERENCES

1. Hollett RB. Canine brucellosis: outbreaks and compliance. Theriogenology 2006; 66(3):575–87.
2. Carmichael LE, Bruner DW. Characteristics of a newly-recognized species of Brucella responsible for infectious canine abortions. Cornell Vet 1968;48(4):579–92.
3. Carmichael LE, Kenney RM. Canine abortion caused by *Brucella canis*. J Am Vet Med Assoc 1968;152(6):605–16.
4. Saegusa J, Ueda K, Goto Y, et al. Ocular lesions in experimental canine brucellosis. Nippon Juigaku Zasshi 1977;39(2):181–5.
5. Riecke JA, Rhoades HE. *Brucella canis* isolated from the eye of a dog. J Am Vet Med Assoc 1975;166(6):583–4.
6. Henderson RA, Hoerlein BF, Kramer TT, et al. Discospondylitis in three dogs infected with *Brucella canis*. J Am Vet Med Assoc 1974;165(5):451–5.
7. Anderson GI, Binnington AG. Discospondylitis and orchitis associated with high Brucella titre in a dog. Can Vet J 1983;24(8):249–52.
8. Hurov L, Troy G, Turnwald G. Diskospondylitis in the dog: 27 cases. J Am Vet Med Assoc 1978;173(3):275–81.
9. Kerwin SC, Lewis DD, Hribernik TN, et al. Diskospondylitis associated with *Brucella canis* infection in dogs: 14 cases (1980–1991). J Am Vet Med Assoc 1992;201(8):1253–7.
10. Serikawa T, Muraguchi T, Nakao N, et al. Significance of urine-culture for detecting infection with Brucella canis in dogs. Nippon Juigaku Zasshi 1978;40(3):353–5.

11. Kauffman L. Detection of Brucellosis canis DNA in canine urine, semen and vaginal cells via QPCR analysis. 2009. Available from: http://www.reeis.usda.gov/web/crisprojectpages/220415.html. Accessed August 9, 2011.

12. Flores-Castro R, Suarez F, Ramirez-Pfeiffer C, et al. Canine brucellosis: bacteriological and serological investigation of naturally infected dogs in Mexico City. J Clin Microbiol 1977;6(6):591–7.

13. Greene CE, Carmichael LE. Canine brucellosis. In: Greene C, editor. Infectious diseases of the dog and cat. Philadelphia (PA): W.B. Saunders Co; 2006. p. 369–90.

14. Carmichael LE, Joubert JC. Transmission of Brucella canis by contact exposure. Cornell Vet 1988;78(1):63–73.

15. Serikawa T, Muraguchi T, Yamada J, et al. Long-term observation of canine brucellosis: excretion of Brucella canis into urine of infected male dogs. Jikken Dobutsu 1981;30(1):7–14.

16. Wanke MM. Canine brucellosis. Anim Reprod Sci 2004;82–83:195–207.

17. Johnson CA, Walker RD. Clinical signs and diagnosis of Brucella canis infection. Compendium Continuing Education Practitioner Veterinary 1992;14(763/767):770–2.

18. Lewis GE Jr, Crumrine MH, Jennings PB, et al. Therapeutic value of tetracycline and ampicillin in dogs infected with Brucella canis. J Am Vet Med Assoc 1973;163(3):239–41.

19. Schoeb TR, Morton R. Scrotal and testical changes in canine brucellosis: a case report. J Am Vet Med Assoc 1978;172(5):598–600.

20. Serikawa T, Muraguchi T, Yamada J, et al. Spermagglutination and spermagglutinating activity of serum and tissue extracts from reproductive organs in male dogs experimentally infected with Brucella canis. Nippon Juigaku Zasshi 1981;43(4): 469–90.

21. Serikawa T, Kondo Y, Takada H, et al. Head-to-head type auto-sperm agglutination with IgA antibody to acrosome induced by Brucella canis infection. Nippon Juigaku Zasshi 1984;46(1):41–8.

22. Carmichael LE, Shin SJ. Canine brucellosis: a diagnostician's dilemma. Semin Vet Med Surg (Small Anim) 1996;11(3):161–5.

23. Keid LB, Soares RM, Vasconcellos SA, et al. A polymerase chain reaction for the detection of Brucella canis in semen of naturally infected dogs. Theriogenology 2007;67(7):1203–10.

24. Keid LB, Soares RM, Vasconcellos SA, et al. A polymerase chain reaction for detection of Brucella canis in vaginal swabs of naturally infected bitches. Theriogenology 2007;68(9):1260–70.

25. Keid LB, Soares RM, Vasconcellos SA, et al. Comparison of a PCR assay in whole blood and serum specimens for canine brucellosis diagnosis. Vet Rec 2010;167(3):96–9.

26. Plang JF, Huddleson IF. Brucella infection in a dog. J Am Vet Med Assoc 1931;79: 251–2.

27. Dillon AR, Henderson RA. Brucella canis in a uterine stump abscess in a bitch. J Am Vet Med Assoc 1981;78(0):087–8.

28. Flores-Castro R, Carmichael LE. Brucella canis infection in dogs: treatment trials. Rev Latinoam Microbiol 1981;23(2):75–9.

29. Jennings PB, Crumrine MH, Lewis GE Jr, et al. The effect of a two-stage antibiotic regimen on dogs infected with Brucella canis. J Am Vet Med Assoc 1974;164(5):513–4.

30. Vinayak A, Greene CE, Moore PA, et al. Clinical resolution of Brucella canis-induced ocular inflammation in a dog. J Am Vet Med Assoc 2004;224(11):1788–9, 1804–7.

31. Wanke MM, Delpino MV, Baldi PC. Use of enrofloxacin in the treatment of canine brucellosis in a dog kennel (clinical trial). Theriogenology 2006;66(6–7):1573–8.

Hepatozoon spp Infections in the United States

Kelly E. Allen, MS, PhD*, Eileen M. Johnson, DVM, MS, PhD,
Susan E. Little, DVM, PhD

KEYWORDS

- Apicomplexa • *Hepatozoon* spp • Phylogeny
- Polymerase chain reaction (PCR) • 18S rRNA
- Vertical transmission

Members of the genus *Hepatozoon* are unique, heteroxenous hemogregarines in their oral routes of infection to vertebrate intermediate hosts and polysporocystic oocyst formation in invertebrate definitive hosts.[1] Conventionally, the accepted primary route of transmission of *Hepatozoon* spp to vertebrate intermediate hosts is by ingestion of hematophagous, arthropod, definitive hosts containing sporulated oocysts.[1,2]

Currently, 2 *Hepatozoon* spp are recognized parasites of domestic dogs (*Canis familiaris*) in the United States: *H canis* and *H americanum*.[3–5] *Hepatozoon canis*, first observed in the blood of domestic dogs in India in 1905, is now documented in many areas of the world including Africa, Southeast Asia, the Middle East, southern Europe, and South America.[2,5,6–8] However, *H canis* was not definitively identified in canids in the United States until 2008, despite the presence of its accepted primary definitive host and tick vector, *Rhipicephalus sanguineus*, throughout North America.[3,5,9,10]

The first natural canine *Hepatozoon* sp infection in the United States was reported in a coyote (*Canis latrans*) in Texas near the Gulf Coast in 1978.[7,11,12] Reports in domestic dogs in Texas and other states bordering the Gulf Coast soon followed, but the etiologic agent, *Hepatozoon americanum*, was not recognized as distinct from *H canis* until 1997.[7,8,13] The accepted primary definitive host and tick vector of *H americanum* is *Amblyomma maculatum*, the Gulf Coast tick.[14,15]

Hepatozoon canis and *H americanum* differ in numerous aspects including geographic distribution, definitive tick hosts, sites of merogony and resulting clinical syndromes in canine intermediate hosts, treatment approaches, and regions of 18S rRNA gene sequence.[6,7,15–20] This chapter reviews much of what is known about canine hepatozoonois in both the Old World and New World. Emphasis is given to

This work was supported by the Krull-Ewing endowment at Oklahoma State University.
The authors have nothing to disclose.
Department of Veterinary Pathobiology, Oklahoma State University Center for Veterinary Health Sciences, 250 McElroy Hall, Stillwater, OK 74078, USA
* Corresponding author.
E-mail address: Kelly.allen10@okstate.edu

Vet Clin Small Anim 41 (2011) 1221–1238
doi:10.1016/j.cvsm.2011.08.006
0195-5616/11/$ – see front matter © 2011 Elsevier Inc. All rights reserved.

more recent research findings that have provided insight into the epizootology of canine hepatozoonosis in North America.

GEOGRAPHIC DISTRIBUTIONS, PREVALENCE ESTIMATIONS, AND POSSIBLE WILDLIFE RESERVOIR HOSTS OF *H CANIS* AND *H AMERICANUM*
Prevalence Estimations in Domestic Dogs in the United States and Possible Wildlife Reservoir Hosts

Hepatozoon canis was first discovered by S.P. James in 1905 in the blood of domestic dogs (*Canis familiaris*) in India.[2,17] Since its discovery, this parasite has been reported in dogs in many areas of the world, including Europe, Asia, Africa, and South America.[2,5,7] *Hepatozoon canis* was not thought to be a parasite infecting domestic dogs in the United States since the recognition of *H americanum*. However, in 2008, 2 separate survey studies evaluating genetic data of *Hepatozoon* spp amplified from domestic dogs in the United States molecularly confirmed the presence of *H canis*.[3,4] Allen and colleagues (2008) obtained 2 identical sequences from 2 dogs housed in an animal control shelter in Oklahoma that were 98.8% identical to a sequence previously documented as *H canis*. Li and colleagues (2008) reviewed quantitative PCR results from 614 dogs with clinical signs of hepatozoonosis from all over the United States and discovered *H canis* infections and coinfections of *H canis* and *H americanum* in approximately 5% of the animals evaluated. *Hepatozoon canis* and *H canis* and *H americanum* coinfections were documented in Alabama, Georgia, Louisiana, Mississippi, Oklahoma, and Virginia. These molecular studies documented evidence of *H canis* infections and *H canis* and *H americanum* coinfections in domestic dogs in the United States for the first time.[3,4] It remains unclear whether *H canis* infections in North America are autochthonous or are the result of introduction through increased international travel practices.

Although *H canis* is mainly identified in domestic dogs, this parasite has been reported in jackals, hyenas, and palm civets in other areas of the world; however, the species of *Hepatozoon* infecting these wild carnivores have not been confirmed.[21] Recently, genetic sequences most identical to those documented as *H canis* were obtained from red foxes (*Vulpes vulpes*) in Italy[22] and Croatia[23] and domestic cats (*Felis catus*) in France,[24] Thailand,[25] and Brazil.[26]

Hepatozoon americanum was first reported by Davis and colleagues in a coyote (*Canis latrans*) in Texas in 1978.[11] Over the next 2 decades, *H americanum* was reported in domestic dogs in several states in North America including Texas, Louisiana, Mississippi, Alabama, Georgia, and Oklahoma.[7,13,16,27] Initially, these infections were attributed to a particularly virulent strain of *H canis*. Further research on the North American parasite indicated that it was distinct from *H canis*, and in 1997, it was recognized as the causative agent of American canine hepatozoonosis (ACH).[10,13,17,28] Although reports of ACH have traditionally occurred in south-central and southeastern states where the accepted tick definitive host and vector of *H americanum* is established, genetic data of *H americanum* infections in clinically presenting dogs in additional states were reported in 2008.[4] *Hepatozoon americanum* infections are now documented in California, Kentucky, Nebraska, North Carolina, Virginia, Vermont, and Washington, in addition to states previously reported.[4]

The overall prevalence of *H americanum* in the United States is not well understood. In the largest survey study published, 614 blood samples collected from clinically presenting dogs from 28 states were submitted to the Molecular Diagnostics Laboratory at Auburn University between 2006 and 2008 for PCR confirmation of *H americanum* infection.[4] Approximately 30% of the specimens tested were positive for *H americanum* DNA, the majority of which were submitted from states in the southeast.[4]

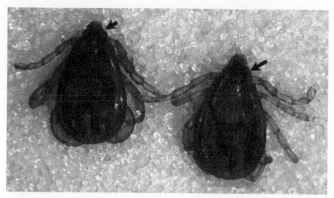

Fig. 1. *Rhipicephalus sanguineus*, the brown dog tick, dorsal view of adult male (*left*) and female (*right*) (magnification ×0.8). Notice the inornate scutum, short palps, and hexagonal basis capituli (*arrows*).

However, this estimation may be lower than the actual infection prevalence because muscle biopsy, rather than whole blood, is considered ideal for detecting *H americanum* infection, as parisitemia in ACH patients and biopsy-confirmed, experimentally infected dogs, is often extremely low.[12,29]

Survey studies in areas of Oklahoma where ACH is enzootic have revealed that approximately half of evaluated coyotes have muscle stages of a parasite that resemble those seen in domestic dogs infected with *H americanum*.[9,19,30,31] Cross-transmission studies between dogs and coyotes indicated that both hosts were likely infected with the same parasite.[32] Based on the prevalence of *H americanum* in coyotes in enzootic areas, some researchers suspect coyotes are an important reservoir host of the parasite,[30,32] while others conjecture that both domestic dogs and coyotes are accidentally inserted into a transmission cycle involving *A maculatum* and another, unidentified reservoir host in nature.[12] Coyotes appear to tolerate *H americanum* infection better than dogs; however, naturally infected coyotes develop pathognomonic muscle and bone lesions, and experimentally infected animals display clinical disease consistent with ACH.[9,19,30–33]

DEFINITIVE TICK HOSTS OF *H CANIS* AND *H AMERICANUM*

The primary definitive host and tick vector of *H canis* was identified by Christophers in 1907 as *Rhipicephalus sanguineus* (**Fig. 1**), the brown dog tick.[2,17] *R sanguineus* nymphs have been experimentally demonstrated to support *H canis* oocyst formation after repletion feeding on infected dogs or after percutaneous injection with buffy coat from infected dogs.[2,34] Larvae are apparently refractory to infection.[10,15] Mature oocysts are found approximately 53 days post-repletion in 66% to 85% of molted adult cohorts infected with *H canis* as nymphs.[2,34] It is not entirely clear where zygote formation and sporogony occur within the tick, or whether these processes take place intracellularly or extracellularly.[2] Experiments assessing transovarial transmission of *H canis* in *R. sanguineus* indicate this route does not occur.[34]

Rhipicephalus sanguineus, a 3-host tick that preferentially feeds on dogs during each instar,[35,36] is capable of establishing in a variety of climates with regard to temperature, relative humidity, and precipitation,[36] including indoor facilities.[35] As it is able to adapt to various environmental conditions, *R sanguineus* is cosmopolitan in its

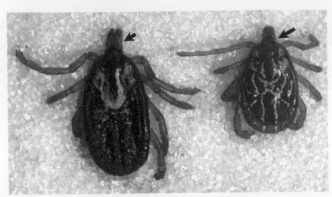

Fig. 2. *Amblyomma maculatum*, the Gulf coast tick, dorsal view of adult female (*left*) and male (*right*) (magnification ×0.8). Notice the diffusely ornate scutum, long palps, and rectangular basis capituli (*arrows*).

geographic distribution.[36] Therefore, the recent discovery of *H canis* in domestic dogs in North America is not entirely surprising.[3,5]

Additional tick species have been reported as potential hosts of *H canis* in other geographic locations. Oocysts have been identified in *Haemaphysalis longicornis* and *Haemaphysalis flava* collected from dogs naturally infected with *H canis* in Japan.[34,37] A molecular survey of organisms in wild-caught *Ixodes ricinus* in Luxumbourg revealed *H canis* DNA in an unfed adult female.[38] In Brazil, an adult *Amblyomma ovale* collected from a naturally infected dog was reported to contain *Hepatozoon* spp oocysts. Sporozoites liberated from these oocysts were injected into an uninfected dog intraperitoneally and circulating gamonts were observed 84 days after inoculation.[39] Another study demonstrated transstadial transmission of *H canis* by *A ovale* to susceptible dogs,[40] implicating *A ovale* as a definitive host and vector of *H canis* in parts of South America.

Although *Hepatozoon* spp oocysts have been recognized in feeding *Amblyomma maculatum* removed from canids in enzootic areas of ACH, such reports are scarce, and the species of parasites were not determined.[13,15] However, *A maculatum* (**Fig. 2**) has experimentally been demonstrated to be an excellent definitive host of *H americanum*, while other common tick species in ACH enzootic areas, including *R sanguineus*, *A americanum*, and *Dermacentor variabilis*, have empirically been refractory to infection.[14,15] Experiments characterizing the development of *H americanum* in *A maculatum* infected via blood meal acquisition have revealed transstadial maintenance in the tick from larvae to nymph, nymph to adult, and larva to adult.[15] Molted cohorts are demonstrated to harbor sporulated oocysts infective to canine hosts after approximately 33 to 42 days postrepletion in the majority (96% to 99%) of those dissected.[14,15] Intermittent microscopic examination of experimentally infected ticks has shown evidence of oocyst formation occurring within gut cells of tick hosts.[14] Experiments assessing transovarial transmission of *H americanum* in *A maculatum* have not been reported; this route is not suspected, as it has not been documented in other known definitive hosts of *Hepatozoon* spp.[21,34]

In the United States, *A maculatum* was traditionally endemic in states bordering the Gulf Coast and several states bordering the Atlantic coast including Georgia, Florida, and the southern portion of South Carolina.[41] However, current data report establishment of the Gulf Coast tick in states farther inland including Oklahoma, Kansas,

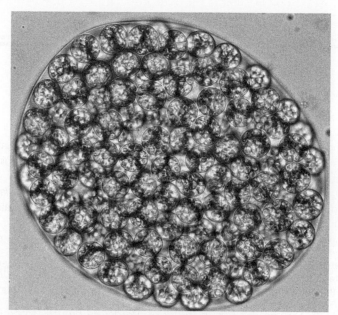

Fig. 3. Sporulated oocyst of *Hepatozoon americanum* collected from the hemocoel of an experimentally infected *Ambylomma maculatum* adult tick (magnification ×60).

Arizona, Arkansas, Missouri, Indiana, Kentucky, and Tennessee and additional states along the Atlantic coast including Maryland, Virginia, and West Virginia.[7,41,42] *A maculatum* is also documented in Central and South American regions that border the Gulf of Mexico and Caribbean Sea including Mexico, Guatemala, Belize, Nicaragua, Honduras, Costa Rica, Colombia, Venezuela, and parts of Ecuador and Peru,[43] although recent evaluations of historical records in these regions from the past 50 years indicate that Gulf Coast ticks had sometimes been confused with *Amblyomma triste*.[44] No confirmed reports of *H americanum* infections have occurred in South America.

Unlike with *H canis*, other invertebrate definitive hosts of *H americanum* have not been implicated. Prior to 2008, reports of ACH generally correlated with the geographic distribution of *A maculatum* in the United States.[3,4,8] Newly reported cases of ACH in areas where *A maculatum* is not established are thought to be instances of patient relocations from confirmed *H americanum* enzootic areas.[3,5]

TRANSMISSION OF *H CANIS* AND *H AMERICANUM* TO CANID INTERMEDIATE HOSTS

It is conventionally accepted that most *Hepatozoon* spp infections are acquired by the consumption of invertebrate hosts carrying sporulated oocysts (**Fig. 3**) of parasite.[1,45] This may occur when vertebrates ingest invertebrates as sustenance,[1] while grooming self or companions,[2,19] or accidentally during predation and/or scavenging.[19,46] The preponderance of knowledge regarding *H canis* infections has been gleaned from observations in naturally infected domestic dogs.[1,2,47] Canid intermediate hosts are thought to primarily become infected by ingesting *R. sanguineus* ticks that contain *H canis* oocysts.[2] However, monozoic cysts of *H canis* have been reported in the spleens of naturally and experimentally infected dogs that are morphologically similar

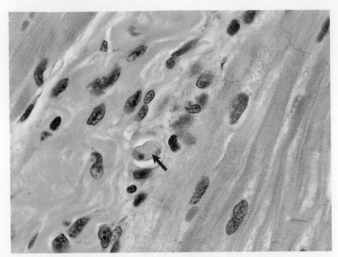

Fig. 4. Hematoxylin-eosin–stained section of skeletal muscle from a laboratory-raised New Zealand White rabbit experimentally infected with *Hepatozoon americanum* showing a cystozoite (*arrow*) (magnification ×100). (*Courtesy of* Dr Roger Panciera, Oklahoma State University.)

to cystozoites, which are arrested zoites encysted in tissues of documented paratenic hosts of other *Hepatozoon* species, that are infective to intermediate hosts ingesting them.[1,2,47] In dogs infected with *H canis*, these cysts are present in tissues in addition to meronts, which may indicate that dogs serve as both intermediate and paratenic hosts,[2,48] although experiments investigating the infectivity of monozoic cysts of *H canis* for dogs consuming them have not been reported.

A tertiary route of congenital transmission, documented initially in natural *Hepatozoon griseisciuri* infections in squirrels, is also reported in *H canis* infections.[49,50] Murata and colleagues (1993) monitored *H canis* infections in 6 litters of beagle pups born of 3 naturally infected dams. Fourteen pups comprising 5 litters from 2 infected dams were positive for circulating parasite after 21 to 31 days. Initially, gamonts were present in 0.02% to 0.04% of leukocytes observed, but after several months were present in as many as 3.3%; the rise in parasitemia suggested active merogony and gamont production. Meronts were also observed in the main visceral organs of 1 of 2 pups that died. Additionally, 4 pups whelped from a third infected dam were positive for gamonts 4 weeks after birth, indicating congenital transmission of *H canis* with subsequent parasite establishment and development in these animals.[50]

The primary documented route of *H americanum* transmission to canid intermediate hosts is by the ingestion of infected *A maculatum*.[7,19,46] However, experiments conducted by Johnson and colleagues in 2008[51] and 2009[29] to establish the susceptibility of several preferred hosts of immature instars of *A maculatum* demonstrated development of cystozoites (**Fig. 4**) in the tissues of cotton rats (*Sigmodon hispidus*), mice (*Mus musculus*), and New Zealand white rabbits (*Oryctolagus cuniculus*), but not rats (*Rattus norvegicus*), after ingestion of *H americanum* oocysts. The cyst-laden tissues were, in turn, infective to dogs ingesting them. Parasite development and clinical disease in dogs occurred as described in infections resulting from sporozoite ingestion.[29,41,46] The susceptibility of other hosts to *H americanum* infection with development of cystozoites within these hosts, although experimental, suggests that paratenic hosts for *H americanum* could be a source of infection for dogs and implies that predation, either of infected prey or prey infested with infected ticks, is a significant epidemiologic factor in natural transmission cycles.[29,46] Focused wildlife survey studies conducted in ACH enzootic areas in Oklahoma have documented *Hepatozoon* spp infections in trapped rodents and hunted rabbits,[46,52] but thus far, confirmed natural *H americanum* infections as evidenced by microscopic and molecular data have only been reported in domestic dogs and coyotes.[3,4,16,31,53]

Although speculated to occur, vertical transmission of *H americanum* in naturally infected dogs has not been reported. Most ACH cases are of singly presenting patients residing in rural areas.[19,46] Patient histories often include behaviors of roaming and predatory tendencies.[46] The youngest reported age of *H americanum* infection is 11 weeks, which is an age allowing enough time from parasite exposure to clinical presentation by either of the 2 established routes of infection.[29] Documented multiple dog outbreaks of ACH have also occurred in rural settings, in animals old enough to roam at will or to be used in recreational hunting pursuits,[46] not in young littermates still relying heavily on their mothers for survival.

A pilot experiment to assess congenital transmission of *H americanum* was conducted at Oklahoma State University in 2008 using a chronically infected, intact female hound.[54] The carrier birthed 8 pups that were monitored for infection weekly for 3 months by complete blood counts, blood smear examination, and PCR of whole blood. None of 7 surviving pups developed clinical signs, laboratory abnormalities, or parasitemia as evidenced by blood film or PCR. One pup died from aspiration pneumonia 4 days after birth; neither histologic lesions nor meronts of *H americanum* were observed in tissues of this pup. At the conclusion of the study, a xenodiagnosis experiment using laboratory-raised *A maculatum* nymphs was performed. None of the molted adult cohorts, dissected approximately 2 months after repletion feeding as nymphs, were found to contain parasite oocysts (Kelly E. Allen, unpublished observations). However, due to only the single dam and litter of pups evaluated, the results of this study cannot be considered definitive evidence for lack of vertical transmission in *H americanum* infections. The timing of infection, whether before or during pregnancy, the stage of parasite by which infected, whether sporozoites or cystozoites, and the clinical phase of disease, whether acute or chronic, may be factors influencing the occurrence of transplacental transmission of *H americanum* in naturally infected dogs.

H CANIS AND *H AMERICANUM* TISSUE TROPISM AND DEVELOPMENT WITHIN CANINE HOSTS

Ingested *Hepatozoon* spp oocysts within tick hosts likely rupture during canid mastication or when introduced into the stomach.[9,34] It remains unclear whether *Hepatozoon* spp sporozoites released from sporocysts in the canine alimentary tract penetrate the gut lining and migrate to target organs or if they are engulfed by phagocytic cells and carried hematogenously to tissues.[2,55] Typical sites of merogony in *H canis* infections include bone marrow, lymph nodes, and spleen.[2,6,56] In a study conducted by Baneth and colleagues (2007),[2] 2 morphologically distinct populations of meronts were observed in the bone marrow of experimentally infected dogs after 26 days. One form contained only 2 to 4 large zoites, termed macromerozoites, randomly arranged within the meront. The role of macromerozoites in *H canis* infections remains to be elucidated, but they are documented to give rise to micromerozoites and perpetuate merogony in other species of *Hepatozoon*.[2] The second type of meront contained 20 to 30 smaller zoites arranged in a "wheel-spoked" configuration (**Fig. 5**) similar to that documented in other species of *Hepatozoon*.[2,7] These zoites, termed micromerozoites, were thought to be the

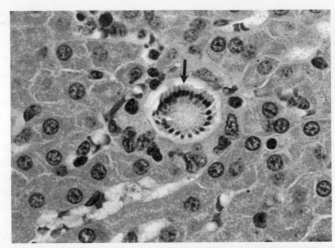

Fig. 5. Hematoxylin-eosin–stained section of liver from a naturally infected, field-trapped, cotton rat showing a mature, "wheel spoke" meront of a *Hepatozoon* sp (magnification ×40). (*Courtesy of* Dr Roger Panciera, Oklahoma State University.)

progenitors of gamonts.[2] Mature gamonts of *H canis* in experimentally infected dogs can be observed in peripheral neutrophils 4 weeks after infection.[2,34] *H canis* infections are often associated with high levels of parasitemia, with gamonts sometimes reported in as many as 100% of neutrophils on blood smears.[57]

In *H americanum* infections, meronts (**Fig. 6**) are found within canine host cells, likely monocytes, principally located between individual fibers of skeletal and cardiac muscle tissues as soon as 3.5 weeks after exposure.[57] Maturing meronts of *H americanum* do not have a characteristic "wheel-spoked" arrangement of zoites but, rather, exhibit blastophore formation[7] and appear to transform host cells.[12,33,55] In

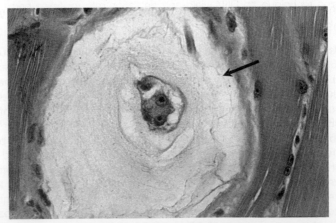

Fig. 6. Hematoxylin-eosin–stained section of skeletal muscle from a dog containing an "onion skinned," early meront of *Hepatozoon americanum* (magnification ×40). (*Courtesy of* Dr Roger Panciera, Oklahoma State University.)

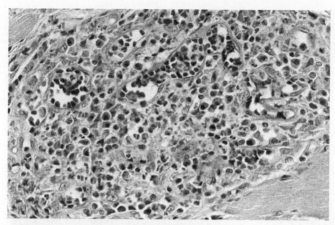

Fig. 7. Hematoxylin-eosin–stained section of skeletal muscle from a *Hepatozoon americanum*–infected dog containing a pyogranuloma (magnification ×40). (*Courtesy of* Dr Roger Panciera, Oklahoma State University.)

histologic preparations of muscle tissue, parasitized cells are surrounded by concentric strata of a mucopolysaccharide-rich material reminiscent of onion skin layers.[12,33] The lesions are aptly termed "onion skin" cysts (**Fig. 7**).[12,55,58] Over time, meronts overtake and rupture host cells, thereby liberating merozoites that breach degenerating cyst walls. Merozoites incite local influxes of inflammatory cells that often progress to granulomata (**Fig. 8**).[12,55,59] Distinct populations of macromerozoites and micromerozoites as are seen in *H canis* infections have not been observed in *H americanum* infections.[28,55,58] It is hypothesized that some merozoites develop into gamonts after invading new leukocytes while others distribute hematogenously to new sites and continue to reproduce asexually.[9,12,55,59] Gamonts (**Fig. 9**), usually

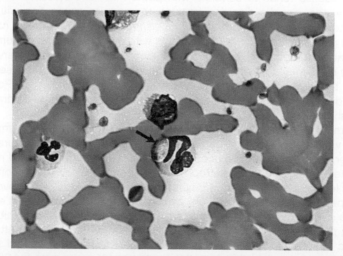

Fig. 8. Giemsa-stained peripheral blood smear from a *Hepatozoon americanum*–infected dog demonstrating a gamont in a peripheral neutrophil (*arrow*) (magnification ×100).

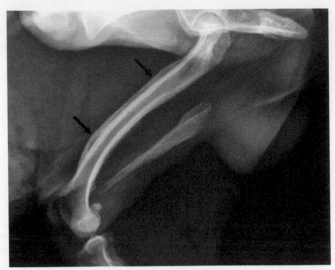

Fig. 9. Radiograph of the hindlimb of a dog with chronic periosteal hypertrophic proliferation commonly detected in *Hepatozoon americanum*–infected dogs. The thickening of the periosteum is most evident in the femur (*arrows*). (*Courtesy of* Dr Robert Bahr, Oklahoma State University.)

present in less than 0.1% of circulating white blood cells, are observable on blood smears as soon as 4 to 5 weeks after exposure to *H americanum* zoites. However, they are primarily found during the acute stage of disease.[12,29]

CLINICAL PRESENTATIONS AND DIAGNOSIS OF CANINE HEPATOZOONOSIS

Disease associated with *H canis* infection may range from subclinical and chronic, especially in the absence of concurrent infections, to severe and life-threatening.[2,34] Severity of disease tends to correlate with patient immune status, which may be impacted by age, genetic disorder, immune therapy, or coinfection with another etiologic agent such as *Ehrlichia canis*, *Leishmania canis*, *Babesia canis*, and *Toxoplasma gondii*.[2,13,34,60–62] In rare patients with overt disease, symptoms including fever, anemia, lethargy, anorexia, and depression may be observed.[2,13,34] *Hepatozoon canis* infections are classically diagnosed by microscopic observation of gamonts in blood films, which sometimes are incidental findings.[2,7,20] Polymerase chain reaction (PCR) methods have recently been developed to detect parasite DNA in peripheral blood.[4,6,63,64]

In experimental *H americanum* infections, dogs often present with symptoms of ACH 4 to 5 weeks after ingesting parasite oocysts.[33] Salient clinical features of ACH include fever, lethargy, copious mucopurulent ocular discharge, pain and reluctance to move, altered gait, and muscle atrophy.[7,9,13,18,33] Laboratory findings often reveal neutrophilic leukocytosis, which may be profound, and anemia.[7,13,33] In severe cases, symmetric periosteal bone proliferation, particularly of the long bones, is evident on radiographs (**Fig. 9**).[7,13,33,65] Dogs infected with *H americanum* may exhibit waxing and waning courses of clinical disease over time, with clinical relapses attributed to the periodic release of merozoites from tissue meronts and associated inflammation.[7,18,59] Although chronically infected animals have been reported, ACH patients often die within 12 to 24 months without supportive therapies.[7,18,19]

Clinical signs, blood count abnormalities (particularly neutrophilia), observation of rare gamonts in blood smears, and characteristic osteal lesions on radiographs are findings that often lead to a diagnosis of ACH.[8,12,13,66] Muscle biopsy, although invasive, is considered the gold-standard method for achieving a definitive diagnosis, as parasite or parasite-induced lesions can readily be observed in histopathologic stained sections of the biopsied sample.[8,12,66,67] PCR methods have been developed for detecting circulating *Hepatozoon* spp but may lack sensitivity in *H americanum* infections due to low levels of parasitemia.[3,4,8]

TREATMENT APPROACHES FOR CANINE HEPATOZOONOSIS

Hepatozoon canis infections are most commonly treated with imidocarb dipropionate twice monthly, administered subcutaneously at 5 to 6 mg/kg, until gamonts are no longer evident in patient blood smears for 2 to 3 consecutive months.[18,20] The mechanism of action of this compound is not well understood.[20] Although clinical improvement of patients may occur, this drug does not clear *H canis* at its currently recommended dose.[20] *Hepatozoon canis* DNA is detectable in peripheral blood by PCR for weeks following treatment end, even though gamonts have not been microscopically observable on blood or buffy coat smears for several months.[20] Still, clinical signs due to *H canis* infection can be well controlled in many patients with this drug compound, although relapses may occur.[18,20]

Currently, the Companion Animal Parasite Council (CAPC) (www.capcvet.org) recommends presenting ACH patients be treated with either a triple combination of trimethoprim-sulfadiazine (15 mg/kg bid), clindamycin (10 mg/kg tid), and pyrimethamine (0.25 mg/kg once daily) or ponazuril (10 mg/kg bid) for 14 days followed by 2 years of twice-daily decoquinate administration (10 to 20 mg/kg). Decoquinate appears to prevent or delay clinical relapse by arresting merogony.[7,18] Supplemental nonsteroidal anti-inflammatory drugs (NSAIDs) may be given for fever and pain control.[7,9,18]

Triple therapy with trimethoprim-sulfadiazine, clindamycin, and pyrimethamine (TCP) is aimed at inhibiting parasite folic–folinic acid metabolism and is used to treat toxoplasmosis in dogs and cats. Decoquinate is classified as a coccidiostat, but in higher concentrations it is coccidiocidal and targets parasite mitochondria. It is commonly used as a preventative of coccidiosis in chickens, sheep, goats, and rabbits.[18] Combined TCP and decoquinate treatment was evaluated in naturally infected dogs in a study conducted by Macintire and colleagues.[18] Although this treatment regimen is not curative, it does extend life expectancy and improve quality of life for many ACH patients.[18] Should clinical relapse occur, it is recommended that TCP or ponazuril treatments be repeated and again followed by long-term decoquinate administration.[7,18]

Ponazuril (toltrazuril sulfone), a recommended alternative to TCP in the treatment of ACH, is approved by the US Food and Drug Administration solely for the treatment of equine protozoal myeloencephalitis (EPM) caused by *Sarcocystis neurona*.[68,69] However, ponazuril is widely used as an effective treatment of *Cystoisospora* spp infections in young dogs and cats[68] as well as a preventative of coccidiosis in chickens.[68,70] Ponazuril has been shown to inhibit development of other tissue-cyst forming protozoans including *Toxoplasma gondii* and *Neospora caninum* in mice and in vitro systems.[70,71] Although a currently accepted alternative to TCP treatment of ACH patients, ponazuril had not been evaluated experimentally in *H americanum* infections for clinical sign alleviation or clearance of parasite until recently. A pilot trial was conducted by Allen and colleagues (2010)[72] to assess the efficacy of ponazuril as a stand-alone 4-week treatment for ACH. Although extended treatment with 10 mg/kg ponazuril twice daily for 4 weeks in combination with NSAID administration (2.2 mg/kg carprofen) for pain ameliorated acute clinical signs, parasite clearance was not achieved. Parasites were detected in both the treated dog and a positive control dog by histopathology and PCR 43 weeks postexposure.[72]

GENETIC CHARACTERIZATION AND PHYLOGENETIC RELATIONSHIPS OF *HEPATOZOON* SPP IN THE UNITED STATES

In addition to canids, a broad range of vertebrate hosts are reported to be infected with *Hepatozoon* species worldwide, with over 300 species observed and named in poikilotherms, other mammals, and some birds.[1,2,8] To date, there are 29 species of *Hepatozoon* reported from North America, of which 24 are in snakes.[73–78] *Hepatozoon* species reported in mammals include *H muris* in rats (*Rattus norvegicus*),[79] *Hepatozoon procyonis* in raccoons (*Procyon lotor*),[80–82] *Hepatozoon griseisciuri* in grey squirrels (*Sciurus carolinensis*),[83] *H americanum* in domestic dogs and coyotes,[12,13,31] and, more recently, *H canis* in domestic dogs.[3–5] Undetermined species have been reported in a domestic cat (*Felis catus*),[84] bobcats (*Lynx rufus*), and ocelots (*Leopardus pardalis*).[84,85]

With discoveries of alternate transmission routes of some *Hepatozoon* spp, the utilization of obligate paratenic hosts by several *Hepatozoon* spp, and the abilities of other *Hepatozoon* spp to infect experimental facultative transport hosts, genetic characterization has become an important criterion in the complete description of established *Hepatozoon* species and the proposition of novel species.[6,17,52,86] There are approximately 200 *Hepatozoon* sequences listed in the National Center for Biotechnology Information database (NCBI), GenBank, with less than 20 sequences collected from North American animals. Prior to 2007, only *Hepatozoon* sequences obtained from domestic dogs were available in the NCBI database.[6,17,87] Since then, 1 sequence collected from cotton rats (*Sigmodon hispidus*), 1 sequence collected from white-footed mice (*Peromyscus leucopus*),[52] 6 additional sequences from domestic dogs (*Canis familiaris*),[3] 1 sequence from a cottontail rabbit (*Sylvilagus floridanus*), 1 sequence from a swamp rabbit (*Sylvilagus aquaticus*),[46] and 1 sequence (GU344682) from a turkey vulture (*Cathartes aura*) have been contributed to the database. The sequences from 6 additional dogs contributed to GenBank by Allen and colleagues in 2008 demonstrated that the *Hepatozoon* spp organisms infecting domestic dogs in the United States are diverse and provided molecular evidence for the existence of multiple species and strains of canid *Hepatozoon* spp in North America.[3]

The dearth of *Hepatozoon* spp sequence contributions to GenBank from the United States and the diversity within the data available led to a collaborative effort with other researchers to obtain, compile, and submit *Hepatozoon* spp sequences from known and previously unrecognized hosts.[88] An approximate 500–base pair fragment of a hypervariable region of the 18S rRNA gene of *Hepatozoon* spp and some other apicomplexans was amplified from blood or tissues of 16 vertebrate host species from the United States. Phylogenetic analyses and comparison with other *Hepatozoon* spp sequences in GenBank revealed distinct taxonomic groupings. In general, sequences obtained from scavengers and carnivores (1 opossum, 1 gray fox, 4 raccoons, 2 bobcats, 1 domestic cat, coyotes, and domestic dogs) grouped together and sequences from rodents formed a separate cluster. However, interestingly, sequences from wild rabbits were most closely related to sequences obtained from carnivores, and sequence from a boa constrictor was most closely related to sequences within the rodent cluster. These data support recent experimental work identifying predator/prey transmission cycles in *Hepatozoon* spp[1,46,47,89] and suggest this particular transmission pattern may be more common than previously recognized. Additionally, the study possibly elucidated sequence data of *Hepatozoon* spp previously identified morphologically in grey squirrels and raccoons,[80–83] provided molecular evidence of *H americanum* infections in coyotes, confirming prior suspicions, and documented possible coinfections of coyotes with different strains of *H americanum*. A sequence obtained from a domestic cat that was nearly identical (99.4%) to *H americanum* indicated that felids are susceptible to *H americanum* infection, especially if immunocompromised.[2] Also, a sequence from a gray fox that was most similar to that reported as *H canis* indicated the possible susceptibility of North American wild carnivores to *H canis* and supported results from 2 previous molecular survey studies in domestic dogs in North America documenting the presence of *H canis* in North America.[3,4]

SUMMARY

It is now clear that 2 *Hepatozoon* species infect domestic dogs in the United States, *H canis* and *H americanum*. *Hepatozoon canis* is documented in several states in the Southeast, and *H americanum*, previously thought to be a parasite of dogs limited to the south central and southeastern states, is now documented in states in other regions of the country. It is important for veterinarians throughout the United States to understand that although canine hepatozoonosis caused by both organisms is incurable, infections can be well managed with different treatment approaches. It is commonly thought that *H canis* is predominantly cycled between *R sanguineus* and dogs, whereas recent experimental evidence has demonstrated the ability of *H americanum* to use several alternate vertebrate species as paratenic hosts, making it reasonable to consider the possible importance of predator/prey relationships in natural transmission cycles of *H americanum*. *Hepatozoon* spp genetic data from canids and other vertebrates in the United States are diverse, and phylogenetic comparisons of previously and recently documented sequences support the assertion of predator–prey relationships of vertebrate hosts of several *Hepatozoon* species. Further research is needed to better understand the *Hepatozoon* organisms cycling in nature in the United States.

REFERENCES

1. Smith TG. The genus *Hepatozoon* (Apicomplexa: Adeleina). J Parasit 1996;82(4): 565–83.
2. Baneth G, Samish M, Shkap V. Life cycle of *Hepatozoon canis* (Apicomplexa: Adeleorina: Hepatozoidae) in the tick *Rhipicephalus sanguineus* and domestic dog (*Canis familiaris*). J Parasit 2007;93(2):283–99.
3. Allen KE, Li Y, Kaltenboeck B, et al. Diversity of *Hepatozoon* species in naturally infected dogs in the southern United States. Vet Parasitol 2008;154(3-4):220–5.
4. Li Y, Wang C, Allen KE, et al. Diagnosis of canine *Hepatozoon* spp infection by quantitative PCR. Vet Parasitol 2008;157:50–8.
5. Little SE, Allen KE, Johnson EM, et al. New developments in canine hepatozoonosis in North America: a review. Parasit Vectors 2009;2 Suppl 1:S5.
6. Baneth G, Barta JR, Shkap V, et al. Genetic and antigenic evidence supports the separation of *Hepatozoon canis* and *Hepatozoon americanum* at the species level. J Clin Microbiol 2000;38(3): 1298–301.
7. Vincent-Johnson NA. American canine hepatozoonosis. Vet Clin North Am Small Anim Pract 2003;33(4):905–20.
8. Potter TM, Macintire DK. *Hepatozoon americanum*: An emerging disease in the south-central/southeastern United States. JVECC 2010;20(1):70–6.

9. Ewing SA, Panciera RJ, Mathew JS, et al. American canine hepatozoonosis. An emerging disease in the New World. Ann N Y Acad Sci 2000;916:81–92.
10. Ewing SA, Mathew JS, Panciera RJ. Transmission of *Hepatozoon americanum* (Apicomplexa: Adeleorina) by ixodids (Acari: Ixodidae). J Med Entomol 2002;39(4): 631–34.
11. Davis DS, Robinson RM, Craig TM. Naturally occurring hepatozoonosis in a coyote. J Wildl Dis 1978;14(2):244–6.
12. Ewing SA, Panciera RJ. American canine hepatozoonosis. Clin Microbiol Rev 2003; 16(4):688–97.
13. Vincent-Johnson NA, Macintire DK, Lindsay DS, et al. A new *Hepatozoon* species from dogs: Description of the causative agent of canine hepatozoonosis in North America. J Parasitol 1997;83(6):1165–72.
14. Mathew JS, Ewing SA, Panciera RJ, et al. Experimental transmission of *Hepatozoon americanum* Vincent-Johnson et al, 1997 to dogs by the Gulf Coast tick, *Amblyomma maculatum* Koch. Vet Parasitol 1998;80(1):1–14.
15. Ewing SA, Dubois JG, Mathew JS, et al. Larval Gulf Coast ticks (*Amblyomma maculatum*) [Acari: Ixodidae] as host for *Hepatozoon americanum* [Apicomplexa: Adeleorina Vet Parasitol 2002;103(1-2):43–51.
16. Panciera RJ, Gatto NT, Crystal MA, et al. Canine hepatozoonosis in Oklahoma. J Am Anim Hosp Assoc 1997;33(3):221–5.
17. Mathew JS, Van Den Bussche RA, Ewing, SA, et al. Phylogenetic relationships of *Hepatozoon* (Apicomplexa: Adeleorina) based on molecular, morphologic, and life-cycle characters. J Parasitol 2000;86(2):366–72.
18. Macintire DK, Vincent-Johnson NA, Kane, CW Lindsay et al. Treatment of dogs infected with *Hepatozoon americanum*: 53 cases (1989-1998). J Am Vet Med Assoc 2001;218(1):77–82.
19. Ewing SA, Panciera RJ, Mathew JS. Persistence of *Hepatozoon americanum* (Apicomplexa: Adeleorina) in a naturally-infected dog. J Parasitol 2003;89(3):611–13.
20. Sasanelli M, Paradies P, Greco B, et al. Failure of imidocarb dipropionate to eliminate *Hepatozoon canis* in naturally infected dogs based on parasitological and molecular evaluation methods. Vet Parasitol 2010;171(3-4):194–9.
21. Levine ND. Veterinary protozoology. Ames (IA): The Iowa State University Press;1985. p. 261–5.
22. Gabrielli S, Kumlien S, Calderini P, et al. The first report of *Hepatozoon canis* identified in *Vulpes vulpes* and ticks from Italy. Vector Borne Zoonotic Dis 2010;10(9): 855–99.
23. Dezdek D, Vojta L, Curković S, et al. Molecular detection of *Theileria annae* and *Hepatozoon canis* in foxes (*Vulpes vulpes*) in Croatia. Vet Parasitol 2010;172(3-4): 333–6.
24. Criado-Fornelio A, Buling A, Pingret JL, et al. Hemoprotozoa of domestic animals in France: Prevalence and molecular characterization. Vet Parasitol 2009;159(1):73–6.
25. Jittapalapong S, Rungphisutthipongse O, Maruyama S, et al. Detection of *Hepatozoon canis* in stray dogs and cats in Bangkok, Thailand. Ann N Y Acad Sci 2006; 1081:479–88.
26. Rubini AS, dos Santos Paduan K, Perez RR, et al. Molecular characterization of feline *Hepatozoon* species from Brazil. Vet Parasit 2006;137(1-2):168–71.
27. Craig TM, Smallwood JE, Knauer KW, et al. *Hepatozoon canis* infection in dogs: Clinical, radiographic, and hematologic findings. J Am Vet Med Assoc 1978;173(8): 967–72.
28. Panciera RJ, Mathew JS, Cummings CA, et al. Comparison of tissue stages of *Hepatozoon americanum* in the dog using immunohistochemical and routine histologic methods. Vet Pathol 2001;38(4):422–46.

29. Johnson EM, Allen KE, Panciera RJ, et al. Experimental transmission of *Hepatozoon americanum* to New Zealand White rabbits (*Oryctolagus cuniculus*) and infectivity of cystozoites for a dog. Vet Parasitol 2009; 164(2-4):162–6.

30. Kocan AA, Breshears M, Cummings C, et al. Naturally occurring hepatozoonosis in coyotes from Oklahoma. J Wildl Dis 1999;35(1):86–9.

31. Kocan AA, Cummings CA, Panciera, RJ, et al. Naturally occurring and experimentally transmitted *Hepatozoon americanum* in coyotes from Oklahoma. J Wildl Dis 2000; 36(1):149–53.

32. Garrett JJ, Kocan AA, Reichard MV, et al. Experimental infection of adult and juvenile coyotes with domestic dog and wild coyote isolates of *Hepatozoon americanum* (Apicomplexa: Adeleorina). J Wildl Dis 2005;41(3):588–92.

33. Panciera RJ, Ewing SA. American canine hepatozoonosis. Anim Health Res Rev 2003;4(1):27–34.

34. Baneth G, Samish M, Alekseev E, et al. Transmission of *Hepatozoon canis* to dogs by naturally-fed or percutaneously-injected *Rhipicephalus sanguineus* ticks. J Parasitol 2001;87(3):606–11.

35. Dantas-Torres F. The brown dog tick, *Rhipicephalus sanguineus* (Latreille, 1806) (Acari: Ixodidae) from taxonomy to control. Vet Parasitol 2008;152(3-4):173–85.

36. Dantas-Torres F. Biology and ecology of the brown dog tick, *Rhipicephalus sanguineus*. Parasit Vectors 2010;3:26.

37. Murata T, Inoue M, Taura Y, et al. Detection of *Hepatozoon canis* oocysts from ticks collected from the infected dogs. J Vet Med Sci 1995;57(1):111–2.

38. Reye AL, Hübschen JM, Sausy A, et al. Prevalence and seasonality of tick-borne pathogens in questing *Ixodes ricinus* ticks from Luxembourg. Appl Environ Microbiol 2010;76(9):2923–31.

39. Forlano M, Scofield A, Elisei C, et al. Diagnosis of *Hepatozoon* spp in *Amblyomma ovale* and its experimental transmission in domestic dogs in Brazil. Vet Parasitol 2005;134(1-2):1–7.

40. Rubini AS, Paduan KS, Martins TF, et al. Acquisition and transmission of *Hepatozoon canis* (Apicomplexa: Hepatozoidae) by the tick *Amblyomma ovale* (Acari: Ixodidae). Vet Parasitol 2009;164(2-4): 324–7.

41. Kasari TR, Miller RS, James AM, et al. Recognition of the threat of *Ehrlichia ruminantium* infection in domestic and wild ruminants in the continental United States. J Am Vet Med Assoc 2010;237(5):520–30.

42. Paddock CD, Finley RW, Wright CS, et al. *Rickettsia parkeri* rickettsiosis and its clinical distinction from Rocky Mountain spotted fever. Clin Infect Dis 2008;47(9):1188–96.

43. Sumner JW, Durden LA, Goddard J, et al. Gulf Coast ticks (*Amblyomma maculatum*) and *Rickettsia parkeri*, United States. Emerg Infect Dis 2007;13(5):751–75-3.

44. Mertins JW, Moorhouse AS, Alfred JT, et al. *Amblyomma triste* (Acari: Ixodidae): new North American collection records, including the first from the United States. J Med Entomol 2010; 47(4):536–42.

45. Smith TG, Desser SS. Ultrastructural features of cystic and merogonic stages of *Hepatozoon sipedon* (Apicomplexa: Adeleorina) in northern leopard frogs (*Rana pipiens*) and northern water snakes (*Nerodia sipedon*) from Ontario, Canada. J Eukaryot Microbiol 1998;45(4):419–25.

46. Johnson EM, Panciera RJ, Allen KE et al. Alternate pathway of infection with *Hepatozoon americanum* and the epidemiologic importance of predation. J Vet Internal Med 2009;23(6):1315–8.

47. Baneth G, Shkap V. Monozoic cysts of *Hepatozoon canis*. J Parasitol 2003;89: 379–81.

48. Baneth G, Mathew JS, Shkap V, et al. Canine hepatozoozosis: 2 disease syndromes caused by separate Hepatozoon spp. Trends Parasitol 2003;19(1): 27–31.

49. Clark GM. Hepatozoon griseisciuri n sp; a new species of Hepatozoon from the grey squirrel (Sciurus carolinensis Gmelin, 1788), with studies on the life cycle. J Parasitol 1958;44(1):52–63.

50. Murata T, Inoue M, Tateyama S, et al. Vertical transmission of Hepatozoon canis in dogs. J Vet Med Sci 1993;55(5):867–8.

51. Johnson EM, Allen KE, Panciera RJ, et al. Infectivity of Hepatozoon americanum cystozoites for a dog. Vet Parasitol 2008;154(1-2):148–50.

52. Johnson EM, Allen KE, Panciera RJ, et al. Field survey of rodents for Hepatozoon infections in an endemic focus of American canine hepatozoonosis. Vet Parasitol 2007;150(1-2):27–32.

53. Macintire DK, Vincent-Johnson N, Dillon AR, et al. Hepatozoonosis in dogs: 22 cases (1989-1984). J Am Vet Med Assoc 1997;210(7): 916–22.

54. Allen KE. Hepatozoon species in North America: Phylogenetic diversity, transmission patterns, and opportunities for control [PhD dissertation]. Stillwater (OK): Oklahoma State University; 2010.

55. Cummings CA, Panciera RJ, Kocan KM, et al. Characterization of stages of Hepatozoon americanum and of parasitized canine host cells. Vet Pathol 2005; 42(6):788–96.

56. Baneth G, Weigler B. Retrospective case-control study of hepatozoonosis in dogs in Israel. J Vet Internal Med 1997;11(6):365–70.

57. Baneth G, Vincent-Johnson N. Hepatozoonosis. In: Shaw WE, Day MJ, editors. Arthropod-borne infectious diseases of the dog and cat. 1st edition. London: Manson Publishing Ltd; 2005. p. 78–88.

58. Panciera RJ, Ewing SA, Mathew JS, et al. Canine hepatozoonosis: Comparison of lesions and parasites in skeletal muscle of dogs experimentally or naturally infected with Hepatozoon americanum. Vet Parasitol 1999;82(4):261–72.

59. Panciera RJ, Ewing SA, Mathew JS, et al. Observations on tissue stages of Hepatozoon americanum in 19 naturally infected dogs. Vet Parasitol 1998;78(4): 265–76.

60. Harmelin A, Dubey JP, Yakobson B, et al. Concurrent Hepatozoon canis and Toxoplasma gondii infections in a dog. Vet Parasitol 1992;43(1-2):132–6.

61. Baneth G, Aroch I, Presentey B. Hepatozoon canis infection in a litter of Dalmatian dogs. Vet Parasitol 1997;70(1-3):201–6.

62. Mylonakis ME, Leontides L, Gonen L, et al. Anti-Hepatozoon canis serum antibodies and gamonts in naturally-occurring canine monocytic ehrlichiosis. Vet Parasitol 2005; 129(3-4):229–33.

63. Oyamada M, Vavoust B, Boni M, et al. Detection of Babesia canis rossi, B canis vogeli, and Hepatozoon canis in dogs in a village of eastern Sudan by using a screening PCR and sequencing methodologies. Clinical and Diagnostic Laboratory Immunology 2005;12:1343–6.

64. Criado-Fornelio A, Buling A, Cunha-Filho NA, et al. Development and evaluation of a quantitative PCR assay for detection of Hepatozoon sp. Vet Parasitol 2007;150(4): 352–6.

65. Panciera RJ, Mathew JS, Ewing SA, et al. Skeletal lesions of canine hepatozoonosis caused by Hepatozoon americanum. Vet Pathol 2000;37(3):225–30.

66. Holman PJ, Snowden KF. Canine hepatozoonosis and babesiosis, and feline cytauxzoonosis. Vet Clin North Am Small Anim Pract 2009;39(6):1035–53.

67. Bowman D. Georgis' parasitology for veterinarians. Philadelphia: Saunders Elsevier; 1985. p. 106–7.

68. Charles SD, Chopade HM, Ciszewski KD, et al. Safety of 5% Ponazuril (Toltrazuril sulfone) oral suspension and efficacy against naturally acquired *Cystoisospora ohioensis*-like infection in beagle puppies. Parasitol Res 2007;101:S137–44.

69. Mackay RJ, Tanhauser ST, Gillis,KD, et al. Effect of intermittent oral administration of ponazuril on experimental *Sarcoystis neurona* infection of horses. Am J Vet Res 2008;69(3):396–402.

70. Mitchell SM, Zajac AM, Davis WL, et al. The effects of ponazuril on development of apicomplexans *in vitro*. J Eukaryot Microbiol 2005;52(3):231–5.

71. Mitchell SM, Zajac AM, Davis WL, et al. Efficacy of ponazuril in *vitro* and in preventing and treating *Toxoplasma gondii* infections in mice. J Parasitol 2004;90(3):639–42.

72. Allen KE, Little SE, Johnson EM, et al. Treatment of *Hepatozoon americanum* infection: review of the literature and experimental evaluation of efficacy. Vet Ther 2010;11(4): E1–8.

73. Telford SR, Wozniak EJ Jr, Butler JF. Haemogregarine specificity in 2 communities of Florida snakes, with descriptions of six new species of *Hepatozoon* (Apicomplexa: Hepatozoidae) and a possible species of *Haemogregarina* (Apicomplexa: Haemogregarinidae). J Parasitol 2001;87(4):890–905.

74. Telford SR Jr, Butler JF, Telford RS. *Hepatozoon* species (Apicomplexa: Hepatozoidae) of the corn snake, *Elaphe guttata* (Serpentes: Colubridae) and the pigmy rattlesnake, *Sistrurus miliarius barbouri* (Serpentes: Viperidae) in south Florida. J Parasitol 2002;88(4):778–82.

75. Telford SR Jr, Butler JF, Moler PE. Two additional *Hepatozoon* species (Apicomplexa: Hepatozoidae) from the southern black racer, *Coluber constrictor priapus* (Serpentes: Colubridae), in northern Florida. J Parasitol 2005a;91(1):139–43.

76. Telford SR Jr, Butler JF, Telford RS. *Hepatozoon polytopis* n sp parasitic in 2 genera and species of colubrid snakes in southern Florida. J Parasitol 2005b;91(1):144–7.

77. Telford SR Jr, Moler PE, Butler JF. *Hepatozoon* species of the timber rattlesnake in northern Florida: description of a new species, evidence of salivary gland oocysts, and a natural cross-familial transmission of an *Hepatozoon* species. J Parasitol 2008; 94(2):520–3.

78. Telford SR Jr. Three new *Hepatozoon* species (Apicomplexa: Hepatozoidae) infecting the Florida kingsnake, *Lampropeltis getula floridana*. J Parasitol 2010;96(1):162–9.

79. Eyles DE. Incidence of *Trypanosoma lewisi* and *Hepatozoon muris* in the Norway rat. J Parasitol 1952;38(3):222–5.

80. Clark GM. *Hepatozoon griseisciuri* n sp;A new species of *Hepatozoon* from the grey squirrel (*Sciurus carolinensis* Gmelin, 1788), with studies on the life cycle. J Parasitol 1958;44(1):52–63.

81. Schaffer GD, Hanson WL, Davidson WR, et al. Hematotropic parasites of translocated raccoons in the southeast. J Am Vet Med Assoc 1978;173(9):1148–51.

82. Pietrzak SM, Pung OJ. Trypanosomiasis in raccoons from Georgia. J Wildl Dis 1998;34(1):132–6.

83. Davidson WR, Calpin JP. *Hepatozoon griseisciuri* infection in gray squirrels of the southeastern Unites States. J Wildl Dis 1976;12(1):72–6.

84. Lane JR, Kocan AA. *Hepatozoon* sp infection in bobcats. J Am Vet Med Assoc 1983;183(11):1323–4.

85. Mercer SH, Jones LP, Rappole JH, et al. *Hepatozoon* sp in wild carnivores in Texas. J Wildl Dis 1988;24(3):574–6.

86. Forlano MD, Teixeira KR, Scofield A. Molecular characterization of *Hepatozoon* sp from Brazilian dogs and its phylogenetic relationship with other *Hepatozoon* spp. Vet Parasitol 2007;145(1-2):21–30.

87. Paludo GR, Friedmann H, Dell'Porto A, et al. *Hepatozoon* spp: Pathological and partial 18S rRNA sequence analysis from three Brazilian dogs. Parasitol Res 2005; 97(2):167–70.

88. Allen KE, Yabsley MJ, Johnson EM, et al. Novel *Hepaotzoon* invertebrates from the southern United States. J Parasitol 2011 97(4):648-53.

89. Desser SS. Tissue "cysts" of *Hepatozoon griseisciuri* in the grey squirrel, *Sciurus carolinensis*: the significance of these cysts in species of *Hepatozoon*. J Parasitol 1990;76(2):257–9.

North American Snake Envenomation in the Dog and Cat

Lyndi L. Gilliam, DVM*, Jill Brunker, DVM

KEYWORDS

- Snakebite • Envenomation • Dog • Cat • Echinocytosis

Venomous snakes are found in 47 of the 50 US states.[1] The majority of venomous snakebites occur in the southwestern United States.[2] Approximately 4700 human exposures to venomous snakes are reported to poison control centers annually.[3] It is estimated that 150,000 animals, primarily dogs and cats, are bitten in the United States every year.[1] Although human mortality following snakebite in the United States is low (0.06%),[3] reported mortality in dogs ranges from 1% to 30%.[4] Snakebite poses a significant risk of morbidity in humans as well as domestic animal species. Veterinarians must be aware of the venomous snakes in their practice area, be able to recognize the clinical picture typical of an envenomation by these snakes, and be equipped to treat these patients.

VENOMOUS SNAKES OF NORTH AMERICA

Venomous snakes in North America that have been reported to cause illness in domestic animals are members of the family Elapidae or Crotalidae. The coral snake species are the only Elapids native to North America. **Table 1** gives a listing of coral snakes located in North America with their approximate geographical distribution. Several nonvenomous snakes are easily mistaken as coral snakes. Coral snakes are marked with broad bands of bright colors and, in contrast to the pit vipers, have round pupils and no pit on their face.[5] The red and yellow bands on a coral snake are in direct contact and completely encircle the body.[6] Coral snakes make up approximately 2% of the envenomations that occur in humans every year.[3] Elapids have small fixed front fangs and they must chew on their prey in order to envenomate, making envenomation by these snakes much less common.[6] Coral snake venom is the most toxic per milligram of dried weight of any snake venom in the United

The authors have nothing to disclose.
Center for Veterinary Health Sciences, Department of Veterinary Clinical Sciences, Oklahoma State University, 1 Farm Road—BVMTH, Stillwater, OK 74078, USA
* Corresponding author.
E-mail address: l.gilliam@okstate.edu

Vet Clin Small Anim 41 (2011) 1239–1259
doi:10.1016/j.cvsm.2011.08.008
0195-5616/11/$ – see front matter © 2011 Elsevier Inc. All rights reserved.

vetsmall.theclinics.com

Table 1
North American snakes in the family Elapidae and their general geographical distribution

Scientific Name	Common Name	Geographical Distribution
Micruroides euryanthus	Sonoran Coral Snake	Central and SE Arizona, SW New Mexico
Micrurus fulvius fulvius	Eastern Coral Snake	N. Carolina, S. Carolina, Georgia, Alabama, Mississippi, Louisiana
Micrurus fulvius tenere	Texas Coral Snake	Texas, Louisiana, Arkansas
Micrurus fulvius barbouri	South Florida Coral Snake	South Florida

States; fortunately, approximately 60% of all coral snakebites do not result in envenomation.[5,6]

Snakes in the family Crotalidae make up the largest percentage of snakebite exposures each year.[3] Snakes in this family are the pit vipers including rattlesnakes, cottonmouths, and copperheads. Pit vipers are distinguished by their diamond-shaped heads, elliptical pupils, heat-sensing pit on their face between their eye and their nose, and retractable front fangs.[1] Pit vipers have the ability to control the amount of venom they inject and can bite without injecting venom, resulting in a "dry bite." Approximately 25% of all pit viper bites are dry bites.[2] A defensive strike may be a "dry bite" or inject very little venom in contrast to an offensive bite, in which they will inject a controlled amount of venom, or an agonal bite, where they will discharge their venom gland entirely.[1]

There are several different species of rattlesnakes in North America (**Figs. 1–3**). **Table 2** provides a listing of rattlesnakes in North America and their approximate geographical locations. Approximately 65% of venomous snakebites are caused by rattlesnakes.[2] Rattlesnake envenomation results in more deaths and a higher morbidity than any of the other pit vipers found in North America.[3] The species of rattlesnakes most commonly reported with bites are the Eastern diamondback rattlesnake, the Western diamondback rattlesnake, the prairie rattlesnake, the Pacific

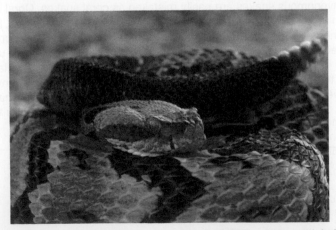

Fig. 1. *Crotalus horridus horridus* (timber rattlesnake). Note the thick, solid dark tail characteristic of the timber rattlesnake. (*Courtesy of* John N. Gilliam, DVM, MS, DACVIM, DABVP, Stillwater, OK.)

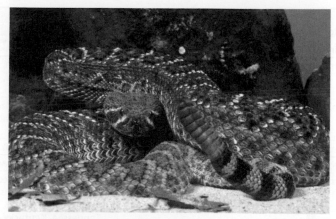

Fig. 2. *Crotalus atrox* (Western diamondback rattlesnake). Notice the black and white bands on the tail. (*Courtesy of* Charlotte L. Ownby, PhD, Stillwater, OK.)

rattlesnake, the timber rattlesnake, and the pygmy rattlesnake. Of these species, the Eastern and Western diamondback rattlesnakes are most often associated with mortality.[2] Rattlesnake venom varies from species to species and within a species; therefore, the clinical picture resulting from rattlesnake envenomation is largely variable.

Copperhead (**Fig. 4**) bites are the second most common snake envenomation in the United States (25%), followed by cottonmouths (about 10%).[3] **Table 2** shows the approximate geographical distribution of these snakes. Cottonmouth moccasins are semiaquatic snakes that are capable of biting while under water.[2] Copperhead and cottonmouth envenomations generally result in significantly less mortality and morbidity than does rattlesnake envenomation.

TOXIC EFFECTS AND CLINICAL SIGNS

Snakes swallow their prey whole; it can take up to 14 days for complete digestion to occur.[2] Putrefaction of the prey may cause the snake to regurgitate before digestion

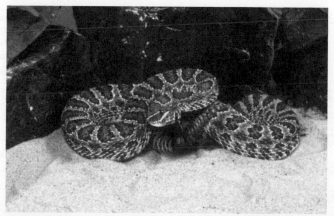

Fig. 3. *Crotalus viridis viridis* (prairie rattlesnake). (*Courtesy of* Charlotte L. Ownby, PhD, Stillwater, OK.)

Table 2
North American pit vipers and their general geographical distribution

Scientific Name	Common Name	Geographical Distribution
Crotalus adamanteus	Eastern Diamondback rattlesnake	N. Carolina, S. Carolina, Georgia, Alabama, Mississippi, Louisiana, Florida
Crotalus atrox	Western Diamondback rattlesnake	California, Nevada, Arizona, New Mexico, Texas, Oklahoma, Arkansas
Crotalus cerastes	Mojave Desert Sidewinder	California, Nevada, Arizona, Utah
Crotalus concolor	Midget Faded rattlesnake	Wyoming, Utah, Colorado
Crotalus horridus	Timber rattlesnake	Texas, Minnesota, Wisconsin, Iowa, Nebraska, Kansas, Oklahoma, Arkansas, Missouri, Tennessee, Kentucky, Illinois, Indiana, Ohio, N. Carolina, S. Carolina, Georgia, Alabama, Mississippi, Louisiana, Florida, Pennsylvania, New Jersey, Maryland, Delaware, Virginia, W. Virginia, New York, New England
Crotalus lepidus	Rock rattlesnake	Arizona, New Mexico, Texas
Crotalus mitchelli	Speckled rattlesnake	California, Nevada, Arizona
Crotalus molossus	Black-tailed rattlesnake	Arizona, New Mexico, Texas
Crotalus pricei	Twin-spotted rattlesnake	Arizona
Crotalus scutulatus	Mojave rattlesnake	Nevada, SW Texas, S. California, Tuscon to Phoenix, Arizona, New Mexico
Crotalus ruber	Red Diamond rattlesnake	Washington, Oregon, Idaho
Crotalus tigris	Tiger rattlesnake	Arizona
Crotalus viridis	Western rattlesnake	Oregon, Idaho, Arizona, New Mexico, Texas, Montana, S. Dakota, N. Dakota, Nebraska, Iowa, Utah, Colorado, Kansas, Oklahoma
Crotalus viridis viridis	Prairie rattlesnake	Oregon, Idaho, Arizona, New Mexico, Texas, Montana, S. Dakota, N. Dakota, Nebraska, Iowa, Utah, Colorado, Kansas, Oklahoma, Wyoming, Alberta Canada
Crotalus viridis abyssus	Grand Canyon rattlesnake	Arizona
Crotalus viridis helleri	Southern Pacific rattlesnake	California
Crotalus viridis lutosus	Great Basin rattlesnake	Oregon, Idaho, California, Nevada, Arizona, Utah
Crotalus viridis oreganus	Northern Pacific rattlesnake	Washington, Oregon, Idaho, California, Nevada
Crotalus willardi	Ridge-nosed rattlesnake	Arizona

(continued on next page)

Table 2 (continued)		
Scientific Name	**Common Name**	**Geographical Distribution**
Sistrurus catenatus	Massasauga rattlesnake	Arizona, New Mexico, Texas, Michigan, Wisconsin, Minnesota, Nebraska, Iowa, Colorado, Kansas, Oklahoma, Arkansas, Missouri, Illinois, Indiana, Ohio, New York, Pennsylvania
Sistrurus miliarius	Pigmy rattlesnake	Texas, Oklahoma, Arkansas, Missouri, Tennessee, Florida, N. Carolina, S. Carolina, Georgia, Alabama, Mississippi, Louisiana
Agkistrodon contortix	Southern Copperhead	Kansas, Oklahoma, Arkansas, Missouri, Tennessee, Kentucky, Illinois, Indiana, Ohio, N. Carolina, S. Carolina, Georgia, Alabama, Mississippi, Louisiana, Pennsylvania, New Jersey, Maryland, Deleware, Virginia, W. Virginia, New York, New England
Agkistrodon piscivorus	Eastern/Western Cottonmouth	Texas, Nebraska, Iowa, Kansas, Oklahoma, Arkansas, Missouri, Tennessee, Kentucky, Illinois, N. Carolina, S. Carolina, Georgia, Alabama, Mississippi, Louisiana, Virginia

Data from Singletary EM, Rochman AS, Bodmer JC, et al. Envenomations. Med Clin N Am 2005;89:1205, and Russell FE. Snake venom poisoning in the United States. Annu Rev Med 1980; 31:250–1.

is complete.[2] The role of venom, therefore, is to predigest the prey, allowing it to be fully digested more rapidly, within 2 to 5 days.[2] The proteins and enzymes that allow for immobilization and predigestion of the prey are responsible for the clinical signs we see in our patients. To better understand the clinical picture of these envenomated patients, it is helpful to have a working knowledge of the individual venom component's effect on the body. It is perhaps easiest to discuss these venom components in conjunction with the clinical signs that they cause.

CLINICAL SIGNS OF ELAPID ENVENOMATION

Close examination of a suspect elapid bite victim, focusing on the lips, muzzle, and distal limbs, should be performed to look for the presence of fang puncture wounds.[7] Coral snake fang punctures are small, looking more like scratches, and are easily missed.[7] Clinical signs of coral snake envenomation are largely attributed to the venom's neurotoxic effects and typically have a delayed onset, making it difficult, initially, to determine if envenomation has occurred.[5] Clinical signs may occur within 1 hour of envenomation but can be delayed up to 18 hours.[5] Interestingly, coral snakebites often do not result in severe pain. Swelling in the area of the bite is not an indicator of severity of envenomation as fatal envenomation can occur with minimal

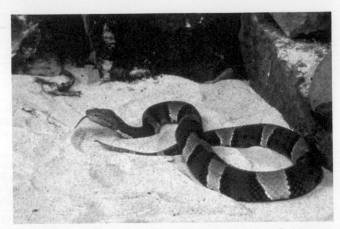

Fig. 4. *Agkistrodon contortrix laticinctus* (broadbanded copperhead). (*Courtesy of* Charlotte L. Ownby, PhD, Stillwater, OK.)

local tissue damage.[5] Dogs envenomated by coral snakes typically become lethargic and exhibit vomiting and ptyalism acutely due to the venom's excitatory effects on the autonomic nervous system.[8] The postsynaptic action of the neurotoxin at the acetylcholine receptor site eventually results in generalized muscle weakness, quadriplegia, and paralysis.[9] The neurotoxicity may manifest itself as ptosis and weakness of the extrinsic musculature of the eyeball.[5] The most common clinical signs seen in 9 dogs envenomated by coral snakes were lethargy and lower motor neuron weakness, marked ptyalism, vomiting, and reddened urine.[5,7] Cardiac arrhythmias have been reported secondary to coral snake envenomation but are not common.[5,7] Death typically occurs secondary to respiratory paralysis.[5] Coral snake envenomation in the cat is not widely reported; however, in one case series of 3 cats suspected of having coral snake envenomation, common clinical signs were sedation, peracute onset of ascending flaccid paralysis, hypothermia, decreased nociception, loss of spinal reflexes, and loss of cutaneous trunci reflex.[9]

CLINICAL SIGNS OF PIT VIPER ENVENOMATION

Clinical signs of pit viper envenomation tend to be more severe in dogs than cats as cats seem to be more resistant to pit viper venom on a milligram of venom–per–kilogram of body mass basis.[1] Species, age, size, location of the bite, postbite excitability, and health status at the time of the bite are all factors that will affect the severity of envenomation in a given individual.[1] Concurrent medications at the time of the bite may also affect the severity of the clinical signs (eg, nonsteroidal anti-inflammatory drugs further inhibit platelet function; beta-blockers may mask early onset of anaphylaxis).[1,6] The primary factors related to the snake that affect severity of envenomation are the quantity and toxicity of the venom.[1] The quantity of venom available for injection can be affected by season, time since last discharge of venom, age and size of the snake, and motivation of the snake (offensive vs defensive vs agonal).[6]

Puncture wounds that are oozing blood or serum are a characteristic clinical sign of pit viper envenomation (**Figs. 5–9**). It is important to note that the presence of fang marks does not confirm envenomation due to the high percentage of "dry bites." If there is absent to minimal swelling observed 1 hour post bite and the animal is not

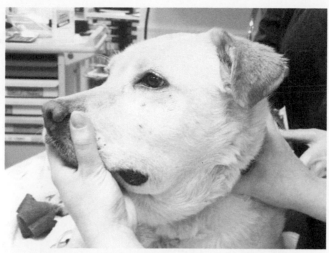

Fig. 5. Fang marks on upper lip of a dog bitten by a copperhead at the time of presentation.

showing any systemic signs of envenomation, it is very unlikely that envenomation occurred.[10,11] With moderate to severe envenomation, local tissue damage is evident within 10 minutes of the bite (exception may be the Mojave rattlesnake), the area is painful, and there is often local hemorrhage.[10,11]

Acute pain, marked swelling and edema, and ecchymosis at the bite site are also characteristic of pit viper envenomation (**Figs. 6** and **8**). Tissue damage and necrosis in the area of the bite is the most commonly recognized clinical sign following North American pit viper envenomation.[12] Tissue damage is most likely a combination of the direct effect of the venom on the tissues and damage caused by inflammation and swelling secondary to edema formation and hemorrhage.

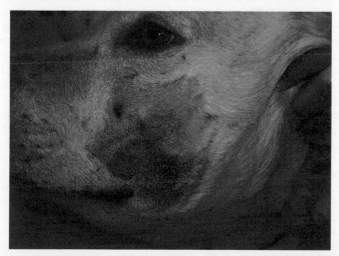

Fig. 6. Dog from **Figs. 5** and **6** at 24 hours postpresentation for copperhead bite. Signs of envenomation are obvious including increased swelling and ecchymosis around the bite site.

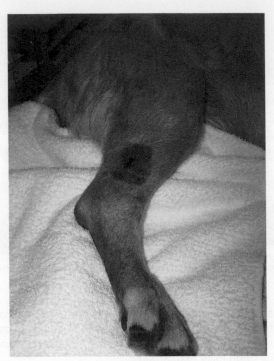

Fig. 7. Fang marks on the distal hind limb of a dog bitten by a copperhead at the time of presentation. Note slight serous discharge at the bite site.

Multiple venom components are involved in causing tissue damage and necrosis. Venom metalloproteinases (VMPs) cause local myonecrosis and skin damage as well as hemorrhage and systemic inflammation.[12] They cleave pro–tumor necrosis factor alpha (pro-TNFα) and release activated TNFα, a normal mediator of the inflammatory response.[12] Activated TNFα results in production of similar human metalloproteinases (HMPs) which break down extracellular matrix proteins, resulting in further tissue damage.[12] HMPs also cleave pro-TNFα and result in a vicious cycle of inflammation.[12] Venom hyaluronidase and collagenase lead to deeper venom penetration through connective tissue.[13] Hyaluronidase decreases connective tissue viscosity by catalyzing the cleavage of internal glycoside bonds and mucopolysaccharides while collagenases digest collagen.[13]

Local tissue reactions are less dramatic with cottonmouth and copperhead snakes than rattlesnakes. There are rare occasions where fatal pit viper envenomation can occur without local tissue effects (**Fig. 9**). This is most likely to occur with one of the snakes that have primarily neurotoxic venoms such as the Mojave rattlesnake.[1,14]

The Mojave rattlesnake, timber rattlesnake, and canebrake rattlesnake all possess a neurotoxin. The Mojave toxin can cause a flaccid paralysis; however, weakness and paralysis are not commonly seen following Mojave rattlesnake envenomation.[12] This toxin is thought to work presynaptically by blocking the calcium channels in the presynaptic motor neuron at neuromuscular junctions.[12] This blockade prevents the release of acetylcholine, preventing the activation of the acetylcholine receptor on skeletal muscle and thus preventing muscle contraction.[12] Calcium channel blockade by the Mojave toxin will not improve with calcium therapy.[12] Effects of Mojave toxin

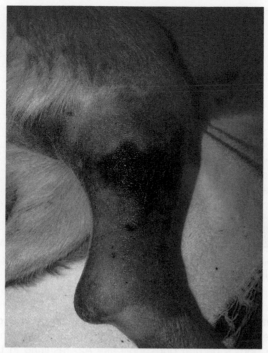

Fig. 8. Dog from Figs. 5 and 6 at 24 hours postpresentation for copperhead bite. Signs of envenomation are obvious including increased swelling and ecchymosis around the bite site.

experimentally are greatest on the motor axon terminals of the diaphragm, which could lead to respiratory paralysis.[15] The venom of the Mojave found near Phoenix is thought to be less neurotoxic than that of the Mojave found in southwestern Arizona and southeastern California.[1]

The primary neurotoxic sign seen with timber rattlesnake envenomation is myokymia, a type of muscle fasciculation that resembles a wave or wormlike movement below the skin. The proposed mechanism also involves calcium channels at the presynaptic neuromuscular junction.[12] Intravenous calcium does result in clinical improvement.[12]

Further clinical signs seen with pit viper envenomation include but are not limited to petechiae, increased salivation, vomiting, diarrhea, urinary and fecal incontinence, excessive thirst, severe hypotension, regional lymphadenopathy, altered respiratory rate, pulmonary edema, cyanosis, cardiac arrhythmias, bleeding, obtundation, shock, coma, and convulsions.[1,4,10,13,16,17]

Indications of coagulopathy such as petechiae or spontaneous bleeding occur with severe envenomations. One retrospective study found that the presence of petechiation was negatively correlated with survival in a group of dogs envenomated by pit vipers.[4]

Lethargy, increased salivation, vomiting, diarrhea, and urinary and fecal incontinence are most likely due to the venom's excitatory effect directly on visceral smooth muscle or indirectly on the autonomic nervous system.[8]

Severe hypotension is multifactorial. A myocardial depressor protein has been demonstrated in Western diamondback venom that could directly result in hypotension.[18]

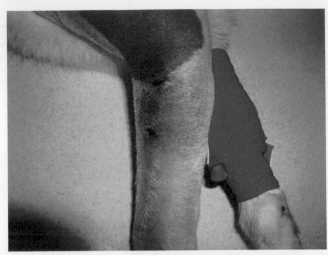

Fig. 9. Fang marks on the distal limb of a cat inflicted by a pit viper. Note the lack of echhymosis or swelling.

Rattlesnake venom contains kininogenases that act on plasma globulins to form bradykinins,[19] potent vasodilators that can result in profound hypotension. Bradykinins can stimulate the body's natural phospholipase A2, resulting in the production of prostaglandins and thromboxane A2.[19] Prostaglandins E2 and I2 cause vasodilation, which results in decreased systemic arterial pressure and contributes to hypotension.[19] Prostaglandins can also cause severe congestion in the lungs, increased vascular permeability and hemorrhage.[19] Indomethacin, a cyclooxygenase inhibitor, has been shown to improve Mojave rattlesnake venom–induced hypotension in a mouse model, suggesting the role of prostaglandins in venom-induced hypotension.[8]

Large amounts of fluid may be lost in acute envenomation, resulting in hypotension. Fluid losses are attributed to third space losses secondary to severe endothelial damage, vomiting, and hemorrhage.[19] A lethal factor in Crotalus venom has been shown to cause lysis of plasma membranes resulting in microangiopathic vascular permeability, which allows plasma proteins and red blood cells to leak into the surrounding tissues.[20] This extravascular fluid loss can lead to volume depletion and hypoperfusion followed by hemoconcentration, lactic acidosis, and hypovolemic shock.

Another contributor to venom-induced hypotension is blood pooling. Crotalidae venom has been shown to cause pooling of blood in the hepatosplanhnic vasculature of dogs and in the lungs of cats.[13] Victims may have an altered respiratory rate, pulmonary edema, and cyanosis.[1]

Cardiac perfusion will suffer with prolonged or untreated hypotension, resulting in a further decrease in cardiac output. Cardiac arrhythmias may be seen.[1,17,21] No direct effect of pit viper venom on the heart has been specifically identified. At present it is uncertain whether cardiac arrhythmias are due to direct or secondary effects of North American pit viper and elapidae venom.

Bites to the head or neck can result in severe edema and swelling of the pharyngeal area resulting in respiratory distress or asphyxia. Dogs are most commonly bitten on the head; second most commonly the legs, and rarely the body.[13] Cats are most commonly bitten on the front legs, followed by the head and then the body.[13] In cases of head bites, there may be epistaxis, which can appear frothy, and swelling of the face may prevent opening of the eyelids, resulting in temporary blindness.[16]

Venom travels via the lymphatics; therefore, regional lymphadenopathy may be recognized. This lymphadenopathy is often mistaken for secondary infection; however, it rarely is associated with infection in human patients.[22] Bites to extremities may continue to have edema for weeks to months due to reduced lymphatic function.[12]

DIFFERENTIAL DIAGNOSES

Differential diagnoses for coral snake envenomation include tick paralysis, polyradiculo-neuritis, botulism, and myasthenia gravis.[5] Differential diagnoses for pit viper envenomation include trauma, angioedema (ie, insect bite or sting), a nonsnake animal bite, abscess, non–snakebite wound–induced cellulitis, or puncture wound.[1,16]

EMERGENCY FIELD TREATMENT/FIRST AID

Over the years many recommendations have been put forth for the field treatment of snakebites. Scientific studies of these methods have proved that many are ineffective and some are even harmful. Keeping the animal as restricted and calm as possible and transporting them the nearest veterinary facility is the best response to a snakebite.[6] In the case of coral snake envenomation, it is ideal to get the animal to a facility that can offer mechanical ventilation in case it is needed.[6] Antivenin availability is also very important. Most medical facilities in areas where poisonous snakes are endemic will have access to antivenin. Therapies that are contraindicated include cryotherapy, hot packs, electroshock therapy, incision and suction of the bite site, and tourniquet application.[1] Compression bandages have been shown to be beneficial in Australian Elapid envenomation; thus, they may have a place in field treatment of coral snake envenomation.[6] They have not, however, been demonstrated to be beneficial in pit viper envenomation. Keeping the venom concentrated in one area may only result in increased tissue necrosis.[1,2,12] Due to the difficulty with appropriate application in the case of coral snake envenomation and the potential contraindication in pit viper envenomation, the authors cannot recommend the use of compression bandages. The Extractor is a negative suction device that has been evaluated for its use as a first aid device with snake envenomation.[23–25] If applied within 3 minutes of envenomation, 23% of venom could be extracted after 3 minutes of suction and 34% after 30 minutes of suction.[24] However, the distance between fang tip punctures in defensive bites of western diamondback rattlesnakes were measured and it was concluded that The Extractor could not simultaneously cover both puncture wounds, indicating that 2 of these devices may be necessary to aspirate venom from a bite site.[25] The Extractor did not reduce local venom induced tissue injury in an artificial model of rattlesnake evenomation in pigs.[26] In addition, this model indicated local skin damage may occur secondary to prolonged application of the device.[26] Application of this device has not been reported in veterinary medicine. Hair-covered skin may present a challenge to establishing negative pressure with the device and more information on the product's application to the veterinary species is needed.

It is not uncommon for cats to be bitten by a snake on the body. A localizing circumferential compression device has been evaluated in pigs experimentally envenomated with Eastern diamondback rattlesnake venom on the torso and was found to be beneficial in delaying the onset of signs of envenomation.[27] This device may or may not be practical in our veterinary patients. Application to feline patients may be very difficult and stressful, making it impractical.

Snakebite victims that are treated appropriately within 2 hours of being bitten have an excellent prognosis.[2] Many attempts at field first aid ultimately delay appropriate care in the hospital. Such a delay was a common denominator in human victims who died secondary to rattlesnake bite.[28]

Although it is helpful to have identification of the snake, owners should not risk capturing the snake for identification purposes. These efforts can result in the owner getting bitten and will delay appropriate treatment for the animal. Owners should be cautioned that dead and decapitated snakes can still envenomate.[1]

DIAGNOSTIC TESTING

A minimum database should be collected on a patient presented for snakebite even if signs of envenomation are not present initially. Laboratory abnormalities may be present that will confirm envenomation prior to clinical signs becoming apparent. A baseline complete blood count (CBC) and blood chemistry panel should be performed. Common CBC findings are nonspecific and include mild to severe anemia, leukocytosis (may or may not have a left shift), and thrombocytopenia. Anemia in dogs bitten by coral snakes may be due to severe hemolysis.[5] The proposed mechanism is the action of venom phospholipase A2 (PLA2) on red blood cell membranes.[6] This has not been documented in cats bitten by coral snakes. In North American pit viper envenomation, the anemia is more commonly due to hemorrhage as hemolysis is uncommon in the absence of disseminated intravascular coagulation. The chemistry panel should include but not be limited to creatine phosphokinase (CPK), creatinine, blood urea nitrogen, sodium, potassium, chloride, calcium, and glucose.[1]

Rhabdomyolysis may occur secondary to envenomation and may, at least in part, be due to the venom protein myotoxin a. Myotoxin a affects calcium regulation within the cell, causing increases in intracellular calcium and eventual skeletal muscle cell necrosis.[8] The exact mechanism of myotoxin a is not known.[12] Myotoxin a is absent in Western diamondback rattlesnake venom.[29] Venom PLA2 may also play a role in rhabdomyolysis by damaging muscle cell membranes, disrupting organelles, and allowing increased influx of calcium.[19] Increased intracellular calcium may result in necrosis. Muscle fiber proteins can be damaged by venom proteolytic enzymes RNase, DNase, and 5′ nucleotidase if the venom is injected directly into a muscle.[2] Profound swelling of an area may result in an ischemic myonecrosis secondary to the envenomation.[30] In veterinary patients, pain indicative of a typical rhabdomyolysis may not be exhibited; therefore, the syndrome may not be recognized without evaluating CPK. A marked early increase in CPK is an indicator of severe envenomation.[13]

Hypokalemia has been documented secondary to pit viper envenomation[1] and may contribute to signs of weakness and cardiac dysfunction.

A blood smear should be examined to look for the presence or absence of echinocytosis. Echinocytosis has been reported in the literature secondary to coral snake and rattlesnake envenomation.[6,31] Although there are no reports of echinocytosis secondary to copperhead envenomation in the literature, it has been seen in at least 2 dogs with documented copperhead envenomation (Robin Allison, DVM, DACVP, Stillwater, OK, personal communication, March 2011) (**Fig. 10**). Exposure of human, canine, equine, and feline red blood cells to Western diamondback rattlesnake venom resulted in echinocytosis in an in vitro study.[32] Low venom concentrations resulted in Type I and Type II echinocytes.[32] Type III echinocytes, spheroechinocytes, and spherocytes occurred with increased venom concentrations.[32] The absence of echinocytosis does not indicate that envenomation did not occur.[1,32]

Rattlesnake venoms are reported to cause more severe coagulopathies than those of other pit vipers[12]; therefore, a coagulation panel including activated clotting time

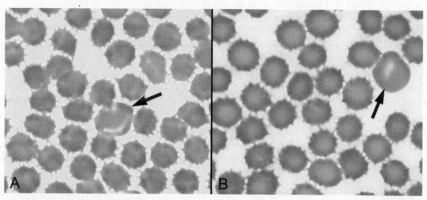

Fig. 10. Blood smears demonstrating type III echinocytes caused by pit viper envenomation. *A,* Dog bitten by a rattlesnake. *B,* Dog bitten by a copperhead. The arrows point to polychromatophils, which are always unaffected. (*Courtesy of* Robin W. Allison, DVM, PhD, DACVP, Stillwater, OK.)

(ACT), prothrombin time (PT), partial thromboplastin time (PTT), fibrinogen, fibrin degradation products (FDPs), and an accurate platelet count should be evaluated.[1] Decreased platelet counts and/or increased ACT, PT, and PTT indicate envenomation has occurred and the degree of change is an indicator of severity of envenomation.[13] Common findings on a coagulation panel from animals with moderate to severe North American pit viper envenomation are hypofibrinogenemia, increased FDPs, and prolonged PT and PTT.[10] In contrast, animals with coral snake envenomation are more likely to have a hyperfibrinogenemia.[6]

Venom disrupts the coagulation process by one or more mechanisms that differ from species to species and even within the same species of snake.[12] Venom fibrinolysins destroy both fibrinogen and fibrin, while venom thrombin-like enzymes result in the construction of a weak fibrin chain by inadequate fibrinopeptide cleavage.[12] In addition, thrombin-like enzymes do not activate factor XIII. The net result of these venom activities is defibrination characterized by inadequate fibrin clot formation, hypofibrinogenemia, increased FDPs, abnormal coagulation profiles, and diminished to absent intravascular clotting.[12] Snake-bitten patients suffering from defibrination alone are often misdiagnosed with disseminated intravascular coagulation (DIC) because of their abnormal coagulation profiles; however, platelet function and numbers are normal, factor VII is unaffected, and clinical bleeding is unusual in these animals.[12]

Phospholipids must be available for use in the clotting cascade—in particular, for the activation of factor X. Venom PLA2 forms complexes with phospholipids, preventing them from being used for clotting protein activation.[19] The result is a dysfunctional clotting cascade and a diminished clotting ability manifested with an increased PT and PTT.

Platelet function and number can be affected in crotalid snake envenomation patients. The mechanisms by which venom-induced thrombocytopenia (VIT) occurs are not understood. Effects of rattlesnake venom on the bone marrow resulting in decreased production have not been demonstrated.[33] Two other basic mechanisms have been proposed: aggregation and consumption/destruction. Several rattlesnake venoms have been noted to cause platelet aggregation resulting in thrombocytopenia.[34] Crotalocytin, a specific serine protease isolated from timber rattlesnake venom, has been shown to cause platelet aggregation in vitro.[33] Venom PLA2 can result in production of prostaglandin E2 and thromboxane A2, which also cause platelet aggregation.[19] Phospholipases have been implicated in damaging platelet membranes and resulting in their ultimate destruction. In addition, envenomation can result in a tremendous amount of endothelial damage, which results in platelet adherence and sequestration at the bite site.[33]

Coagulopathies may exist in the face of normal platelet number due to abnormal platelet function. A protein found in Western diamondback rattlesnake venom, catrocollastatin, inhibits platelet adhesion to collagen, resulting in abnormal platelet function in the face of normal platelet numbers.[35] Crovidisin, a toxin found in prairie rattlesnake venom, binds to collagen fibers and prevents platelets from interacting with collagen. This prevents platelet adhesion, release reaction, thromboxane formation, and aggregation.[36]

Hemorrhagic toxins damage capillary endothelial cells and vessel wall basement membranes resulting in extravasation of erythrocytes.[22] The smaller blood vessels tend to be more susceptible to these toxins.[22] Upon necropsy of animals that have died from snake envenomation, there is often a large amount of hemorrhage in the tissues surrounding the bite site.

When evaluating the pit viper envenomated patient for coagulopathies, it is important to realize that DIC rarely occurs in snakebite victims and abnormal coagulation profiles as well as observed increased bleeding are more likely due to one or more of the many direct effects of the venom.[12]

A baseline urinalysis should be performed to look for hematuria, hemoglobinuria, myoglobinuria, proteinuria, or glucosuria.[1] The presence of pigmenturia is an indicator of severe envenomation.[13] Renal compromise can occur in snakebite patients and is most likely a secondary rather than primary effect of envenomation.[30] Hypotension, hypoperfusion, microthrombosis, myglobinuria, and hemoglobinuria may all contribute to renal compromise and/or damage in these patients.

Electrocardiograms are indicated in any patient with severe envenomation or with suspect cardiac toxicity. Measuring cardiac troponin I may be beneficial in detecting myocardial damage.

Animals bitten on an extremity should have circumferential measurements taken of the limb just above and just below the bite site at presentation.[1] These measurements should be repeated every 15 minutes until they are static over 4 measurements.

Snakebite severity scores have been developed to aid in determining if antivenin is indicated.[37] These scores may aid the clinician in evaluating not only the severity of the envenomation but also the progression. They can assist in determining the necessity of antivenin therapy. **Table 3** shows a human snakebite severity score that has been adapted for use in veterinary patients.

IN HOSPITAL TREATMENT

Treatment of a snakebite victim should first involve determining whether envenomation has occurred followed by a combination of supportive care and therapy aimed at reversing the adverse effects of the venom. Snakebite victims should be hospitalized for a minimum of 8 hours to determine the severity of a potential envenomation.[1] The snakebite severity score sheet should be filled out on presentation and repeated 6 hours after presentation. It is imperative to have a baseline and at least one comparison to be certain subtle changes are not occurring that would indicate the patient's impending decline.[1] Circumferential measurements should also be made at this time (see section on diagnostic testing).

Some clinicians may choose to treat patients with diphenydramine at presentation for its sedative effects. Keeping the animals as calm as possible is necessary.

Table 3
Snakebite severity score
Scoring should occur at presentation and at 6-hour intervals thereafter. Maximum possible score is 20. Risk of mortality increases with increasing scores

Snakebite Severity Score		
System	**Score**	**Signs**
Respiratory	0	Normal
	1	Minimal: slight dyspnea
	2	Moderate: respiratory compromise, tachypnea, use of accessory muscles
	3	Severe: cyanosis, air hunger, extreme tachypnea, respiratory insufficiency or respiratory arrest from any cause
Cardiovascular	0	Normal
	1	Minimal: tachycardia, general weakness, benign dysrhythmia, hypertension
	2	Moderate: tachycardia, hyptension (tarsal pulse still palpable)
	3	Severe: extreme tachycardia, hypotension (nonpalpable tarsal pulse or systolic blood pressure <80 mmHg), malignant dysrhythmia or cardiac arrest
Local Wound	0	Normal
	1	Minimal: pain, swelling, ecchymosis, erythema limited to bite site
	2	Moderate: pain, swelling, ecchymosis, erythema involves less than half of extremity and may be spreading slowly
	3	Severe: pain, swelling, ecchymosis, erythema involves most or all of one extremity and is spreading rapidly
	4	Very severe: pain, swelling, ecchymosis, erythema extends beyond affected extremity, or significant tissue necrosis
Gastrointestinal	0	Normal
	1	Minimal: abdominal pain, tenesmus
	2	Moderate: vomiting, diarrhea
	3	Severe: repetitive vomiting, diarrhea, or hematemesis
Hematological	0	Normal
	1	Minimal: coagulation parameters slightly abnormal, PT < 20 sec, PTT < 50 sec, platelets 100,000 to 150,000/mm3
	2	Moderate: coagulation parameters abnormal, PT 20-50 sec, PTT 50–75 sec, platelets 50,000 to 100,000/mm3
	3	Severe: coagulation parameters abnormal, PT 50–100 sec, PTT 75–100 sec, platelets 20,000 to 50,000/mm3
	4	Very severe: coagulation parameters markedly abnormal with bleeding present or the threat of spontaneous bleeding, including PT unmeasurable, PTT unmeasurable, platelets <20,000/mm3
Central Nervous System	0	Normal
	1	Minimal: apprehension
	2	Moderate: chills, weakness, faintness, ataxia
	3	Severe: lethargy, seizures, coma

Modified from Peterson ME. Snake bite: Pit vipers. Clin Techn Small Anim Pract 2006;21:177–8; with permission.

Antihistamines have no direct effect on the venom or its effects[1]; however, its administration has been positively associated with survival in dogs envenomated by pit vipers.[4]

Therapy for coral snake envenomation in the United States is currently supportive as coral snake antivenin is not available. Supportive care of these patients involves maintaining hydration, appropriate care for the paralyzed patient, and prevention of aspiration pneumonia.[6] Intravenous crystalloid fluids are indicated to maintain hydration and should be initiated early since clinical signs are often delayed. If significant hemolysis or rhabdomyolysis occurs, animals should be maintained on intravenous fluids until evidence of hemolysis and muscle damage have diminished in order to prevent renal damage.

Antivenom is a key component of most severe pit viper envenomation treatments. Not all envenomated patients will require antivenom. One hundred cases of prairie rattlesnake envenomation in dogs found most dogs did not require antivenin for resolution of clinical signs.[21] Very few copperhead bites require treatment with antivenom.[38] It has been widely accepted that the smaller the victim, the more severe the envenomation and thus the higher the dose of antivenom. A study of 31 dogs bitten by the Eastern diamondback rattlesnake showed that the smaller dogs had a worse prognosis.[17] However, a study of 114 cases of snake envenomation in children refuted this fact as all children did well with conservative treatment and did not require antivenom therapy.[39] These conflicting facts confirm that the outcome of each individual envenomation is dependent on several things, size being only one of them. The choice to administer antivenom should be made based on the clinical picture of the patient. The Snakebite Severity Score may aid in this decision. Four common indications for antivenom administration are[12]:

1. Rapid progression of swelling
2. Significant coagulopathy, defibrination, or thrombocytopenia
3. Neuromuscular toxicity
4. Shock

It is important for clinicians and owners to remember that antivenom will not prevent all the effects of the venom. Currently available veterinary antivenom[a] does not have antibodies against myotoxin a and, if not administered within 20 minutes of envenomation, will not reverse or block the effects of venom metalloproteinases. Thrombocytopenia induced by timber rattlesnake venom is not responsive to antivenom.[1] These facts do not, however, preclude the use of antivenom as it is very beneficial in reversing most systemic effects of the venom such as coagulation deficits, fluid loss, neurologic signs, and cardiac dysrhythmias.[1] Specific doses for antivenom have not been established. In the veterinary patient, cost is often the greatest factor in determining a dose of antivenom. Any amount of venom that is bound is less venom in circulation causing detrimental effects. The inability to give a large dose of antivenom should not discourage the clinician from giving what is feasible. The average dose for dogs and cats is 1 to 2 vials; however, resolution of clinical signs could require as many as 12 vials.[1] Antivenom is most effective when administered early on, but there is evidence that as long as there is circulating venom, antivenom will be beneficial.[1,11] Larger doses of antivenom have been associated with a lower chance of survival, although this may be due to the fact that the most severe envenomations are most likely to receive the higher doses of antivenom.[4]

---

[a]Crotalidae Polyvalent Antivenin, Boehringer Ingelheim Vetmedica, Inc.

The human literature describes skin testing prior to antivenom administration; however, this is not practiced in veterinary medicine. The slow administration of antivenom coupled with the diligent observation of the patient should allow early identification of an allergic reaction. Hyperemia of the inner pinna is a good indicator of early systemic reactions.[13] It is very important to have all items necessary to treat anaphylaxis immediately available while administering antivenom.[12] When reconstituting antivenom it should not be shaken but can be swirled and warmed to body temperature in order to facilitate more rapid dissolution.[1] Recommended dilution is 1 vial of antivenom to 100 to 250 ml of crystalloid fluid.[1] This dilution may have to be adjusted for very small patients to avoid volume overload when administering the entire antivenom dose.[1] Antivenom should be administered intravenously and should not be administered directly at the bite site.

If an anaphylactoid reaction is noted during antivenom administration, the drug should be stopped and the animal should be treated, most commonly with diphenydramine. The infusion can typically then be resumed after a short period of time.[1] If anaphylaxis is noted the antivenom administration is stopped and the animal is treated typically with epinephrine plus or minus corticosteroids and intravenous crystalloid fluids.[1] In a group of 218 pit viper envenomated dogs, 7% experienced acute reactions to antivenom,[4] which is much lower than the 23% to 56% rate reported in humans.[40]

A patient that receives antivenom should remain in the hospital for at least 24 hours.[22] If laboratory abnormalities were noted initially, these tests should be repeated after antivenom therapy before discharging the patient.

A newer antivenom is available that is a purified and lyophilized ovine Fab immunoglobulin fragment product.[1] This product does not contain the Fc immunoglobulin fragment, making it much less likely to cause an allergic reaction. Currently this product is cost prohibitive for the veterinary patient. A recurrence phenomenon has been well documented with this ovine antivenom.[41] Patients receive antivenom and clinical signs improve and 2 to 14 days later clinical signs of envenomation recur.[42] It is thought that venom is sequestered in the tissues and is released slowly over time as reperfusion and healing to the envenomated area occur. Venom has been detected in a human patient up to 6 days after envenomation, indicating a prolonged elimination time.[43] The smaller Fab fragments are thought to be cleared from circulation rapidly and are then not available to continue to bind venom that is released over time.[41] The whole IgG equine antivenom (veterinary product) stays in circulation longer and has been found in urine 4 months post administration.[41]

Colloids are controversial in the treatment of snakebite patients. As described earlier, the venom has profound effects on the vasculature resulting in large amounts of fluids leaking into the extravascular fluid spaces. If colloids are leaked outside the vascular space, they will act as an osmotic draw for more fluid to exit the vasculature. One location this is likely to occur, particularly in cats, is the pulmonary vasculature, resulting in pulmonary edema.[1] Whole blood transfusions, however, may be necessary if hemorrhage or hemolysis is severe.[44]

Snakebite patients are often very painful. Care must be taken when manipulating these patients. Initial analgesia should consist primarily of narcotics. NSAIDs are contraindicated as long as a coagulopathy is present. Morphine-induced histamine release can be confused with antivenom anaphylaxis so other opiates such as fentanyl are preferred.[1]

Corticosteroids have been very controversial in snakebite victims over the years. Work in humans has failed to show any beneficial effect of steroids with envenomation.[45] Use of steroids in some species has been reported to be detrimental even increasing mortality.[1]

Heparin has been used to inhibit the venom thrombin-like enzymes; however, they are not inhibited by heparin and therefore its use is not indicated.[1]

Broad-spectrum antibiotics are often administered to animals suffering from snake envenomation. This is a controversial practice in human medicine. Regional lymphadenopathy as a result of venom traveling up the lymphatics is often misdiagnosed as a sign of infection in the area of the bite. Infections secondary to snake envenomation in human patients are not common[22]; however, the nature of our patients and the environment in which they live are quite different, perhaps leading to a bigger concern about wound infection. Venom is thought to be sterile but the snake's mouth contains a variety of aerobes and anaerobes that are undoubtedly inoculated at the time of a bite.[46] When dogs envenomated by pit vipers were treated with fluoroquinolone antimicrobials the odds of survival were greater.[4] Interestingly, dogs treated with other antimicrobials had no increased odds of survival over those untreated.[4] It is the general consensus among the veterinary literature that broad-spectrum antibiotics are still indicated in snake envenomation patients.

Fasciotomy is rarely indicated in snake envenomation patients. In order to determine if fasciotomy will be beneficial, one must first diagnose compartment syndrome. This is challenging and not frequently done in the veterinary patient. Compartment syndrome does not commonly occur in snakebite victims.

Tetanus antitoxin has been advocated in the treatment of canine snake envenomation. Tetanus is rare in dogs and C tetani has not been isolated from the snakes mouth, so its necessity is questioned.[10,17]

A rattlesnake vaccine (Red Rock Biologics, Woodland, CA, USA) is marketed for the dog and the horse. Empirical data have been conflicting, with some veterinarians reporting much lesser degrees of illness secondary to envenomation in vaccinated dogs (Stacey McLoud, DVM, Spearman, TX, personal communication, March 2011) and others reporting no difference.[1] Efficacy studies with this product are in vitro and an in vivo challenge study has not been published. Safety data on the vaccine indicate the product is safe. One author's personal experience is that animals that are bitten more than once typically have a milder reaction with each subsequent bite (L.G.). This could support the theory of naturally protective titers. More peer-reviewed research needs to be presented on this product in order to determine its in vivo efficacy.

COMPLICATIONS

It is not uncommon for aspiration pneumonia to occur secondary to coral snake envenomation. This is most likely due to dysphagia from neurologic dysfunction to the larynx and pharynx.[5] The hypersalivation that occurs secondary to envenomation further complicates the picture.

Serum sickness secondary to antivenom administration has been reported in a dog.[47] In people it can occur in up to 50% of patients who receive more than 8 vials of antivenom and is characterized by fever, malaise, nausea, diarrhea, arthralgia, myalgia, lymphadenopathy, peripheral edema, and dermatopathy.[47] In the dog, serum sickness was manifest as fever, chemosis, urticaria, focal purpura, and limb edema, which was responsive to steroids. These signs occurred at the third day after antivenom administration, which is earlier than what is typically seen in people (1 to 2 weeks post administration).[12,47]

SUMMARY

North American snake envenomation can result in significant morbidity in the veterinary patient. An understanding of the mechanisms of the snake's venom endemic to your practice area will facilitate appropriate treatment of these patients. Client education on field treatment of snakebites may result in the patient being transported for medical attention in a timely manner. Envenomation does not occur with every snakebite. Victims should be monitored closely for 8 hours for signs of envenomation. If signs do not occur in this time period, it is very unlikely that envenomation occurred. Attempts should be made to evaluate severity of envenomation by physical examination, calculation of serial Snakebite Severity Scores, and evaluation of hematology and blood chemistry values with particular attention paid to the presence/absence and severity of echinocytosis. The foundation of snake envenomation treatment is supportive care and antivenom. Antivenom is typically only necessary with cases of severe envenomation. Patients receiving prompt and appropriate care have an excellent prognosis for recovery.

REFERENCES

1. Peterson ME. Snake bite: pit vipers. Clin Techn Small Anim Pract 2006;21:174–82.
2. Gold BS, Wingert WA. Snake venom poisoning in the United States: a review of therapeutic practice. South Med J 1994;87:579–89.
3. Seifert SA, Boyer LV, Benson BE, et al. AAPCC database characterization of native U.S. venomous snake exposures, 2001–2005. Clin Toxicol (Phila) 2009;47:327–35.
4. McCown JL, Cooke KL, Hanel RM, et al. Effect of antivenin dose on outcome from crotalid envenomation: 218 dogs (1988–2006). J Vet Emerg Crit Care 2009;19: 603–10.
5. Marks SL, Mannella C, Schaer M. Coral snake envenomation in the dog: report of four cases and review of the literature. J Am Anim Hosp Assoc 1990;26:629–34.
6. Peterson ME. Snake bite: coral snakes. Clin Techn Small Anim Pract 2006;21:183–6.
7. Kremer KA, Schaer M. Coral snake (Micrurus fulvius fulvius) envenomation in five dogs: present and earlier findings. J Vet Emerg Crit Care 1995;5:9–15.
8. Tu AT. Rattlesnake Venoms: Their actions and Treatment. New York: Marcel Dekker; 1982.
9. Chrisman CL, Hopkins AL, Ford SL, et al. Acute, flaccid quadriplegia in three cats with suspected coral snake envenomation. J Am Anim Hosp Assoc 1996;32:343–9.
10. Mansfield PD. The management of snake venom poisoning in dogs. Comp Cont Educ Pract Vet 1984;6:988–92 4.
11. Russell FE. Snake venom poisoning in the United States. Annu Rev Med 1980;31: 247–59.
12. Holstege CP, Miller MB, Wermuth M, et al. Crotalid snake envenomation. Crit Care Clin 1997;13:889–921.
13. Peterson ME, Meerdink GL. Current Veterinary Therapy. Philadelphia: WB Saunders; 1989.
14. Farstad D, Thomas T, Chow T, et al. Mojave rattlesnake envenomation in southern California: a review of suspected cases. Wilderness Environ Med 1997;8:89–93.
15. Gopalakrishnakone P, Hawgood BJ, Holbrooke SE, et al. Sites of action of Mojave toxin isolated from the venom of the Mojave rattlesnake. Br J Pharmacol 1980;69: 421–31.
16. Garland T. Recognition and Treatment for Snake Bites. 18th American College of Veterinary Internal Medicine Forum, 2000;48–9.
17. Willey JR, Schaer M. Eastern Diamondback Rattlesnake (Crotalus adamanteus) envenomation of dogs: 31 cases (1982–2002). J Am Anim Hosp Assoc 2005;41: 22–33.

18. Bonilla CA, Rammel OJ. Comparative biochemistry and pharmacology of salivary gland secretions. III. Chromatographic isolation of a myocardial depressor protein (MDP) from the venom of Crotalus atrox. J Chromatogr 1976;124:303–14.
19. Hudelson S, Hudelson P. Pathophysiology of snake envenomization and evaluation of treatments: part 1. Comp Cont Educ Pract Vet 1995;17:889–97.
20. Ownby CL, Bjarnason J, Tu AT. Hemorrhagic toxins from rattlesnake (Crotalus atrox) venom. Pathogenesis of hemorrhage induced by three purified toxins. Am J Pathol 1978;93:201–18.
21. Hackett TB, Wingfield WE, Mazzaferro EM, et al. Clinical findings associated with prairie rattlesnake bites in dogs: 100 cases (1989–1998). J Am Vet Med Assoc 2002;220:1675–80.
22. Singletary EM, Rochman AS, Bodmer JC, et al. Envenomations. Med Clin North Am 2005;89:1195–224.
23. Bronstein AC, Russell FE, Sullivan JB. Negative pressure suction in the field treatment of rattlesnake bite victims. Vet Hum Toxicol 1986;28:485.
24. Bronstein AC, Russell FE, Sullivan JB, et al. Negative pressure suction in field treatment of rattlesnake bite. Vet Hum Toxicol 1985;28:297.
25. Zamudio KR, Hardy DL Sr, Martins M, et al. Fang tip spread, puncture distance, and suction for snake bite. Toxicon 2000;38:723–8.
26. Bush SP, Hegewald KG, Green SM, et al. Effects of a negative pressure venom extraction device (Extractor) on local tissue injury after artificial rattlesnake envenomation in a porcine model. Wilderness Environ Med 2000;11:180–8.
27. Hack JB, Orogbemi B, DeGuzman JM, et al. A localizing circumferential compression device delayed death after artificial Eastern diamondback rattlesnake envenomation to the torso of an animal model in a pilot study. J Med Toxicol 2010;6:207–11.
28. Hardy DL Sr. Fatal ratllesnake envenomation in Arizona: 1969–1984. J Toxicol Clin Toxicol 1986;24.
29. Bober MA, Glenn JL, Straight RC, et al. Detection of myotoxin alpha-like proteins in various snake venoms. Toxicon 1988;26:665–73.
30. Hudelson S, Hudelson P. Pathophysiology of snake envenomization and evaluation of treatments: part II. Comp Cont Educ Pract Vet 1995;17:1035–40.
31. Brown DE, Meyer DJ, Wingfield WE, et al. Echinocytosis associated with rattlesnake envenomation in dogs. Vet Pathol 1994;31:654–7.
32. Walton RM, Brown DE, Hamar DW, et al. Mechanisms of echinocytosis induced by Crotalus atrox venom. Vet Pathol 1997;34:442–9.
33. Offerman SR, Barry JD, Schneir A, et al. Biphasic rattlesnake venom-induced thrombocytopenia. J Emerg Med 2003;24:289–93.
34. Hudelson S, Hudelson P. Pathophysiology of snake envenomization and evaluation of treatments, part III. Comp Cont Educ Pract Vet 1995;17:1385–94.
35. Zhou Q, Smith JB, Grossman MH. Molecular cloning and expression of catrocollastatin, a snake-venom protein from Crotalus atrox (western diamondback rattlesnake) which inhibits platelet adhesion to collagen. Biochem J 1995;307(Pt 2):411–7.
36. Liu CZ, Huang TF. Crovidisin, a collagen-binding protein isolated from snake venom of Crotalus viridis, prevents platelet-collagen interaction. Arch Biochem Biophys 1997; 337:291–9.
37. Dart RC, Hurlbut KM, Garcia R, et al. Validation of a severity score for the assessment of crotalid snakebite. Ann Emerg Med 1996;27:321–6.
38. Russell FE. AIDS, cancer, and snakebite: what do these three have in common? West J Med 1988;148:84–5.
39. Campbell BT, Corsi JM, Boneti C, et al. Pediatric snakebites: lessons learned from 114 cases. J Pediatr Surg 2008;43:1338–41.

40. Dart RC, McNally J. Efficacy, safety, and use of snake antivenoms in the United States. Ann Emerg Med 2001;37:181–8.
41. Seifert SA, Boyer LV. Recurrence phenomena after immunoglobulin therapy for snake envenomations, part 1. Pharmacokinetics and pharmacodynamics of immunoglobulin antivenoms and related antibodies. Ann Emerg Med 2001;37:189–95.
42. Cox MR, Reeves JK, Smith KM. Concepts in crotaline snake envenomation management. Orthopedics 2006;29:1083–7.
43. Ownby CL, Reisbeck SL, Allen R. Levels of therapeutic antivenin and venom in a human snakebite victim. South Med J 1996:803–6.
44. Schaer M. Eastern diamondback rattlesnake envenomation of 20 dogs. Comp Cont Educ Pract Vet 1984;6:997–1007.
45. Reid H. Specific antivenin and prednisone in viper bite poisoning: a controlled trial. Br Med J 1963:1378.
46. Goldstein EJ, Citron DM, Gonzalez H, et al. Bacteriology of rattlesnake venom and implications for therapy. J Infect Dis 1979;140:818–21.
47. Berdoulay P, Schaer M, Starr J. Serum sickness in a dog associated with antivenin therapy for snake bite caused by Crotalus adamanteus. J Vet Emerg Crit Care 2005;15:206–12.

Disease Transmission from Companion Parrots to Dogs and Cats: What is the Real Risk?

Jamie M. Bush, DVM, MS[a]*, Brian Speer, DVM[b], Noel Opitz, DVM[c]

KEYWORDS

• Disease transmission • Parrot • Dog • Cat

Numerous pet caregivers harbor unwarranted concerns regarding the potential of disease transmission from companion parrots to their dogs and cats. Such concerns may result in an overemphasis on testing and treatment for some of these potential pathogens in companion parrots, rehoming of companion parrots, or prevention of the adoption of parrots because of concern over the health of the household dogs and cats. A number of bacterial, viral, fungal, and parasitic diseases are postulated to undergo transmission from parrots to dogs and cats. In reality, transmission of *Pasteurella multocida* from companion cats to parrots is of greater concern. The following discussion reviews common conditions presumed to undergo such transmission and demonstrates the lack of data to support such concerns.

Mycobacterium spp

Infections with *Mycobacterium avium* or *Mycobacterium genavense* are not uncommon in psittacine species.[1,2] *M genavense* is an atypical mycobacterium that is an important source of infection in parrots.[2] Rare reports of infection with *Mycobacterium tuberculosis* or *Mycobacterium bovis* exist, and such infections probably occur secondary to close contact with infected humans.[2]

Mycobacterium spp are ubiquitous in the environment and are found in soil with heavy fecal contamination or other organic debris.[2] Additional sources include surface water or marshy shaded areas.[2] Transmission occurs by ingestion or inhalation of soil or water contaminated by feces or, less commonly, urine, and vertical transmission is also possible.[2] In parrots, the primary site of entry and initial colonization is the gastrointestinal tract.[2] Inhalation may lead to direct colonization of

[a] IDEXX Laboratories, 6100 East Shelby Drive, Memphis, TN 38103, USA
[b] Medical Center for Birds, 3805 Main Street, Oakley, CA 94561, USA
[c] The Gabriel Foundation, 39520 County Road 13, Elizabeth, CO 80107, USA
* Corresponding author.
E-mail address: Jamie-Bush@idexx.com

Vet Clin Small Anim 41 (2011) 1261–1272
doi:10.1016/j.cvsm.2011.07.004
0195-5616/11/$ – see front matter © 2011 Elsevier Inc. All rights reserved.

respiratory tract, and focal skin disease secondary to inoculation into mucosal or dermal tissues or by contaminated needles may also occur.[2] There is no apparent gender predilection.[2]

Clinically, affected birds demonstrate muscle wasting, loss of subcutaneous and intracoelomic adipose tissue, and poor quality feathers.[2] Initially the bird has a good appetite, followed by anorexia as the disease progresses. Other findings include wasting with increased appetite, poor feather quality, lethargy, weakness, pallor, chronic or intermittent diarrhea, abdominal distension, and rarely, ascites or pericardial effusion.[2] Bone disease is reported to have a wide prevalence (2%–93%) and can result in acute or chronic lameness or a shifting leg lameness.[2] Respiratory disease and reproductive failure are less commonly described.

Grossly, hepatosplenomegaly is commonly reported.[2] Granulomatous lesions occur in the gastrointestinal tract and liver.[2] Tubercles are white, tan, or yellow.[2] Miliary foci to nodules several centimeters in diameter may occur within the gastrointestinal wall, liver, spleen, and bone but may occur in other viscera.[2] Generalized disease may be associated with diffuse enlargement of affected organs.[2] The gastrointestinal tract is often distended and thickened, and the intestinal mucosa may display a shaggy-carpet appearance.[2] The carpometacarpal and elbow joints are most commonly involved, and the skin overlying joints may be thickened and ulcerated.[2] Granulomas in the lungs or compression of air sacs secondary to hepatomegaly can lead to dyspnea or exercise intolerance.[2] Rare nodules are reported within the infraorbital sinus, nares, and syrinx.[2] Tubercles in the skin are rare, and dermatitis results in diffuse nonpruritic thickening and subcutaneous masses.[2] Infections of the eyelids, nictitating membranes, retrobulbar tissue and pecten, and cornea are also reported in birds.[2] Additional reports of lesions in the oropharynx, larynx, and external auditory canal exist.[2] Reproductive failure due to infection of the adrenal glands, pancreas, and gonads resulting in subsequent endocrine abnormalities have infrequently been reported.[2] Pulmonary necrosis, as well as granulomatous cardiopulmonary arteritis, are less common presentations.[2]

Histologically, mycobacterial infections typically present as a granulomatous enteritis, splenitis, or hepatitis with variable intracytoplasmic acid-fast bacteria.[2] Additionally, macrophages within the dermis, mucous membranes, and subserosa of the peritoneum and air sacs are reported.[2] Granulomatous intestinal lesions are associated with expansion of the intestinal villi by diffuse infiltrates of epithelioid macrophages, multinucleated giant cells, fewer lymphocytes, and proliferation of epithelial cells within the glands of Lieberkühn.[2] Infection with M avium typically results in large numbers of acid-fast bacilli, whereas M bovis and M tuberculosis result in small numbers of acid-fast bacilli. In parrots, granulomas do not possess regions of central calcification or extensive necrotic centers.[2] The diffuse form is more difficult to recognize with resultant diffuse infiltration with large foamy histiocytes.[2]

In dogs and cats, mycobacterial infections may be caused by a number of different but closely related bacteria. Relevant members of the tuberculosis complex group in dogs and cats include M tuberculosis, M bovis, and Mycobacterium microti.[3] Other mycobacteria that can be potentially pathogenic in cats and dogs include Mycobacterium lepraemurium and opportunistic nontuberculous mycobacteria such as members of the Mycobacterium chelonae-abscessus group, Mycobacterium fortuitum group, Mycobacterium smegmatis group, and others.[3] In general, mycobacterial infections are rare in both cats and dogs. The majority of cases are seen in cats and present as skin lesions.[3] Most infections in dogs and cats are due to M bovis or, in the case of cats, M microti.[3] Infection with M tuberculosis is increasingly rare.[3] Many cases in dogs and cats are subclinical. Infection usually occurs after prolonged exposure, and disease is seen mainly in adult animals.[3] No gender predisposition is seen in dogs, but male cats seem to be overrepresented.[3] Certain breeds seem to be predisposed, including Siamese, Abyssinian, Bassett hounds, and Miniature Schnauzers.[3]

Depending on the route of infection, infected dogs and cats may present with systemic signs related to the alimentary or respiratory tract or with localized disease affecting the skin.[3] The usual presentation for tuberculosis in cats is cutaneous.[3] These lesions probably arise from infected bite wounds, local spread, or hematogenous dissemination to the skin.[3] The lesions often involve the face, extremities, tail base, or perineum. Less frequently, lesions involve the ventral thorax.[3] Lesions typically appear as firm, raised dermal nodules. Ulceration may be present, as well as nonhealing wounds with draining tracts. Granulomatous inflammation may extend into adjacent subcutaneous tissues, muscle, and bone. Skin lesions are commonly associated with localized or generalized lymphadenomegaly.[3] On occasion, submandibular or prescapular lymphadenomegaly may be the only clinical finding.[3]

When the infection spreads to the lungs, tubercles arise in the lungs and hilar lymph nodes, and affected animals present with weight loss, anorexia, dyspnea, and cough.[3] Additionally, there may be associated sneezing and nasal discharge.[3] Pneumothorax and pleurisy may also occur with pleural and pericardial effusions.[3] Pulmonary cases in dogs have occasionally presented with hypertrophic pulmonary osteopathy.[3]

In the alimentary form, tubercles arise in the intestines and mesenteric lymph nodes.[3] Animals often develop intestinal malabsorption and present with weight loss, anemia, vomiting, and diarrhea.[3] Occasionally, tubercles arise in the tonsils.[3]

In dogs and cats, a range of clinical signs may develop with disseminated disease including splenomegaly, hepatomegaly, generalized lymphadenomegaly, weight loss, and fever.[3] With bone involvement, lameness may develop. Ocular involvement may result in granulomatous uveitis, retinal detachment, and central nervous signs due to extension along the optic nerve.[3] Mycobacterial conjunctivitis may also be seen alone or associated with more generalized changes.[3]

To the authors' knowledge, there are no known published cases of transmission of *Mycobacterium* spp from parrots to dogs and cats. It is more likely that companion pets acquire such infections from living with infected people or through opportunistic infections from environmental exposure.

Chlamydophila psittaci

Chlamydophila psittaci is a zoonotic intracellular bacterial organism that was first reported in humans and psittacine birds in 1895.[4] Most parrots and over 130 species in other taxonomic orders of birds have been found to be capable of being infected by this agent. The potential host spectrum of *C psittaci* also includes practically all domestic mammals including humans and many wild mammals, some amphibians, and arthropods. *Chlamydophila* spp have an intracellular life cycle and are periodically shed by infected birds.[4] Carriers can shed the organism intermittently and typically do not demonstrate any clinical signs.[1] The organism propagates in the epithelial cells of the respiratory tract and then generalizes to other organs.[5]

Clinical signs of disease are quite variable and are dependent on the virulence of the infecting strain as well as the host. Young birds with an incompletely developed immune system may develop acute systemic infections when exposed to particularly virulent strains of *C psittaci*. Most commonly, clinical signs noted in psittacine birds may include respiratory and/or gastrointestinal abnormalities. Clinical signs associated with liver disease are not uncommon in psittacine bird species (lime green diarrhea, biliverdinuria). Some birds may occasionally develop central nervous system abnormalities, keratoconjunctivitis, nasal discharge, and in the cockatiel, flaccid paresis and paralysis have been reported. Multisystemic disease can also develop in cockatiels and other species of parrots.[5]

Gross lesions include hepatic and splenic enlargement.[5] In parrots, infections of the air sacs result in diffuse cloudy opacification with occasional tan-yellow plaques.[5] Affected livers may have minimal gross changes, but many are enlarged and discolored, containing foci of necrosis.[5] The spleen may range from dark red to purple, or the spleen may be pale as a result of increased inflammatory infiltrates.[5] The conjunctiva may be diffusely reddened with serous or purulent exudates.[5]

Histologically, there is a fibrinous air sacculitis.[5] Within the gastrointestinal tract, infection may result in diffuse mucosal necrosis and a moderate lymphoplasmacytic and histiocytic inflammatory infiltrate.[5] C psittaci can also result in marrow granulocytic hyperplasia.[5] Within the liver, there is a mononuclear inflammatory infiltrate, which may be diffuse within the sinusoids.[5] Many of the macrophages contain green-brown pigment consistent with bile pigment and/or hemosiderin.[5] Multifocal to confluent hepatic necrosis is also common.[5] In chronic disease, portal fibrosis and bile duct hyperplasia occurs.[5] Urinary tract lesions include lymphoplasmacytic and histiocytic interstitial inflammation.[5] The most consistent lesion seen in the spleen is histiocytosis.[5] There is hyperplasia of histiocytes of the perivascular sheaths and a diffuse proliferation of plasma cells.[5] Arthritis and nonsuppurative meningitis may also occur.[5] There is typically conjunctival necrosis with a lymphohistiocytic infiltrate.[5] Organisms can be recognized as basophilic punctuate structures within the cytoplasm of macrophages or hepatocytes.[5] These organisms can be visualized with Gimenez stains and other special stains.[5] Uncommon conditions associated with chlamydophilosis include otitis media, bursitis, and solitary nephritis.[6]

In cats, Chlamydophila felis, previously known as C psittaci, is a primary conjunctival pathogen.[7] Cats may also shed this organism from other nonocular sites as well.[7] Infection with this organism is not documented in dogs.

To the authors' knowledge, there are no known published cases of transmission of C psittaci from parrots to other domestic animals.

SALMONELLOSIS

Salmonella spp are gram-negative bacteria that typically function as primary pathogens in parrots. Salmonella spp are members of the large family of Enterobacteriaceae and are widely distributed geographically.[5] Some serotypes have been shown to penetrate the mucosal barrier, and noninvasive serotypes result in carrier states.[5] Salmonella typhimurium is the most common psittacine isolate.[5] Previously, the disease was a significant problem among wild-caught birds that were closely confined in quarantine stations.[5] Currently, this infection is more likely to be identified in parrots from aviaries that have a significant rodent problem.[5]

Affected birds typically die suddenly due to septicemia.[1] Clinically, affected birds develop profuse watery diarrhea, polyuria and polydipsia, dyspnea, pneumonia, depression, inappetance, and neurologic signs.[1]

The classic lesions of salmonellosis include hepatomegaly, splenomegaly, pneumonia, and a catarrhal to hemorrhagic enteritis.[5] Gastrointestinal gross lesions include intestinal redness, exudation, and mucosal ulceration to varying degrees of severity.[5] Gas or fluid distension of the gastrointestinal tract may occur, and there is generally fecal soiling of the feathers of the vent consistent with diarrhea.[5] Systemic infections with Salmonella spp may result in multifocal white nodules within the hepatic parenchyma (paratyphoid nodules).[5]

Histologically, intestinal necrosis with fibrin and heterophilic infiltrates are suggestive of a bacterial enteritis.[5] There may be extension of the inflammatory process into the submucosa as well as the tunica muscularis, and crypt dilatation and abscess formation may be seen.[5] Within the liver, paratyphoid nodules consist of randomly distributed nodular accumulations of histiocytes with fewer numbers of lymphocytes and plasma cells and variable necrosis.[5] In most cases there is a multifocal to coalescing necrotizing splenitis with nodular aggregates of lymphocytes, macrophages, and heterophils.[5] Additionally, salmonellosis may result in lymphohistiocytic meningitis, encephalitis, and myelitis, as well as osteoarthritis associated with bacterial septicemia.[5] Bacteria are not always readily identifiable upon histologic examination, and additional special stains, bacterial culture, or molecular diagnostics may be necessary.[5]

In dogs and cats, infections typically begin with ingestion of organisms in contaminated food or water with subsequent invasion of M cells in the Peyer patches.[8] Clinical signs in these species are often associated with acute disease characterized by fever, malaise, anorexia, diarrhea, and vomiting.[8] The diarrhea is often watery or mucoid and can be bloody.[8] Most animals, though, are asymptomatic, and in rare cases systemic sepsis may occur.[8]

To the authors' knowledge, there are no known published cases documenting disease transmission of *Salmonella* spp between parrots and dogs and cats.

Yersinia pseudotuberculosis

Yersiniosis is rare in parrots and is typically transmitted via the fecal-oral route.[1] Following ingestion, bacteria invade the intestinal mucosa by attaching to and penetrating the mucus layer overlying mucosal epithelial cells then adhere to and colonize intestinal brush border membranes. After penetrating the mucosa, bacteria are phagocytized by neutrophils and macrophages in the mucosa and submucosa. The organisms are able to survive within the cytoplasm of these phagocytic cells and are subsequently systemically spread.

In parrots, yersiniosis results in acute illness, diarrhea, and general ill health.[1] Weight loss, decreased physical activity, and lethargy may be noted.

Gross lesions include hepatomegaly, discoloration of the liver, and miliary white spots throughout the liver, kidneys, and spleen.[1] There may be variable associated foci of necrosis with associated accumulations of caseous material and necrotic debris.[5]

Histologically, yersiniosis results in multifocal random foci of necrosis with variable associated accumulations of neutrophils and macrophages with fewer numbers of lymphocytes and plasma cells.[5] Foci of necrosis may develop associated foci of mineralization and can be variable in size with some foci becoming quite large.[5] Associated with foci of necrosis, there are large colonies of coccobacilli, which are suggestive of infection with *Yersinia* spp.[5] Confirmatory bacterial culture is warranted in such cases.

Yersinia pseudotuberculosis can be ingested by cats eating infected rodents or birds. The bacteria then infect the gastrointestinal tract, liver, and lymph nodes.[9] Clinically, affected cats demonstrate marked weight loss, diarrhea, anorexia, lethargy, jaundice, and mesenteric lymphadenomegaly.[9]

To the authors' knowledge, there are no known published cases documenting disease transmission of *Yersinia* spp from companion parrots to other companion animals in the household.

AVIAN INFLUENZA

Influenza viruses come in three groups: groups B and C affect humans and rarely birds, whereas group A affects birds and rarely humans.[1] The primary reservoir is thought to be wild aquatic birds.[6] Avian influenza has affected parrots, causing no illness to sudden death.[1] There are no pathognomonic clinical signs for this condition, and clinical signs may vary depending on the age and species, presence of concurrent infectious disease, and environmental factors.[10] Affected birds may demonstrate depression, diarrhea, or neurologic signs.[1] Avian influenza virus should be considered as a differential diagnosis for clinical signs of gastrointestinal tract disease in psittacines.[10] This virus is rarely seen in parrots, and most psittacine infections occur either in quarantine stations where it was contracted from other birds or has been caused experimentally.[1] Avian influenza virus varies in its pathogenicity, and the serotypes that affect poultry are not usually a great risk to parrots.[1]

Gross findings include dehydration and evidence of regurgitation such as occluded nares and feed material on the beak, head, and within the oral cavity.[10] The crop may be full of feed material upon evaluation.[10] Evidence of vent soiling consistent with diarrhea is also evident.[6] Additionally, hemorrhagic enteritis is a common finding.[10] Occasionally, a nonsuppurative meningoencephalitis is identified.[5] Polymerase chain reaction with matrix gene as target is needed for confirmation of infection.[10]

Dogs are susceptible to highly pathogenic avian influenza (H5N1) infection. Affected dogs typically develop fever but not fatal disease.[11] Contact exposure experiments of influenza virus–infected cats with uninfected dogs did not result in interspecies transmission.[11] There is a single report of a domestic cat infected with highly pathogenic avian influenza (H5N1) following ingestion of an infected pigeon carcass.[12] Affected cats often demonstrate many of the following: necrotizing pneumonia with hyaline membrane formation, necrotizing and lymphoplasmacytic meningoencephalitis with gliosis, necrotizing myocarditis, necrotizing hepatitis, and necrotizing adrenalitis.[13]

The potential for transmission of avian influenza from parrots to cats remains unsubstantiated. The only documented case of bird-to-cat transmission evidently required ingestion of an infected, nonpsittacine carcass. To the authors' knowledge, there are no known published cases of such transmission from birds to dogs.

ASPERGILLOSIS

Aspergillosis fumigatus is a noncontagious opportunistic angioinvasive fungus that results in acute and chronic respiratory and systemic disease.[14] *A fumigatus* is a ubiquitous fungus found in nature and in the companion bird environment. Soil, moldy litter, moldy grain, and bedding material contaminated with feces are common sources of environmental *Aspergillus* isolates.[14]

Like any infectious disease, the pathogenesis of aspergillosis is a function of interactions between the host, the agent, and the environment. Host factors commonly implicated include immunosuppression, stress, trauma, and toxicoses. Overall, it seems to be uncommon for immunocompetent birds to develop aspergillosis. Stress seems to be a significant contributor to immunocompentency in both wild and captive birds. Some common stressors may include capture, travel, importation, reproductive activity, overcrowding, and excessive human traffic. Host factors that are commonly associated with risk of aspergillosis include malnutrition (hypovitaminosis A), preexisting disease, and prolonged antibiotic or steroid treatments. Agent factors that can have a role in the development of disease include challenge with a large number of spores or increased invasiveness of the organism because of its capability of being highly invasive given the right set of circumstances. Gliotoxins produced by *A fumigatus* are immunosuppressive (cytotoxic to lymphocytes). Lipo-polysaccharide of bacteria, inhaled along with spores of *A fumigatus* in particulate matter, may reduce pulmonary function and the ability to clear debris from the respiratory tract, potentiating fungal colonization. *A fumigatus* is unique among other members of the genus for its thermotolerance; it can grow at a wide range of temperatures (20°C–50°C). Environmental factors contribute to risk of disease through chronic exposure to a small number of spores or acute exposure to a massive number of spores. If the environment is conducive to fungal growth and spore production, the stage is set for increased exposure and increased likelihood of disease. Fungal growth and sporulation are promoted by environmental conditions of warmth and high humidity, followed by a drying period. Poor husbandry practices, allowing the accumulation of debris, discarded feed, feces, and litter support fungal growth. Poor ventilation increases the concentration of spores in the environment. Types of bedding frequently implicated in promoting the growth of *Aspergillus* spp include corncob, walnut shell, and eucalyptus leaves.

Aspergillus spp thrive in high humidity and warm temperatures.[14] Immunosuppres-sion, stress, and other factors related to confinement, poor husbandry, malnutrition, preexisting disease, and prolonged use of antibiotics and/or steroids predisposes to disease in companion birds.[14] Disease is common in overpopulated, poorly venti-lated, and dusty environments.[14] Infection is often a common sequel to other respiratory tract disease.[14] Predominantly seed diets may result in vitamin A defi-ciency and subsequent squamous metaplasia of the oral and respiratory epithelium with secondary establishment of fungal growth.[14] Gray parrots and Pionus species demonstrate increased susceptibility and are commonly represented in the litera-ture.[14] Localized infections of the nasal passages are common in Amazons.[14] Parrots may carry spores in their lungs and air sacs without ill effect.[14]

Infection develops because of inhalation of fungal spores or penetration of broken skin and eggshells, resulting in infection of developing embryos during the incubation process.[14] Disease of the lower respiratory tract, lungs, and air sacs develop typically secondary to the trachea, syrinx, and bronchi being affected.[10] Infections may spread from the respiratory tract to pneumatized bone or enter the peritoneal cavity by direct extension through air sac walls.[14] Vascular invasion and embolism results in systemic spread of the organism.[14]

Clinical disease may be acute or chronic.[1] Acute onset typically results in fatal respiratory disease.[14] Dyspnea, tail bobbing, cyanosis, lethargy, anorexia, polyuria and polydipsia, sudden death, tachypnea, open-mouth breathing, gurgling respira-tions and vomiting may occur.[14] Weight loss is common.[1] Chronic disease results in a change of behavior, reduced level of activity, decreased appetite, exercise intoler-ance, weight loss even with good appetite, respiratory compromise, and tachypnoa and dyspnea late in disease.[14] Biliverdinuria, polyuria and polydipsia, ascites, regurgitation, diarrhea, and abnormal droppings also occur in chronic disease.[14] Ataxia and torticollis may occur with involvement of the central nervous system.[14] Ocular disease may result in blepharospasm, photophobia, severe periorbital swell-ing, and conjunctival hyperemia.[14] The time from onset of clinical signs to death may be less than 1 week to 6 weeks.[14]

Acute disease results in whitish mucoid exudates in the respiratory tract and marked congestion of the lungs with thickening of air sac membranes and miliary foci of inflammation within the caudal thoracic and abdominal air sacs and peripheral lung fields.[14] Abdominal enlargement due to ascites may also occur.[14] Mycotic tracheitis results in granuloma formation within the trachea, syrinx, and primary bronchi with resultant change in vocalization ability or obstructive airway disease.[14] Chronic disease results in multiple nodules, which may coalesce into plaques and larger granulomatous lesions.[14] Adhesions between air sac membranes, lungs, and abdominal viscera are common.[14]

Air sacculitis is the most frequently encountered form of disease with extension to the lungs, most commonly with the posterior thoracic and abdominal air sacs affected.[14] Chronic rhinitis and sinusitis, distension of the infraorbital sinus, and periobital soft tissue swellings are common.[14] Unilateral or bilateral nasal discharge that is serous to purulent with rhinoliths and oronasal granulomas and subsequent upper airway obstruction causing wheezing and secondary bacterial sinus infections is common.[14]

Infection of the central nervous system with encephalitic and meningoencephalitic lesions may occur.[14] Ocular disease is rare and develops secondary to preexisting upper respiratory infection.[14] Corneal epithelial erosions and stromal necrosis with perforation of the cornea or panophthalmitis with functional loss of eye may develop.[14]

Histologically, infections with *Aspergillus* spp result in multifocal granulomas primarily in the respiratory tracts of parrots, including the trachea, syrinx, bronchi, lungs, and air sacs.[5] Lesions consist of multifocal-coalescing variable accumulations of epithelioid macrophages with associated multinucleated giant cells, occasional fibroblasts depending upon the degree of chronicity, and intralesional fungal hyphae.[5] Fungal hyphae are 2 to 4 μm in diameter with parallel cell walls and septae and demonstrate acute angle dichotomous branching.[5] Histologically, fungal hyphae of *Aspergillus* spp are quite characteristic and can be used to diagnose aspergillosis with a degree of confidence.[5]

Aspergillus spp are a common cause of upper respiratory infection in dogs. Canine sinonasal aspergillosis is characterized by colonization and invasion of the nasal passages and frontal sinuses by *A fumigatus*.[15] The disease primarily affects young to middle-aged dogs and is progressive.[15] German Shepherds and Rottweilers are at increased risk.[15] Colonization and invasion of the nasal mucosa results in destruction and necrosis of the nasal turbinates and often results in frontal sinus osteomyelitis.[15] Facial pain, anorexia, sneezing, and mucoid to hemorrhagic nasal discharge and crusting are common.[15] Life-threatening epistaxis and secondary meningoencephalitis may occur.[15]

Disseminated infections typically involve multiple organ systems with no history of nasal or pulmonary involvement.[15] *Aspergillus terreus*, *Aspergillus deflectus*, *Aspergillus flavipes*, and rarely *A fumigatus* have been reported in association with these cases.[15] Dissemination occurs following inhalation of spores and subsequent hematogenous dissemination.[15] German Shepherds seem predisposed to systemic disease.[15] Associated clinical signs are variable and based upon the organ system involved. Uveitis, ophthalmitis, and chorioretinitis may precede the onset of generalized disease.[15] The most common clinical signs are bone pain, paraparesis, draining sinus tracts, weight loss, pyrexia, lethargy, muscle wasting, and fever.[15] Infections with *Aspergillus* spp are often associated with immune suppression in the patient.[15]

To the authors' knowledge, there are no known published cases documenting disease transmission of aspergillosis from parrots to dogs and cats.

Cryptococcus neoformans

Cryptococcus neoformans var *neoformans* is an encapsulated saprophytic fungus with worldwide distribution and is often found in soils contaminated with bird droppings.[14] This organism rarely causes disease in birds, but disseminated infections have been reported in a green wing macaw, Moluccan cockatoo, thick-billed parrot, and North Island brown kiwi.[14]

Clinical signs are based upon location of the infection. Infections of the respiratory tract may result in dyspnea, tail bobbing, or increased respiratory noise, whereas infections of the digestive tract may result in weight loss, diarrhea, or the passing of whole seed in the feces. Finally, central nervous system infections may result in neurologic signs such as ataxia, disorientation, impaired mutation, or even seizures. Infections may sometimes be inapparent clinically and only diagnosed upon post-mortem examination.

Infection of the respiratory tract, digestive tract, and central nervous system results in necrotic granulomatous lesions and thick, pale gelatinous exudates.[14] The lower temperature of the upper respiratory tract makes it more susceptible to infection.[14] Upper respiratory tract involvement may produce facial granulomas that distort the rhamphotheca.[14] Chronic rhinosinusitis has been reported in a Major Mitchell's cockatoo due to *Cryptococcus neoformans* var *gate* with resultant encephalitis and meningitis causing blindness and paralysis.[14]

Histologically, infections with *C neoformans* does not typically incite much of an inflammatory response because of the thick mucopolysaccharide capsule of the organism.[5] When present, inflammatory infiltrates consist of macrophages with possibly associated multinucleated giant cells, lymphocytes, and plasma cells.[5] Organisms may be intracellular or extracellular and are 5 to 7 μm in diameter with a 2- to 3-μm clear capsule, which stains positive with mucicarmine and a central 3- to 4-μm spherical basophilic body. Organisms are numerous and are readily identifiable with fungal stains such as periodic acid–Schiff or silver stains.

Infection occurs via inhalation of the yeast from the environment and is not considered contagious.[16] Debris and droppings in and around avian habitats, especially pigeon habitats, contain large numbers of yeasts.[16] Lesions consist of either granulomatous inflammation with few organisms or gelatinous masses of organisms with little inflammation.[16] Cats are more commonly affected, and there is no breed, age, or sex predilection noted.[16] Clinical findings are typically associated with upper respiratory, nasopharyngeal, cutaneous, ocular, or central nervous system involvement.[16] The lungs are not typically affected. Upper respiratory signs include bilateral mucopurulent nasal discharge with or without blood. Proliferative lesions result in destruction of the nasal turbinates and tissue overlying the bridge of the nose.[16] Oral ulcerations may occur, and granulomatous chorioretinitis variably with retinal detachment and meningoencephalitis is common.[16]

In dogs, disease typically affects young dogs under the age of 4.[16] American Cocker Spaniels, Labrador Retrievers, Great Danes, and Doberman Pinschers are overrepresented.[16] Central nervous system, upper respiratory, ocular, and cutaneous clinical signs are common.[16] The brain is affected in most dogs.[16] The upper respiratory tract is the second most common site with resultant upper airway stridor, nasal discharge, sneezing, epistaxis, or firm swellings over the bridge of the nose.[16] Optic neuritis may result in blindness, and granulomatous chorioretinitis often occurs.[16] The skin is less likely to be affected in dogs.[16]

To the authors' knowledge, there are no known published cases documenting disease transmission for companion birds to dogs and cats.

HISTOPLASMOSIS

Histoplasma capsulatum is an infectious but not contagious fungal organism reported in poultry and zoo parrots only.[14] The organism is soilborne and endemic in the eastern and central United States.[14] *H capsulatum* is commonly associated with fecal material from pigeons and gallinaceous birds.[14] The organism has the ability to grow within dirt substrates of enclosed aviaries and results in disease similar to *Cryptococcus* spp.[14]

An initial pneumonia can progress to disseminated disease with formation of necrotic granulomas in multiple organs.[14] Osteomyelitis and mineralized soft tissue granulomas within the shoulder and antebrachium in a Moluccan cockatoo have been reported.[14]

Histologically, histoplasmosis results in multifocal granulomatous inflammation composed of nodular accumulations of epithelioid macrophages, multinucleated giant cells, and fewer lymphocytes, plasma cells, and heterophils.[5] Variable numbers of intracellular fungal yeast may be identified within macrophages and multinucleated giant cells. Fungal yeasts are 2 to 4 μm in diameter and spherical with a 1- to 2-μm central basophilic body surrounded by a clear halo that develops because of artifactual shrinkage.[5]

In dogs and cats, this infection typically originates in the lungs and potentially the gastrointestinal tract with subsequent dissemination to the lymphatics, liver, spleen, bone marrow, eyes, and other organs.[17] Cats seem more susceptible to infection than dogs.[17] This organism is not contagious, and infection is via ingestion or inhalation.[17] Following phagocytosis by macrophages, where they grow as facultative intracellular organisms, hematogenous and lymphatic dissemination results in multisystemic disease.[17] In dogs the lungs, gastrointestinal system, lymph nodes, liver, spleen, bone marrow, eyes, and adrenal glands are commonly infected.[17] In cats the lungs, liver, lymph nodes, eyes, and bone marrow are commonly affected.[17] Lesions consist of multiorgan granulomas with intrahistiocytic fungal yeasts.

To the authors' knowledge, there are no known published cases of transmission of *H capsulatum* from companion parrots to dogs and cats.

Cryptosporidium spp

Cryptosporidium spp are protozoa that function as an intracellular but extracytoplasmic parasite. Transmission occurs via the fecal-oral route. *Cryptosporidium* infections usually result in disease in immunocompromised birds, more specifically enteritis in small birds such as cockatiels, budgerigars, and lovebirds.[14] Upper respiratory tract disease is described in birds of prey.

Histologically, a mild-moderate lymphoplasmacytic proventriculitis with mucosal, glandular, and ductular hyperplasia has been documented.[17] Organisms are described as intracellular but extracytoplasmic and are histologically identified as apical 1-μm spherical basophilic structures intimately associated with the surface of mucosal epithelial cells.

Cryptosporidium parvum infection in dogs and cats is typically asymptomatic but has been associated with self-limiting diarrhea in cats.[9] In immunocompromised animals, severe hemorrhagic diarrhea has been reported.[9]

There are no published cases documenting disease transmission of *Cryptosporidium* spp from companion parrots to dogs and cats in the same household.

GIARDIASIS

Giardia sp is an intestinal protozoa identified in a number of different species. Morphologically identical cysts are identified in the feces of a number of different species including dogs, cats, and parrots.[18] Despite their similar morphologic appearance, infectivity studies have demonstrated a lack of cross-infectivity among different species.[18,19] *Giardia lamblia* is typically isolated from mammals, whereas *Giardia psittaci* is recognized in birds.[18]

Giardia spp are an infrequent cause of diarrhea and have been associated with feather-destructive behavior in cockatiels.[1] Giardial organisms may be difficult to identify antemortem because they are typically found in the upper small intestine.[1]

Giardiasis often results in minimal grossly visible changes at necropsy, although excessive fluid and mucus and mucosal hyperemia may be noted.[5] Histologically, lesions range from nonexistent to villous atrophy and lymphoplasmacytic inflammation.[5] Organisms may be found within the intestinal crypts but can extend the entire length of the villi.[5] Giardiasis is described as very common in budgerigars, although most infected animals are asymptomatic.[5] Infection is also common in cockatiels.[5]

In dogs and cats, diarrhea and abdominal discomfort are the most commonly recognized clinical signs.[18] Infection is typically asymptomatic, and clinical signs range from mild self-limiting acute diarrhea to severe or chronic diarrhea associated with weight loss.[9] Diagnosis is typically made by identification of the characteristic trophozoites or cysts in fecal samples, although ELISA antigen capture assays are also commercially available.

To the authors' knowledge, there are no known published cases documenting disease transmission of *Giardia* spp from parrots to companion dogs and cats.

SUMMARY

In conclusion, there are a number of bacterial, viral, fungal, and parasitic diseases that are presumed to be transmittable from companion parrots to dogs and cats. Such disease transmission has not been documented to occur; therefore, concerns for such transmission are apparently unwarranted, and pet caregivers should feel comfortable introducing a companion parrot into their household without increased risk of disease to their pet dogs and cats.

UNCITED REFERENCES

This section consists of references that are included in the reference list but are not cited in the article text. Please either cite each of these references in the text or, alternatively, delete it from the reference list. If you do not provide further instruction for this reference, we will retain it in its current form and publish it as an "un-cited reference" with your article.[19]

REFERENCES

1. Tully TN, Dorrestein GM, Jones AK. Handbook of avian medicine. Edinburgh (United Kingdom): Saunders Elsevier; 2009.
2. Pollock CG. Implications of mycobacteria in clinical disorders. In: Harrison GJ, Lightfoot TL, editors. Clinical avian medicine, vol. 2. Palm Beach (FL): Spix Publishing Inc; 2006. p. 681–90.
3. Gunn-Moore DA. Mycobacterial infections in cats and dogs. In: Ettinger SJ, Feldman EC, editors. Textbook of veterinary internal medicine, vol. 1. St. Louis (MO): Saunders Elsevier; 2010. p. 875–81.
4. Tully TN. Update on Chlamydophila psittaci: a short comment. In: Harrison GJ, Lightfoot TL, editors. Clinical avian medicine, vol. 2. Palm Beach (FL): Spix Publishing Inc; 2006. p. 679–80.
5. Schmidt RE, Reavill DR, Phalon DN. Pathology of pet and aviary birds. Ames (IA): Iowa State Press; 2003.
6. Shivaprasal HL. Unusual cases of Chlamydiosis in psittacines. In: Proceedings of the Association of Avian Veterinarians 31st Annual Conference. San Diego (CA): 2010; p. 67–8.

7. Maggs DJ. Ocular manifestations of systemic disease. In: Ettinger SJ, Feldman EC, editors. Textbook of veterinary internal medicine, vol. 1. St. Louis (MO): Saunders Elsevier; 2010. p. 137–42.

8. Marks SL. Enteric bacterial disease. In: Ettinger SJ, Feldman EC, editors. Textbook of veterinary internal medicine, vol. 1. St. Louis (MO): Saunders Elsevier; 2010. p. 917–22.

9. Hall EJ, German AJ. Diseases of the small intestine. In: Ettinger SJ, Feldman EC, editors. Textbook of veterinary internal medicine, vol. 2. St. Louis (MO): Saunders Elsevier; 2010. p. 1526–72.

10. Hawkins MG, Crossley BM, Osofsky A, et al. Avian influenza A virus subtype H5N2 in a red-lored Amazon parrot. J Am Vet Med Assoc 2006;228(2):236–41.

11. Giese M, Harder TC, Teifke JP, et al. Experimental infection and natural contact exposure of dogs with avian influenza virus (H5N1). Emerg Infec Dis 2008;14(2): 308–10.

12. Songserm T, Amonsin A, Jam-on R, et al. Avian influenza H5N1 in naturally infected domestic cat. Emerg Infec Dis 2006;12(4):681–3.

13. Rimmelzwaan GF, van Riel D, Baars M, et al. Influenza A virus (H5N1) infection in cats causes systemic disease with potential novel routes of virus spread within and between hosts. Am J Pathol 2006;168(1):176–83.

14. Dahlhausen RD. Implications of mycoses in clinical disorders. In: Harrison GJ, Lightfoot TL, editors. Clinical avian medicine, vol. 2. Palm Beach (FL): Spix Publishing Inc; 2006. p. 691–704.

15. Davidson AP. Aspergillosis. In: Ettinger SJ, Feldman EC, editors. Textbook of veterinary internal medicine, vol. 1. St. Louis (MO): Saunders Elsevier; 2010. p. 996–1002.

16. Taboada J, Grooters AM. Cryptococcosis. In: Ettinger SJ, Feldman EC, editors. Textbook of veterinary internal medicine, vol. 1. St. Louis (MO): Saunders Elsevier; 2010. p. 988–92.

17. Taboada J, Grooters AJ. Histoplasmosis, blastomycosis, sporotrichosis, candidiasis, pythiosis, and lagenidiosis. In: Ettinger SJ, Feldman EC, editors. Textbook of veterinary internal medicine, vol. 1. St. Louis (MO): Saunders Elsevier; 2010. p. 971–88.

18. Messenger GA, Garner MM. Proventricular cryptosporidiosis in small psittacines. In: Proceedings of the Association of Avian Veterinarians 31st Annual Conference. San Diego (CA), 2010. p. 77–8.

19. Lindsay DS. Giardia and cryptosporidium: really zoonotic? In: Proceedings of the Western States Veterinary Conference. Las Vegas (NV), 2004.

Feline Respiratory Disease Complex

Leah A. Cohn, DVM, PhD

KEYWORDS

- Feline calicivirus • Feline herpes virus • Rhinotracheitis
- *Chlamydophila felis* • *Bordetella bronchiseptica*
- Upper respiratory infection

Feline respiratory disease complex (FRDC) refers to the characteristic acute presentation of a contagious respiratory or ocular disease caused by one or multiple pathogens. The complex is also referred to simply as feline upper respiratory tract infection. Although the presentation of FRDC is usually an acute illness, chronic disease sequelae are possible either from infection or an immune-mediated response to the infection.

Because FRDC is initiated by contagious pathogens, the acute manifestations are exceedingly rare in singly housed indoor cats. Rather, FRDC is a major problem in animal shelters; cats in outdoor colonies; and occasionally in cats housed in catteries, multiple cat households, boarding facilities, or cats that travel to shows. Although pathogens are crucial in initiation of FRDC, it is complicated by a number of factors related to the environment and host. For example, not only are cats housed in animal shelters exposed to contagious pathogens, but also the illness caused by these pathogens may be complicated by factors such as poor air quality or immunosuppression related to stress.[1]

Respiratory disease complex remains a major challenge to veterinarians, shelter operators, and cat owners alike. Although morbidity greatly exceeds mortality, cats and especially young kittens may die as a result of infection. Outbreaks in animal shelters may prevent adoption of homeless cats and increase rates of euthanasia. Costs associated with treatment and prevention may impact the ability of shelters to function effectively.[2–5] Although vaccines are available for several of the pathogens involved in FRDC, they do not prevent infection or pathogen transmission entirely. Although eradication of FRDC is not a realistic goal, studious efforts to minimize transmission and manage infections will result in reduced morbidity and mortality.

The author has been a consultant and speaker for Intervet/Schering Plough Animal Health and Pfizer, both of which produce vaccines against some of the pathogens in this syndrome, as well as for IDEXX, a company that offers a polymerase chain reaction panel (PCR) for diagnosis of these pathogens. The author does not believe these positions present a conflict of interest relevant to this manuscript.
Department of Veterinary Medicine and Surgery, University of Missouri-Columbia, 900 East Campus Drive, Columbia, MO 65211, USA
E-mail address: cohnl@missouri.edu

Vet Clin Small Anim 41 (2011) 1273–1289
doi:10.1016/j.cvsm.2011.07.006
0195-5616/11/$ – see front matter © 2011 Elsevier Inc. All rights reserved.

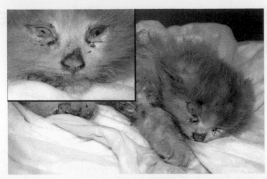

Fig. 1. A young kitten, found as a stray, affected by FRDC. A combination of lethargy, fever, and ocular and nasal discharge is typical, and kittens are usually more severely affected than adult cats.

CLINICAL PRESENTATION

The clinical presentation of kittens and cats with FRDC is similar regardless of the pathogen(s) involved (**Fig. 1**). Clinical signs may be quite mild or extremely severe. Secondary bacterial infections can lead to major complications including lower respiratory infections (ie, pneumonia). Simultaneous viral infections are also possible, especially in the setting of animal shelters. The concurrent presence of two or more infections can greatly complicate the clinical disease picture.[6–8] For instance, although neither feline immunodeficiency virus or feline panleukopenia are respiratory viruses, cats with either of these and simultaneous calicivirus infections would demonstrate a much more severe systemic illness than cats with a typical calicivirus infection alone.

The most common signs of FRDC include serous, mucoid, or mucopurulent nasal discharge; sneezing; conjunctivitis and ocular discharge; ulcerations of the lips, tongue, gums, or nasal planum; salivation; coughing; fever; lethargy; and inappetence. Although there are no truly pathognomonic signs of any particular underlying agent, the presence of certain clinical findings can offer a potential clue to the pathogen involved (**Table 1**).

Table 1	
FRDC: Clinical clues to pathogen incriminated	
Clinical Clue	**Pathogens**
Limping	FCV
Oral ulceration	FCV
	FHV-1
Keratitis, corneal (dendritic) ulcers	FHV-1
Conjunctivitis without nasal signs	*C felis*
	Mycoplasma spp
Dermatitis, dermal ulcers	VS-FCV
	FHV-1
Cough	*B bronchiseptica*

PATHOGENS OF FRDC

A variety of viral and bacterial pathogens have been identified in cats with FRDC, often in combinations of two or more. Simultaneous infection with multiple pathogens exacerbates the severity of illness. Unpublished data from two commercial diagnostic laboratories offering a respiratory diagnostic panel found that 45.6% (CM Leutenegger, unpublished data, IDEXX Laboratories, Inc, 2011) and 48% (David Aucoin, ANTECH, unpublished data, 2011) of cats positive for a given pathogen were positive for at least one additional pathogen. The most common viral pathogens are feline calicivirus (FCV) and feline herpesvirus-1 (FHV-1, or feline viral rhinotracheitis); the bacteria *Chlamydophila felis* and *Bordetella bronchiseptica* are also potential primary pathogens in FRDC. *Mycoplasma* species are normal commensal organisms of the upper respiratory tract, but some species may serve as pathogens. Although extremely rare, certain influenza viruses (H5N1) can cause upper respiratory signs in cats and are of concern due to the theoretical potential for zoonotic infection.[9,10] It is possible that the contribution of other pathogens to FRDC has yet to be recognized.[8] Secondary gram-positive and gram-negative bacterial infections may accompany either viral or bacterial FRDC.

Feline Calicivirus

Feline calicivirus is a single-stranded, nonenveloped RNA virus that is widespread among cat populations worldwide. Great antigenic differences exist within the single serotype.[11,12] The virus is not zoonotic, nor is it an important pathogen in nonfelid species.

Both acutely infected cats and chronic carriers shed the highly contagious virus from bodily secretions and especially in respiratory, ocular, and oral secretions. Cats that recover from the acute infection often clear the virus over a period of weeks, but some cats shed for much longer, and perhaps even for life.[13] The virus is quite stable in the environment and may persist for a month or longer.[14] Although aerosol transmission from cat to cat certainly occurs, contact with contaminated surfaces is a more likely route of transmission.[2,15]

After contact with viral particles, the susceptible cat will develop a transient viremia with the primary site of viral replication in the oropharynx. Clinical disease severity depends on a number of factors including the virulence of the pathogen as well as the response of the host. Cats with a preexisting immunity may remain healthy, whereas naïve cats become ill, partially explaining why kittens are more often severely affected by FCV than adult cats. In general, a single strain of FCV tends to cause a similar disease severity and presentation in most infected cats. Oral ulcers are the classic presentation of FCV; vesicles form on the tongue margins of infected cats due to epithelial necrosis (**Fig. 2**).[15] Sneezing and nasal discharge are less common than in FHV-1–infected cats but are still frequent findings. Less commonly, viral pneumonia and lameness occur as well. Although most manifestations of FCV are acute, it has also been associated with chronic stomatitis. Although the condition has not been reproduced by experimental infection, it is believed that an immune-mediated reaction to FCV may cause chronic lymphoplasmacytic gingivitis/stomatitis.[16]

Occasionally, a highly virulent viral mutation causes a more severe, systemic manifestation rather than typical upper airway disease; these infections are said to be "virulent systemic-FCV," or VS-FCV. Routine FCV vaccination does not mitigate VS-FCV, and unlike many other infectious diseases, VS-FCV may be a more severe disease in adult cats than in kittens.[17] Peripheral edema; hair loss; ulcers of the skin as well as the mucosal surfaces; and even necrosis of the ears, toes, and tail tip may

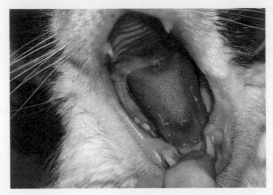

Fig. 2. Lingual ulcers, as seen here, are a characteristic physical examination finding consistent with feline calicivirus. However, not all cats with clinical disease due to FCV will demonstrate oral ulcers, and oral ulcers can occur in the absence of FCV infection.

occur as a result of a profound vasculitis (**Fig. 3**).[17–20] Mortality from VS-FCV is high, and often more than half of infected cats will die from severe vasculitis, hepatocellular necrosis, disseminated intravascular coagulation, or other disease complications.[17,20] Outbreaks of VS-FCV tend to be sporadic. Although a veterinary clinic, shelter, or cattery may be affected widely, the severe disease manifestation does not seem to become endemic in a community over time. Rather, these outbreaks tend to

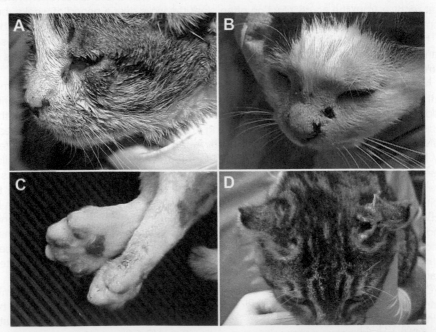

Fig. 3. Virulent-systemic calicivirus results in systemic disease, with manifestations not only of nasal and ocular discharge (A), but also dermal ulceration due to vasculitis (B, D), and peripheral edema (C). (*Courtesy of* Kate F. Hurley, DVM, MPVM, University of California, Davis, CA.)

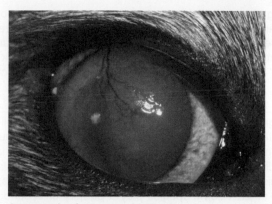

Fig. 4. Extraocular photograph of a 3-year-old FS DSH cat with eosinophilic keratitis. Prominent superficial corneal neovascularization and raised, yellowish plaques are seen. This corneal disease may be associated with FHV-1. (*Courtesy of* Elizabeth A. Giuliano, DVM, MS, University of Missouri, Columbia, MO.)

"burn out" over a relatively short period of time. Not all severe manifestations of FCV are due to a mutated VS-FCV; severe manifestations of routine FCV may also result in mortality, especially when coinfections exist.

Feline Herpesvirus-1

Feline herpesvirus 1 (FHV) is a double-stranded, enveloped DNA virus that is distributed worldwide. It is an important cause of rhinotracheitis in cats but, although antigenically similar to other herpesviruses, is neither zoonotic nor does it cause disease in nonfelid species. The virus replicates in upper respiratory and ocular epithelium as well as in neurons. Viral shedding through nasal, oral, and ocular secretions begins very soon after infection. Although the virus can persist in the environment for a few days, direct exposure to infected cats is believed to be a more important route of infection than are fomites.[21,22] Unlike FCV, FHV-1 is readily destroyed by most disinfectants.

Lytic proliferation in the respiratory and ocular epithelium follows infection. The virus follows sensory nerves to reach neurons, with the trigeminal ganglia being particularly likely to harbor the virus. Although cats generally recover from acute FRDC signs within 2 to 3 weeks, most remain infected for life and can experience intermittent viral reactivation with disease recrudescence during times of stress or during immunosuppression.[23–25] In the absence of recrudescence, some cats develop chronic ocular pathology, including corneal ulcers and stromal keratitis (**Fig. 4**).[26] It is theorized that herpes infection, even when inactive, can predispose cats to chronic rhinosinusitis later in life as a result of damage to nasal turbinates or due to a proinflammatory state.[27]

Chlamydophila felis

An obligate intracellular gram-negative bacterium, *Chlamydophila felis* does not survive for any length of time outside the host. This bacterium is primarily a cause of conjunctivitis with only mild respiratory signs.[28] Because it is shed in ocular secretions, transmission requires close contact between infected and noninfected cats. Infected cats may initially demonstrate unilateral signs but these usually become bilateral. Resulting conjunctivitis can be severe, with hyperemia, ocular discharge, blepharospasm, and chemosis.[28] Unlike FHV-1, *C felis* seldom results in corneal ulceration. It is rare to find *C felis* in healthy cats, quite unlike FCV and FHV-1, which are routinely identified in healthy cats.[29] Although there is a risk for infection of exposed humans, it does not seem to be a common zoonotic infection.[30]

Mycoplasma *spp*

Mycoplasma are gram-negative pleomophic bacteria that lack a cell wall. Compared to most bacteria, they are difficult to culture and speciate. As a result, knowledge of the importance of members of this genus as contributing pathogens in respiratory and ocular disease is limited. It is known that many species of *Mycoplasma* are normal commensal organisms in the upper respiratory tract.[31] Nonetheless, there is mounting evidence that at least some species play a primary or secondary role in upper respiratory disease and conjunctivitis.[32–34] In at least one study, *Mycoplasma* were the organism most commonly identified in cats with conjunctivitis.[34] In several studies, *M felis* was isolated from cats with FRDC or in their housemates but not from healthy cats in noninfected households.[27,29,35,36]

Bordetella bronchiseptica

Most commonly thought of as a cause of canine infectious respiratory disease complex, *B bronchiseptica* can infect cats as well. In fact, this gram-negative coccobacillus can infect many other species of animals but only rarely causes human infections, and then mostly in immunocompromised people.[37,38] The bacterium is shed in oral and nasal secretions of infected animals, and transmission to naïve cats might occur via direct exposure to infected dogs or cats, or possibly through exposure to contaminated environments.[39–41]

Bordetella bronchiseptica colonizes the respiratory epithelium and may remain there without causing disease, or may instigate clinical illness. Although it is likely clinical disease in infected cats is worsened by coinfection, *B bronchiseptica* alone is capable of inducing respiratory disease.[38,39,42] Coughing may be a more common manifestation of FRDC caused by bordetellosis compared to the other common pathogens.

Influenza Virus

Influenza A viruses are single-stranded negative-sense RNA viruses in the family Orthomyxoviridae, and they are named numerically according to the hemagglutinin (H) and neuraminidase (N) expressed. These viruses become adapted to a particular species but are highly susceptible to genomic change and may be able to infect multiple different species or add species affinity through mutation.[43,44] Naturally occurring infections with both the virulent avian influenza H5N1 and the H1N1 reassortment virus (swine flu) have been identified during the last decade. However, as of yet no well adapted feline influenza virus has become established in cat populations.[43]

Influenza remains very rare in cats. Nevertheless, it is important for veterinarians to be aware that cats are susceptible to infection as some influenza A viruses (eg, H5N1 virulent avian influenza, H7N7) have the potential to be zoonotic infections associated with high morbidity or even high mortality in humans.[44–47] Most feline infections with H5N1 are acquired when the cat eats infected birds, but cat-to-cat transmission is also possible via feco–oral or respiratory routes.[48] Experimental inoculation of domestic cats with H5N1 can cause fever, depression, elevation of the third eye lid, conjunctivitis, increased respiratory effort, and nasal discharge as well as icterus, ataxia, seizures, and death.[10,49,50] A few pet cats in the United States have been naturally infected with the H1N1 reassortment virus.[51,52] For at least some of these cats, close contact with the infected owner was reported. The infected cats developed respiratory signs ranging from a relatively mild, self-limiting disease to a fatal infection. In no instance has human infection been confirmed to be the result of exposure to an influenza-infected cat.

PATHOGEN PREVALENCE

The incidence and prevalence of the various pathogens that cause FRDC varies widely. In general, cats in dense housing are most likely to be infected.[1,15] Combined with the rotating populations and inherent stress of animal shelters, shelter-housed cats are most likely to develop illness and to become carriers of FRDC pathogens.[1,5,23] A large number of studies have documented the prevalence of the pathogens in a variety of settings, most often in catteries or animal shelters but also among cats with a variety of specific clinical illnesses including respiratory signs, conjunctivitis, uveitis, chronic stomatitis, nasal polyps, and others.[1,34,53–55] According to most studies, FCV and FVH-1 are overwhelmingly the most common pathogens involved in FRDC with nasal and oral manifestations. In shelter settings where FRDC has been identified, the prevalence of these pathogens is often 20% to 50% or even higher.[1,4,13,23,54,56] In contrast, B bronchiseptica is typically found in fewer than 15% of cats with FRDC.[1,4,57] Predominantly ocular manifestations are usually attributed to FHV-1, C felis, or Mycoplasma infections; no single one of these is clearly demonstrated to be most consistently implicated.[33,34,36,58,59] Of 4772 feline submissions from the United States in 2010, a large commercial laboratory offering multiplex polymerase chain reaction (PCR) panel testing for FRDC pathogens identified at least one pathogen in 66.6% of samples submitted. The positive samples included 41.8% with Mycoplasma felis, 22% positive for FCV, 25.3% positive for FHV-1, 10% positive for B bronchiseptica, and 8.1% with C felis (C.M. Leutenegger, unpublished data, IDEXX Laboratories, Inc, 2011). From 2310 feline sample from 35 states submitted to a second such large commercial laboratory, at least one FRDC pathogens was identified in 57% of samples. The positive samples included 6% with FCV, 58% with FHV-1, 14% with B bronchiseptica, and 13% with C felis (David Aucoin, ANTECH, unpublished data, 2011).

DIAGNOSIS

Any cat with an acute onset of upper respiratory signs or conjunctivitis or both and a history of recent exposure to other cats should be suspected to have infectious FRDC, and the suspicion is increased in kittens and poorly vaccinated cats. Nevertheless, not all cats with typical signs have FRDC. For example, cattery or shelter cats might develop oral ulcers as a result of topical exposure to caustic disinfectants such as quaternary ammonium compounds or phenols (eg, Lysol). For individual cats with upper respiratory signs believed to be due to FRDC, the specific causative agent need not be determined because supportive treatment is similar regardless of the pathogens involved. For individual cats with lower respiratory signs or evidence of secondary bacterial pneumonia, it is appropriate to collect airway lavage samples for bacterial culture and susceptibility testing.

Diagnostic testing aimed at detection of primary pathogens underlying FRDC is of the most use in the setting of a cattery or animal shelter experiencing an increased incidence or severity of upper respiratory infections. Other reasons for specific testing might include evaluation of protocols for disease prevention (eg, when changes to vaccine or disinfection protocols are being considered), to detect a disease carrier before movement from one cattery to another, or for investigation of liability or other legal issues.

Unfortunately, the diagnosis of a specific pathogen as the cause of FRDC is not simple. An educated guess can be useful when clinical signs seem to favor one pathogen over another; for example, prominent oral ulceration suggests FCV. When a guess is inadequate, PCR, bacterial cultures, viral isolation, and serologic assays can all be useful but false-negative and false-positive tests occur often. The most common pathogens can be identified in many healthy cats, so simply finding these pathogens does not prove disease causation. Conventional PCR, nested PCR, and real-time reverse-transcriptase PCR (RT-PCR) have all been used to test for pathogens of FRDC. These tests vary in sensitivity depending on a variety of factors including sampling site and method and the chosen primers; primer choice is especially problematic for pathogens with wide genetic variability such as calicivirus.[54,60–64] Bacterial culture proves a viable bacteria is present in the sample, but as with PCR, it does not prove that the pathogen is the cause of illness. A negative culture does not eliminate a role for bacterial infection either; for instance, B bronchiseptica is best recovered after transport in charcoal Ames medium and growth on selective agar and might be missed if these conditions are not satisfied. Viral isolation depends on the presence of replicative virus such that in vitro inactivation due to neutralizing antibody in the sample or sample handling can cause false-negative results. Antibody detection confirms exposure or vaccination, but again, not disease causation. Prior vaccination not only causes long-lasting seropositivity, but recent use of modified live vaccines can also produce false-positive PCR results.

Differentiation between routine FCV outbreaks and those caused by VS-FCV is not possible with a single test.[65] Instead, the diagnosis depends on a combination of findings. When the outbreak involves more severe disease manifestations with multiple systemic signs and when vaccinated and adult cats are affected to the same degree as are young and naïve cats, VS-FCV is likely. Although no molecular test can demonstrate that a given strain is more virulent than another, such testing will confirm that a single virus strain is involved in an outbreak caused by VS-FCV. Ideally, immunohistochemical evidence of calicivirus in affected tissues (eg, liver) would also be used to confirm a diagnosis of VS-FCV.[18]

Commercially offered respiratory pathogen "profiles" have become increasingly available and can be useful in the investigation of typical FRDC outbreaks. Usually, swab specimens from the oropharynx are submitted for PCR, although other samples, including tissues obtain at necropsy, can also be tested. The saying "buyer beware" applies to laboratories conducting PCR testing; it is incumbent on the veterinarian to use only reputable laboratories with validated testing results. Both false-negative and false-positive results are possible on any one test. Identification of the causative pathogens in an outbreak setting should be based on sampling multiple involved animals (ideally 10%–30%, or a minimum of three to five cats). Cats should be sampled early in the course of disease to reduce the likelihood that complicating rather than inciting pathogens will be identified. Because of the vicissitude involved in causation and diagnosis of FRDC, it is expected that individual cats will test positive for more than one pathogen, and that some ill cats may test negative for any of these pathogens. Only by recognizing which pathogens are common to multiple involved cats can the cause of a disease outbreak be identified confidently.

TREATMENT

The most important aspect of treatment for most cats with FRDC remains supportive care, including nutritional and nursing care. Cats are often unwilling to eat due not only to systemic illness but also to nasal congestion, which interferes with the ability to smell food, and the pain of oral ulcers. Offering highly palatable, aromatic, soft foods is attempted first; warming the food sometimes helps also. Analgesia should be provided for cats with oral ulcers. Mirtazapine (1/8 to ¼ of a 15-mg tablet PO every other day to every third day) can be used as an appetite stimulant. Should these efforts fail, placement of a nasoesophageal or an esophagostomy tube becomes necessary; feeding tubes also facilitate maintenance of systemic hydration. For some cats, parenteral crystalloid fluids may be required to maintain hydration. Nursing care includes removal of nasal discharge. Humidifiers or saline nebulization may loosen thick, tenacious mucus discharge.

Antimicrobial therapy is often beneficial either to address the disease pathogen directly, or to address secondary bacterial infections. Doxycycline is a good first choice to treat infections with C felis, B bronchiseptica, and Mycoplasma spp and the drug achieves good airway penetration. However, if tablets stick in the esophagus, strictures can form; therefore either a liquid doxycycline should be used or the tablet should be followed with oral administration of water.[66] Despite the fact that C felis causes localized ocular infection, systemic antimicrobials are more effective than topical treatments alone.[67] Although azithromycin or fluoroquinolones are good alternatives to doxycycline for the treatment of FRDC, they are less likely to effectively clear infection with C felis.[68-71] Cats with C felis are usually treated for 4 weeks, or 2 weeks past clinical disease resolution to improve the chances of eliminating the pathogen entirely, and cats with close contact to infected cats should be treated simultaneously even if they do not have obvious conjunctivitis.[29,71] Longer treatment periods, up to 42 days, have been suggested for M felis infection.[69] Even cats with primary viral infections may benefit from antibiotics to treat or prevent secondary bacterial infections. For this purpose, beta-lactams (eg, amoxicillin, amoxicillin-clavulanic acid) and azithromycin are reasonable choices, and duration of treatment is often only 7 to 10 days.[3]

Antiviral therapies have also been considered for use in cats with FRDC, but of the many antiviral drugs that are used to treat humans, several are quite toxic in cats. For instance, the FCV inhibitor ribavirin and the FHV-1 inhibitor valacyclovir (the prodrug of acyclovir) are both toxic when systemically administered to cats, precluding routine use.[72,73] On the other hand, oral administration of famciclovir to cats with FHV-1 infection appears to be safe and effective.[74,75] L-Lysine is an oral amino acid supplement that reduces viral shedding in cats with latent FHV-1 infection. Although the treatment is safe and inexpensive, the efficacy in reducing severity or duration of the acute signs of FRDC has not been convincingly demonstrated.[5,76-78] In an interesting trial, lysine was used as a dietary supplement in the food of cats housed in an animal shelter. Although the cats receiving the supplement had neither a reduced incidence nor severity of FHV-1 infection, the study did not directly administer the L-lysine, so intake may not have been adequate to demonstrate an effect.[5] Feline interferon-omega is licensed for use in Europe and should theoretically be useful as an antiviral therapy, but controlled field studies are not available as of yet.[15,22,79,80] Human interferon-α has also been suggested as potentially beneficial, but benefits have not been substantiated in clinical trials.[81]

Other types of care may be required for specific disease manifestations. For example, cats with ocular lesions may require mucinomimetic therapy, topic antibiotics, or mydriatic treatment.[75,82] For cats that develop pneumonia, supplemental oxygen may be required. Cats with pain related to lameness, severe dermatitis, or other complications of infection may require analgesia.

PREVENTION

Although there is no way to eliminate FRDC completely, there are multiple methods to reduce the likelihood and severity of infection. These include vaccination programs and efforts to reduce stress on individual cats as well as efforts to reduce pathogen exposure through population management and sanitation protocols. Some of these methods are readily applied to some cat populations but are not applicable to others. For instance, it is essentially impossible to control exposure to new cats or to disinfect and sanitize surfaces in the setting of a feral or barn cat colony.

Vaccination

Vaccinations have resulted in a tremendous reduction of morbidity and even mortality resulting from feline respiratory infections, but vaccinations are not perfect. Most FRDC vaccines do not provide sterilizing immunity. That is, vaccination can reduce disease severity and perhaps the risk of transmission but will not prevent infection altogether. Severe infection sometimes occurs despite vaccination, and adverse reactions to vaccination occur (albeit rarely). Decisions regarding vaccination should always be based on an understanding of the situation of the individual cat, including environment and risk for exposure as well as comorbidities and owner preferences. For example, although modified live vaccines against FCV and FHV-1 are often recommended, they may not be appropriate in immunocompromised or in pregnant cats. Some cat owners would prefer to forgo vaccination at regular intervals and instead test for antibody titers to gauge when vaccine boosters are appropriate. Titers directly demonstrate humoral immunity but imply that cell-mediated immunity, and more importantly disease protection, may exist also.[83] Vaccine recommendations are available from both the American Association of Feline Practitioners (http://www.catvets.com/professionals/guidelines/publications) and the European Advisory Board on Cat Diseases (http://www.abcd-vets.org/guidelines/index.asp).

Vaccination of cats for FCV and FHV-1 is recommended unless there is a compelling reason not to vaccinate, but neither vaccine provides sterilizing immunity. For most cats, modified live vaccines (MLV) are administered in combination with feline panleukopenia vaccination. In kittens, vaccination is initiated as a series beginning at 6 to 9 weeks of age, then boostered every 3 to 4 weeks until 16 weeks of age, again at 1 year, and then again every 3 years thereafter. Intranasal MLV vaccines offer the advantage of a more rapid onset of protection with the disadvantage that some vaccinated cats display mild respiratory signs after vaccination. Even mild signs can be important in shelters where policies may exist preventing adoption of cats with any signs of respiratory disease. Regardless, MLV for these pathogens is recommended upon entry to any rescue shelter. Inactivated vaccines should be considered in cats with compromised immune responses (eg, cats with retroviral infections, cats on chronic immunosuppressive therapy). Breeding cats should be vaccinated before breeding rather than during pregnancy.

Vaccination against FCV offers special challenges.[84,85] Variability in virus strains can result in vaccine resistance and therefore vaccine failures.[86,87] The VS-FCV has not been mitigated by traditional MLV for FCV.[17] For this reason, a new vaccine has been developed that incorporates strains known to have caused virulent systemic infection (CaliciVax, Boehringer Ingelheim). Although the new vaccine protects from the strain from which it was derived, there has not yet been proof that it protects from other strains that might cause virulent infection. Because the vaccine is a killed product, it requires a booster at 3 weeks and protection is delayed, thus making it unsuitable (by itself) in shelter settings. For now, special vaccines for VS-FCV should be considered conditional rather than core vaccines.

Vaccines also exist for *C felis* and *B bronchiseptica*, but neither is considered a core vaccine. Both MLV and killed vaccines are available for *C felis* but vaccination has only moderate efficacy and a relatively short duration of immunity. It is not recommended for pet cats, but it may be considered in shelters or catteries where recognition of such infections remains common despite intensified efforts aimed at environmental modification. Similarly, although not routinely recommended, vaccination of cats for *B bronchiseptica* may be appropriate in animal shelters with documented outbreaks of this common cause of canine infectious respiratory disease complex.

Stress Reduction

Stress results in the release of excessive cortisol and negatively impacts the ability of the immune response to counter infection.[88] Clinical disease is often worsened in stressed cats, and quiescent FHV-1 infections can be activated through stress.[24,77] Shelter-housed cats are placed under conditions of enormous stress; simple measures may help mitigate such stress. For instance, providing hiding places, visual and auditory segregation of feline and canine populations, providing for environmental enrichment through scratching materials and toys, and group housing of compatible cats can all reduce stress.[89–91] However, measures such as group housing that might reduce stress for one cat might increase stress for another, less social cat. In addition, some of the same measures that reduce stress can increase the potential for pathogen transmission (eg, group housing) or make surface disinfection more challenging (eg, toys and scratching materials).

Population Management

Because FRDC is induced by contagious pathogens, direct or indirect exposure to previously infected cats is required for disease development. When cats with suspected FRDC are presented to the veterinary hospital, they should be taken immediately into a private examination room. Hospitalization should be avoided if at all possible, and if hospitalization is required infected cats should be isolated from all other cats. Any areas where infected cats are kept must be thoroughly disinfected before other cats are brought into the same area. Owners contemplating bringing a new cat into their household or cattery should be sure that all existing family cats are vaccinated against FCV and FHV-1. The new cat should be free of obvious respiratory signs and ideally should be kept isolated from other cats for 1 to 2 weeks after arrival.

The greater dilemmas occur in the setting of animal shelters where there is often no choice but to accept new cats, even cats already demonstrating respiratory signs. When possible, cats demonstrating signs already should be segregated from all other cats. However, routine quarantine of all cats may simply lengthen their stay in a shelter situation and increase stress, which can actually lead to more FRDC manifestations. Often shelters are overcrowded, which contributes to the incidence of FRDC both through simple exposure and because of the stress attendant when cats are kept in crowded situations. The realities of most shelters make the ideals of population management extraordinarily difficult to achieve.[4] By reducing the number of cats in the shelter and the length of time they stay in the shelter through measures such as the use of foster care homes, the incidence of FRDC should be reduced.

Sanitation

Besides limiting contact with infected cats, strict attention to sanitation and disinfection of surfaces and potential fomites can help reduce the incidence of FRDC. Hand washing between handling cats and the use of clean coveralls or laboratory coats is helpful. Because even cats that appear quite healthy may shed pathogens, these simple measures should be practiced between handling any and all cats. Cleaning of caging to remove organic debris followed by disinfection will destroy most of the pathogens associated with FRDC. Only FCV is difficult to inactivate; like other nonenveloped virus types (eg, parvovirus), it is resistant to chlorhexidine, quaternary ammonium, and several other disinfectants.[92] Either potassium peroxymonosulfate or household bleach (5% sodium hypochlorite) diluted 1:32 are good options to destroy FCV.[92,93]

SUMMARY

Infectious viral and bacterial respiratory diseases cause tremendous morbidity and occasional mortality in domestic cats. Although these FRDC-associated illnesses cannot be eradicated, their occurrence can be minimized and mitigated through the judicious use of appropriate diagnosis, treatment, vaccination, and husbandry.

REFERENCES

1. Helps CR, Lait P, Damhuis A, et al. Factors associated with upper respiratory tract disease caused by feline herpesvirus, feline calicivirus, Chlamydophila felis and Bordetella bronchiseptica in cats: experience from 218 European catteries. Vet Rec 2005;156(21):669–73.
2. Coyne KP, Edwards D, Radford AD, et al. Longitudinal molecular epidemiological analysis of feline calicivirus infection in an animal shelter: a model for investigating calicivirus transmission within high-density, high-turnover populations. J Clin Microbiol 2007;45(10):3239–44.
3. Ruch-Gallie RA, Veir JK, Spindel ME, et al. Efficacy of amoxycillin and azithromycin for the empirical treatment of shelter cats with suspected bacterial upper respiratory infections. J Feline Med Surg 2008;10(6):542–50.
4. Bannasch MJ, Foley JE. Epidemiologic evaluation of multiple respiratory pathogens in cats in animal shelters. J Feline Med Surg 2005;7(2):109–19.
5. Drazenovich TL, Fascetti AJ, Westermeyer HD, et al. Effects of dietary lysine supplementation on upper respiratory and ocular disease and detection of infectious organisms in cats within an animal shelter. Am J Vet Res 2009;70(11):1391–400.
6. Reubel GH, George JW, Higgins J, et al. Effect of chronic feline immunodeficiency virus infection on experimental feline calicivirus-induced disease. Vet Microbiol 1994; 39(3–4):335–51.
7. Dawson S, Smyth NR, Bennett M, et al. Effect of primary-stage feline immunodeficiency virus infection on subsequent feline calicivirus vaccination and challenge in cats. AIDS 1991;5(6):747–50.
8. Johnson MS, Martin M, Stone B, et al. Survival of a cat with pneumonia due to cowpox virus and feline herpesvirus infection. J Small Anim Pract 2009;50(9):498–502.
9. Thiry E, Addie D, Belak S, et al. H5N1 avian influenza in cats. ABCD guidelines on prevention and management. J Feline Med Surg 2009;11(7):615–18.
10. Marschall J, Hartmann K. Avian influenza A H5N1 infections in cats. J Feline Med Surg 2008;10(4):359–65.
11. Coyne KP, Reed FC, Porter CJ, et al. Recombination of feline calicivirus within an endemically infected cat colony. J Gen Virol 2006;87(Pt 4):921–6.

12. Radford AD, Dawson S, Ryvar R, et al. High genetic diversity of the immunodominant region of the feline calicivirus capsid gene in endemically infected cat colonies. Virus Genes 2003;27(2):145–55.

13. Coyne KP, Dawson S, Radford AD, et al. Long-term analysis of feline calicivirus prevalence and viral shedding patterns in naturally infected colonies of domestic cats. Vet Microbiol 2006;118(1–2):12–25.

14. Duizer E, Bijkerk P, Rockx B, et al. Inactivation of caliciviruses. Appl Environ Microbiol 2004;70(8):4538–43.

15. Radford AD, Addie D, Belak S, et al. Feline calicivirus infection. ABCD guidelines on prevention and management. J Feline Med Surg 2009;11(7):556–64.

16. Knowles JO, McArdle F, Dawson S, et al. Studies on the role of feline calicivirus in chronic stomatitis in cats. Vet Microbiol 1991;27(3–4):205–19.

17. Hurley KE, Pesavento PA, Pedersen NC, et al. An outbreak of virulent systemic feline calicivirus disease. J Am Vet Med Assoc 2004;224(2):241–9.

18. Coyne KP, Jones BR, Kipar A, et al. Lethal outbreak of disease associated with feline calicivirus infection in cats. Vet Rec 2006;158(16):544–50.

19. Hurley K, Sykes E. Update on feline calicivirus: new trends. Vet Clin North Am Small Anim Pract 2003;33:759–72.

20. Foley J, Hurley K, Pesavento PA, et al. Virulent systemic feline calicivirus infection: local cytokine modulation and contribution of viral mutants. J Feline Med Surg 2006;8(1):55–61.

21. Gaskell R, Dawson S, Radford A, et al. Feline herpesvirus. Vet Res 2007;38(2): 337–54.

22. Thiry E, Addie D, Belak S, et al. Feline herpesvirus infection. ABCD guidelines on prevention and management. J Feline Med Surg 2009;11(7):547–55.

23. Pedersen NC, Sato R, Foley JE, et al. Common virus infections in cats, before and after being placed in shelters, with emphasis on feline enteric coronavirus. J Feline Med Surg 2004;6(2):83–8.

24. Gaskell RM, Povey RC. Experimental induction of feline viral rhinotracheitis virus re-excretion in FVR-recovered cats. Vet Rec 1977;100(7):128–33.

25. Gaskell RM, Dennis PE, Goddard LE, et al. Isolation of felid herpesvirus I from the trigeminal ganglia of latently infected cats. J Gen Virol 1985;66(Pt 2):391–4.

26. Maggs DJ. Update on pathogenesis, diagnosis, and treatment of feline herpesvirus type 1. Clin Tech Small Anim Pract 2005;20(2):94–101.

27. Johnson LR, Foley JE, De Cock HE, et al. Assessment of infectious organisms associated with chronic rhinosinusitis in cats. J Am Vet Med Assoc 2005;227(4): 579–85.

28. Gruffydd-Jones T, Addie D, Belak S, et al. Chlamydophila felis infection. ABCD guidelines on prevention and management. J Feline Med Surg 2009;11(7):605–9.

29. Holst BS, Hanas S, Berndtsson LT, et al. Infectious causes for feline upper respiratory tract disease—a case-control study. J Feline Med Surg 2010;12(10):783–9.

30. Browning GF. Is Chlamydophila felis a significant zoonotic pathogen? Aust Vet J 2004;82(11):695–6.

31. Randolph JF, Moise NS, Scarlett JM, et al. Prevalence of mycoplasmal and ureaplasmal recovery from tracheobronchial lavages and of mycoplasmal recovery from pharyngeal swab specimens in cats with or without pulmonary disease. Am J Vet Res 1993;54(6):897–900.

32. Randolph JF, Moise NS, Scarlett JM, et al. Prevalence of mycoplasmal and ureaplasmal recovery from traceobronchial lavages and of mycoplasmal recovery from pharyngeal swab specimens in cats with or without pulmonary disease. Am J Vet Res 1993;54(6):897–900.

33. Hartmann AD, Hawley J, Werckenthin C, et al. Detection of bacterial and viral organisms from the conjunctiva of cats with conjunctivitis and upper respiratory tract disease. J Feline Med Surg 2010;12(10):775–82.

34. Low HC, Powell CC, Veir JK, et al. Prevalence of feline herpesvirus 1, *Chlamydophila felis*, and *Mycoplasma* spp. DNA in conjunctival cells collected from cats with and without conjunctivitis. Am J Vet Res 2007;68(6):643–8.

35. Shewen PE, Povey RC, Wilson MR. A survey of the conjunctival flora of clinically normal cats and cats with conjunctivitis. Can Vet J 1980;21(8):231–3.

36. Haesebrouck F, Devriese LA, van Rijssen B, et al. Incidence and significance of isolation of Mycoplasma felis from conjunctival swabs of cats. Vet Microbiol 1991; 26(1–2):95–101.

37. Dworkin MS, Sullivan PS, Buskin SE, et al. *Bordetella bronchiseptica* infection in human immunodeficiency virus-infected patients. Clin Infect Dis 1999;28(5):1095–9.

38. Egberink H, Addie D, Belak S, et al. *Bordetella bronchiseptica* infection in cats. ABCD guidelines on prevention and management. J Feline Med Surg 2009;11(7):610–4.

39. Coutts AJ, Dawson S, Binns S, et al. Studies on natural transmission of *Bordetella bronchiseptica* in cats. Vet Microbiol 1996;48(1–2):19–27.

40. Dawson S, Jones D, McCracken CM, et al. *Bordetella bronchiseptica* infection in cats following contact with infected dogs. Vet Rec 2000;146(2):46–8.

41. Foley JE, Rand C, Bannasch MJ, et al. Molecular epidemiology of feline bordetellosis in two animal shelters in California, USA. Prev Vet Med 2002;54(2):141–56.

42. Jacobs AA, Chalmers WS, Pasman J, et al. Feline bordetellosis: challenge and vaccine studies. Vet Rec 1993;133(11):260–3.

43. Harder TC, Vahlenkamp TW. Influenza virus infections in dogs and cats. Vet Immunol Immunopathol 2009;134(1–2):54–60.

44. Shinya K, Makino A, Kawaoka Y. Emerging and reemerging influenza virus infections. Vet Pathol 2010;47(1):53–7.

45. van Riel D, Rimmelzwaan GF, van Amerongen G, et al. Highly pathogenic avian influenza virus H7N7 isolated from a fatal human case causes respiratory disease in cats but does not spread systemically. Am J Pathol 2010;177(5):2185–90.

46. Desvaux S, Marx N, Ong S, et al. Highly pathogenic avian influenza virus (H5N1) outbreak in captive wild birds and cats, Cambodia. Emerg Infect Dis 2009;15(3): 475–8.

47. Chutinimitkul S, Payungporn S, Chieochansin T, et al. The spread of avian influenza H5N1 virus; a pandemic threat to mankind. J Med Assoc Thai 2006;89(Suppl 3): S218–33.

48. Vahlenkamp TW, Teifke JP, Harder TC, et al. Systemic influenza virus H5N1 infection in cats after gastrointestinal exposure. Influenza Other Respi Viruses 2010;4(6):379–86.

49. Rimmelzwaan GF, van Riel D, Baars M, et al. Influenza A virus (H5N1) infection in cats causes systemic disease with potential novel routes of virus spread within and between hosts. Am J Pathol 2006;168(1):176–83 [quiz: 364].

50. Kuiken T, Rimmelzwaan G, van Riel D, et al. Avian H5N1 influenza in cats. Science 2004;306(5694):241.

51. Sponseller BA, Strait E, Jergens A, et al. Influenza A pandemic (H1N1) 2009 virus infection in domestic cat. Emerg Infect Dis;16(3):534–7.

52. Lohr CV, DeBess EE, Baker RJ, et al. Pathology and viral antigen distribution of lethal pneumonia in domestic cats due to pandemic (H1N1) 2009 influenza A virus. Vet Pathol 2010;47(3):378–86.

53. Maggs DJ, Lappin MR, Nasisse MP. Detection of feline herpesvirus-specific antibodies and DNA in aqueous humor from cats with or without uveitis. Am J Vet Res 1999;60(8):932–6.
54. Veir JK, Ruch-Gallie R, Spindel ME, et al. Prevalence of selected infectious organisms and comparison of two anatomic sampling sites in shelter cats with upper respiratory tract disease. J Feline Med Surg 2008;10(6):551–7.
55. Klose TC, MacPhail CM, Schultheiss PC, et al. Prevalence of select infectious agents in inflammatory aural and nasopharyngeal polyps from client-owned cats. J Feline Med Surg 2010;12(10):769–74.
56. Binns SH, Dawson S, Speakman AJ, et al. A study of feline upper respiratory tract disease with reference to prevalence and risk factors for infection with feline calicivirus and feline herpesvirus. J Feline Med Surg 2000;2(3):123–33.
57. Binns SH, Dawson S, Speakman AJ, et al. Prevalence and risk factors for feline *Bordetella bronchiseptica* infection. Vet Rec 1999;144(21):575–80.
58. Sykes JE, Anderson GA, Studdert VP, et al. Prevalence of feline *Chlamydia psittaci* and feline herpesvirus 1 in cats with upper respiratory tract disease. J Vet Intern Med 1999;13(3):153–62.
59. Cai Y, Fukushi H, Koyasu S, et al. An etiological investigation of domestic cats with conjunctivitis and upper respiratory tract disease in Japan. J Vet Med Sci 2002;64(3): 215–9.
60. Sjodahl-Essen T, Tidholm A, Thoren P, et al. Evaluation of different sampling methods and results of real-time PCR for detection of feline herpes virus-1, *Chlamydophila felis* and *Mycoplasma felis* in cats. Vet Ophthalmol 2008;11(6):375–80.
61. Westermeyer HD, Kado-Fong H, Maggs DJ. Effects of sampling instrument and processing technique on DNA yield and detection rate for feline herpesvirus-1 via polymerase chain reaction assay. Am J Vet Res 2008;69(6):811–7.
62. Clarke HE, Kado-Fong H, Maggs DJ. Effects of temperature and time in transit on polymerase chain reaction detection of feline herpesvirus DNA. J Vet Diagn Invest 2006;18(4):388–91.
63. Maggs DJ, Clarke HE. Relative sensitivity of polymerase chain reaction assays used for detection of feline herpesvirus type 1 DNA in clinical samples and commercial vaccines. Am J Vet Res 2005;66(9):1550–5.
64. Sykes JE, Allen JL, Studdert VP, et al. Detection of feline calicivirus, feline herpesvirus 1 and *Chlamydia psittaci* mucosal swabs by multiplex RT-PCR/PCR. Vet Microbiol 2001;81(2):95–108.
65. Ossiboff RJ, Sheh A, Shotton J, et al. Feline caliciviruses (FCVs) isolated from cats with virulent systemic disease possess in vitro phenotypes distinct from those of other FCV isolates. J Gen Virol 2007;88(Pt 2):506–17.
66. German AJ, Cannon MJ, Dye C, et al. Oesophageal strictures in cats associated with doxycycline therapy. J Feline Med Surg 2005;7(1):33–41.
67. Sparkes AH, Caney SM, Sturgess CP, et al. The clinical efficacy of topical and systemic therapy for the treatment of feline ocular chlamydiosis. J Feline Med Surg 1999;1(1):31–5.
68. Owen WMA, Sturgess CP, Harbour DA, et al. Efficacy of azithromycin for the treatment of feline chlamydophilosis. J Feline Med Surg 2003;5(6):305–11.
69. Hartmann AD, Helps CR, Lappin MR, et al. Efficacy of pradofloxacin in cats with feline upper respiratory tract disease due to *Chlamydophila felis* or *Mycoplasma* infections. J Vet Intern Med 2008;22(1):44–52.
70. Gerhardt N, Schulz BS, Werckenthin C, et al. Pharmacokinetics of enrofloxacin and its efficacy in comparison with doxycycline in the treatment of *Chlamydophila felis* infection in cats with conjunctivitis. Vet Rec 2006;159(18):591–4.

71. Dean R, Harley R, Helps C, et al. Use of quantitative real-time PCR to monitor the response of *Chlamydophila felis* infection to doxycycline treatment. J Clin Microbiol 2005;43(4):1858–64.

72. Povey RC. Effect of orally administered ribavirin on experimental feline calicivirus infection in cats. Am J Vet Res 1978;39(8):1337–41.

73. Nasisse MP, Dorman DC, Jamison KC, et al. Effects of valacyclovir in cats infected with feline herpesvirus 1. Am J Vet Res 1997;58(10):1141–4.

74. Malik R, Lessels NS, Webb S, et al. Treatment of feline herpesvirus-1 associated disease in cats with famciclovir and related drugs. J Feline Med Surg 2009;11(1): 40–8.

75. Thomasy SM, Lim CC, Reilly CM, et al. Evaluation of orally administered famciclovir in cats experimentally infected with feline herpesvirus type-1. Am J Vet Res 2011;72(1): 85–95.

76. Maggs DJ. Antiviral therapy for feline herpesvirus infections. Vet Clin North Am Small Anim Pract 2010;40(6):1055–62.

77. Maggs DJ, Nasisse MP, Kass PH. Efficacy of oral supplementation with L-lysine in cats latently infected with feline herpesvirus. Am J Vet Res 2003;64(1):37–42.

78. Maggs DJ, Sykes JE, Clarke HE, et al. Effects of dietary lysine supplementation in cats with enzootic upper respiratory disease. J Feline Med Surg 2007;9(2):97–108.

79. Ohe K, Takahashi T, Hara D, et al. Sensitivity of FCV to recombinant feline interferon (rFeIFN). Vet Res Commun 2008;32(2):167–74.

80. Gutzwiller ME, Brachelente C, Taglinger K, et al. Feline herpes dermatitis treated with interferon omega. Vet Dermatol 2007;18(1):50–4.

81. Sandmeyer LS, Keller CB, Bienzle D. Effects of interferon-α on cytopathic changes and titers for feline herpesvirus-1 in primary cultures of feline corneal epithelial cells. Am J Vet Res 2005;66(2):210–6.

82. Stiles J. Treatment of cats with ocular disease attributable to herpesvirus infection: 17 cases (1983–1993). J Am Vet Med Assoc 1995;207(5):599–603.

83. Lappin MR, Andrews J, Simpson D, et al. Use of serologic tests to predict resistance to feline herpesvirus 1, feline calicivirus, and feline parvovirus infection in cats. J Am Vet Med Assoc 2002;220(1):38–42.

84. Radford AD, Dawson S, Coyne KP, et al. The challenge for the next generation of feline calicivirus vaccines. Vet Microbiol 2006;117(1):14–8.

85. Poulet H, Jas D, Lemeter C, et al. Efficacy of a bivalent inactivated non-adjuvanted feline calicivirus vaccine: relation between in vitro cross-neutralization and heterologous protection in vivo. Vaccine 2008;26(29–30):3647–54.

86. Radford AD, Dawson S, Wharmby C, et al. Comparison of serological and sequence-based methods for typing feline calicivirus isolates from vaccine failures. Vet Rec 2000;146(5):117–23.

87. Radford AD, Sommerville L, Ryvar R, et al. Endemic infection of a cat colony with a feline calicivirus closely related to an isolate used in live attenuated vaccines. Vaccine 2001;19(31):4358–62.

88. Singer LM, Cohn LA. Immune deficiency, stress, and infection. In: Little S, editor. The cat: clinical medicine and management, vol. 1. St. Louis (MO): Elsevier; 2011, in press.

89. Gourkow N, Fraser D. The effect of housing and handling practices on the welfare, behaviour and selection of domestic cats (*Felis sylvestris catus*) by dopters in an animal shelter. Anim Welfare 2006;15:371–7.

90. Kessler MR, Turner DC. Effects of density and cage size on stress in domestic cats (*Felis sylvestris catus*) housed in animal shelters and boarding catteries. Anim Welfare 1999;8:259–67.

91. Kessler MR, Turner DC. Stress and adaptation of cats (*Felis silvestris catus*) housed singly in pairs and in groups in boarding catteries. Anim Welfare 1997;6:243–54.
92. Eleraky NZ, Potgieter LN, Kennedy MA. Virucidal efficacy of four new disinfectants. J Am Anim Hosp Assoc 2002;38(3):231–4.
93. Radford AD, Gaskell RM, Hart CA. Human norovirus infection and the lessons from animal caliciviruses. Curr Opin Infect Dis 2004;17(5):471–8.

Index

Note: Page numbers of article titles are in **boldface** type.

A

Acute-phase proteins
  in FCoV diagnosis, 1146–1149
Aspergillosis
  in companion parrots
    transmission to dogs and cats, 1266–1268
Astroviruses (AstVs)
  causes of, 1087–1088
  described, 1087–1089
  in dogs, **1087–1095**
    causes of, 1087–1088
    cultivation in vitro, 1090
    diagnosis of, 1093
    genome organization of, 1090–1091
    pathogenesis of, 1091–1092
AstVs. *See* Astroviruses (AstVs)
Avian influenza
  in companion parrots
    transmission to dogs and cats, 1266

B

Biochemical profile
  in FCoV diagnosis, 1146
Bordetella bronchiseptica
  FRDC due to, 1278
Brucella canis
  canine brucellosis due to, 1209
Brucellosis
  canine, **1209–1219**. *See also* Canine brucellosis

C

Calicivirus(es)
  in cats
    FRDC due to, 1275–1277
  described, 1171–1172
  in dogs, 1172–1173
Canine brucellosis, **1209–1219**
  causative agent, 1209
  clinical signs of, 1210–1211
  diagnosis of, 1212–1216

Vet Clin Small Anim 41 (2011) 1291–1300
doi:10.1016/S0195-5616(11)00181-1
0195-5616/11/$ – see front matter © 2011 Elsevier Inc. All rights reserved.
vetsmall.theclinics.com

United States Postal Service

Statement of Ownership, Management, and Circulation
(All Periodicals Publications Except Requestor Publications)

1. Publication Title	2. Publication Number	3. Filing Date
Veterinary Clinics of North America: Small Animal Practice	0 0 3 – 1 5 5 0	9/16/11

4. Issue Frequency	5. Number of Issues Published Annually	6. Annual Subscription Price
Jan, Mar, May, Jul, Sep, Nov	6	$262.00

7. Complete Mailing Address of Known Office of Publication (Not printer) (Street, city, county, state, and ZIP+4®)

Elsevier Inc.
360 Park Avenue South
New York, NY 10010-1710

Contact Person
Stephen Bushing

Telephone (Include area code)
215-239-3688

8. Complete Mailing Address of Headquarters or General Business Office of Publisher (Not printer)

Elsevier Inc., 360 Park Avenue South, New York, NY 10010-1710

9. Full Names and Complete Mailing Addresses of Publisher, Editor, and Managing Editor (Do not leave blank)

Publisher (Name and complete mailing address)

Kim Murphy, Elsevier, Inc., 1600 John F. Kennedy Blvd. Suite 1800, Philadelphia, PA 19103-2899

Editor (Name and complete mailing address)

John Vassallo, Elsevier, Inc., 1600 John F. Kennedy Blvd. Suite 1800, Philadelphia, PA 19103-2899

Managing Editor (Name and complete mailing address)

Barbara Cohen-Kligerman, Elsevier, Inc., 1600 John F. Kennedy Blvd. Suite 1800, Philadelphia, PA 19103-2899

10. Owner (Do not leave blank. If the publication is owned by a corporation, give the name and address of the corporation immediately followed by the names and addresses of all stockholders owning or holding 1 percent or more of the total amount of stock. If not owned by a corporation, give the names and addresses of the individual owners. If owned by a partnership or other unincorporated firm, give its name and address as well as those of each individual owner. If the publication is published by a nonprofit organization, give its name and address.)

Full Name	Complete Mailing Address
Wholly owned subsidiary of	4520 East-West Highway
Reed/Elsevier, US holdings	Bethesda, MD 20814

11. Known Bondholders, Mortgagees, and Other Security Holders Owning or Holding 1 Percent or More of Total Amount of Bonds, Mortgages, or Other Securities. If none, check box   ☐ None

Full Name	Complete Mailing Address
N/A	

12. Tax Status (For completion by nonprofit organizations authorized to mail at nonprofit rates) (Check one)
The purpose, function, and nonprofit status of this organization and the exempt status for federal income tax purposes:
☐ Has Not Changed During Preceding 12 Months
☐ Has Changed During Preceding 12 Months (Publisher must submit explanation of change with this statement)

PS Form 3526, September 2007 (Page 1 of 3 (Instructions Page 3))   PSN 7530-01-000-9931   PRIVACY NOTICE: See our Privacy policy in www.usps.com

---

13. Publication Title		14. Issue Date for Circulation Data Below
Veterinary Clinics of North America: Small Animal Practice		July 2011

15. Extent and Nature of Circulation		Average No. Copies Each Issue During Preceding 12 Months	No. Copies of Single Issue Published Nearest to Filing Date
a. Total Number of Copies (Net press run)		2388	2297
b. Paid Circulation (By Mail and Outside the Mail)	(1) Mailed Outside-County Paid Subscriptions Stated on PS Form 3541. (Include paid distribution above nominal rate, advertiser's proof copies, and exchange copies)	1332	1211
	(2) Mailed In-County Paid Subscriptions Stated on PS Form 3541 (Include paid distribution above nominal rate, advertiser's proof copies, and exchange copies)		
	(3) Paid Distribution Outside the Mails Including Sales Through Dealers and Carriers, Street Vendors, Counter Sales, and Other Paid Distribution Outside USPS®	356	337
	(4) Paid Distribution by Other Classes Mailed Through the USPS (e.g. First-Class Mail®)		
c. Total Paid Distribution (Sum of 15b (1), (2), (3), and (4))	▶	1688	1548
d. Free or Nominal Rate Distribution (By Mail and Outside the Mail)	(1) Free or Nominal Rate Outside-County Copies Included on PS Form 3541	94	85
	(2) Free or Nominal Rate In-County Copies Included on PS Form 3541		
	(3) Free or Nominal Rate Copies Mailed at Other Classes Through the USPS (e.g. First-Class Mail)		
	(4) Free or Nominal Rate Distribution Outside the Mail (Carriers or other means)		
e. Total Free or Nominal Rate Distribution (Sum of 15d (1), (2), (3) and (4))	▶	94	85
f. Total Distribution (Sum of 15c and 15e)	▶	1782	1633
g. Copies not Distributed (See instructions to publishers #4 (page #3))	▶	606	664
h. Total (Sum of 15f and g)	▶	2388	2297
i. Percent Paid (15c divided by 15f times 100)	▶	94.73%	94.79%

16. Publication of Statement of Ownership

☐ If the publication is a general publication, publication of this statement is required. Will be printed
in the November 2011 issue of this publication.   ☐ Publication not required.

17. Signature and Title of Editor, Publisher, Business Manager, or Owner	Date
Stephen R. Bushing —Inventory Distribution Coordinator	September 16, 2011

I certify that all information furnished on this form is true and complete. I understand that anyone who furnishes false or misleading information on this form or who omits material or information requested on the form may be subject to criminal sanctions (including fines and imprisonment) and/or civil sanctions (including civil penalties).

PS Form 3526, September 2007 (Page 2 of 3)

Moving?

Make sure your subscription moves with you!

To notify us of your new address, find your **Clinics Account Number** (located on your mailing label above your name), and contact customer service at:

Email: journalscustomerservice-usa@elsevier.com

800-654-2452 (subscribers in the U.S. & Canada)
314-447-8871 (subscribers outside of the U.S. & Canada)

Fax number: 314-447-8029

Elsevier Health Sciences Division
Subscription Customer Service
3251 Riverport Lane
Maryland Heights, MO 63043

*To ensure uninterrupted delivery of your subscription, please notify us at least 4 weeks in advance of move.

Printed and bound by CPI Group (UK) Ltd, Croydon, CR0 4YY

03/10/2024

01040442-0005